Caring for the Dying at Home

Companions on the journey

Keri Thomas

General Practitioner
Macmillan GP Advisor
National Lead for Macmillan Gold Standards
Framework Programme

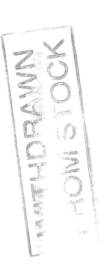
Forewords by

David Colin-Thomé
and
Jane Maher

Radcliffe Medical Press

Radcliffe Medical Press Ltd
18 Marcham Road
Abingdon
Oxon OX14 1AA
United Kingdom

www.radcliffe-oxford.com
The Radcliffe Medical Press electronic catalogue and online ordering facility.
Direct sales to anywhere in the world.

British Library Cataloguing in Publication Data

A catalogue record for this book is available from the British Library.

ISBN 1 85775 946 X

Typeset by Advance Typesetting Ltd, Oxfordshire
Printed and bound by TJ International Ltd, Padstow, Cornwall

Contents

Foreword

It gives me great pleasure in recommending this book to all who are interested and involved in palliative care and, specifically, to all of us who work in primary care, as it is an excellent framework for our clinical practice. Primary care remains the most popular part of the NHS as it provides a local skilled generalist and holistic service. The USA academic Barbara Starfield has long extolled the virtues of British primary care in offering a personal continuity of service that is coordinated and longitudinal. Good palliative care that extends beyond cancer alone, although cancer is the commonest cause of death, reaffirms the centrality of primary care, and yet to achieve excellence in this area requires us to focus on a systematic approach to care. The Gold Standards Framework, described here with its seven 'Cs', is an excellent template for systematic and yet holistic care, a gold standard indeed for all aspects of our care. This book of course offers far more in exploring wider aspects of palliative care including aspects of spiritual, holistic care, and it leaves me far better informed and enlightened. I am certain you will feel the same.

Professor David Colin-Thomé
National Clinical Director of Primary Care
Department of Health
General Practitioner
Castlefields Practice
Runcorn
January 2003

Looking after the dying is often seen as an unpleasant and emotionally distressing aspect of working in primary care. Many have been registered at the practice for years and witnessing them stagger from one crisis to the next is really upsetting. And afterwards, we are there to try and help the family and friends come to terms with what happened. All too often, a colleague would visit a dying patient in their home and stay for 40 minutes or more. They would come away, shaking their heads in sorrow, saying there was nothing they could do. But they did a great deal for the patient and their families just by being there and supporting them.

The Gold Standards Framework has transformed our practice's approach to the care of the dying. The whole team no longer perceives palliative care as all doom and gloom and is more confident that we can make a positive contribution. The teamworking, care coordination and anticipation of problems mean that our patients experience fewer crises and have a much better outcome. We are so pleased that we have decided to start applying the principles of the Gold Standards Framework to all of our cancer patients from the point of referral onwards.

David Lyon
General Practitioner
Castlefields Health Centre
Runcorn

It is with pleasure that I recommend Dr Thomas' book and the use of the Gold Standards Framework in primary care. Caring for dying patients has to be one of the most rewarding and challenging elements of community nursing and is an aspect of my district nursing role that gives me immense personal and professional satisfaction. Whilst welcoming the shift towards community-based provision for cancer patients, it cannot be ignored that this has made a significant impact on district nursing resources. Often, when a patient has died the team has questioned whether things could have been done better, could more support have been given to the patient and carers; could planning have been improved; could the team have thought further ahead about medication, home equipment, symptom control? We knew that cancer services in the community needed to be improved if the challenges of the NHS Cancer Plan (2000) were to be fulfilled.

When our primary healthcare team were introduced to the Gold Standards Framework we found our answers. Here was a structure on which our clinical practice could be based to significantly improve the experience of a dying patient in our care. As a coordinator for GSF in my practice, I have found that the framework has provided the opportunity for the whole team to communicate on aspects of care and to explore and change, where necessary, our ways of working with cancer patients. These changes have had a profound effect. Patient and carer are better supported and the team are strengthened in the knowledge that they are providing the best possible quality of care. We will certainly continue to use this excellent framework to support our services to cancer patients in the community.

Jane Melvin BSc (Hons), RGN
District Nurse and Primary Care Cancer Nurse
Castlefields Health Centre
Runcorn

Foreword

As Chief Medical Officer for Macmillan Cancer Relief it has been my privilege to work with Keri Thomas for the last three years and to see the birth and development of the Gold Standards Framework.

It will be of interest to anybody who is involved with the care of people with incurable illness and as an oncologist I found much to inspire, learn and apply.

This book not only describes matters needed but has many examples and stories to inspire along the way. It is truly the head, hands and heart of care. As Don Berwick says, the system is important but people make the difference. I'm sure this book will inspire more people to do just that.

Jane Maher
Chief Medical Officer
Macmillan Cancer Relief
January 2003

Preface

There are many reasons for writing this book, some professional and some personal. Professionally, I have been a GP for 20 years and have always nurtured a passion for palliative care from within general practice, seeing its holistic and loving approach as encompassing some of the best of medical care. I undertook further training as an SHO in Palliative Medicine, and as a GP took the Diploma in Palliative Care and the MSc (Cardiff), continuing to work part-time in hospices for over 12 years and witnessing first-hand the inspirational care provided. The natural development of this interest was crystallised in the sessional role of Macmillan GP Facilitator, which I undertook from 1998 for Calderdale and Kirklees Health Authority, West Yorkshire. This involved visiting practices, running workshops and teaching sessions, examining the barriers to improvement for community palliative care and exploring ways of overcoming them.

Later, I became Regional Macmillan GP Advisor, supporting other Facilitators and linking in with various national strategic developments – the NHS Cancer Plan, primary care representative on the Commission for Health Improvement's *Cancer Report*, Supportive Care Strategy Editorial Board member, Deputy National Lead for Primary Care in the Cancer Services Collaborative of the NHS Modernisation Agency, National Council for Hospice and Specialist Palliative Care member, etc.). But the mainstay of this work was derived from my discussions with GPs, district nurses and specialists across the country about ways to improve palliative care service provision in the community, based on their own grass-roots practice and experience. In response to the commonly voiced need to improve out-of-hours palliative care, we developed an award-winning local out-of-hours palliative care protocol which led to the Macmillan *Out-of-Hours Palliative Care Report* in March 2000, since used in the development of guidance by the Department of Health. In a similar way, the Gold Standards Framework (GSF) detailed here, firmly rooted in primary care, was derived from a local desire to improve round-the-clock palliative care for patients in the community, and was later extended from West Yorkshire across the UK.

The second area of contribution is on a more personal level. I am a working mum with five children at home and a brilliant, long-suffering husband, so I am constantly juggling demands and prioritising, whilst attempting to keep perspective and balance amidst the ordinary demands of family life, from sorting the socks to delousing the twins. This also maintains a rootedness and reminds me of what it is all for, and of the one thing in life I know to be true above all else – love. As a clergy wife, I am indirectly in touch with the needs and suffering of many within a community, and am privileged perhaps to benefit from many discussions at a deeper level than usual. I live in the context of the fact that there is more to life than this visible outer shell – the inner life, the spiritual, is vitally important. I write as someone also personally affected by death, as I was widowed at the age of 25 when my first husband, Andrew, was killed in a car crash in Africa. So the recognition of the briefness of our lives, the perspective of living always in the knowledge of our dying, has sharpened my keenness to live life to the full, to contribute and to better support others as they face their own death.

Rooted in primary care and in real-life experience, my hope is that this book will make a practical contribution to improving the care of the seriously ill in their final months of life at home, and that it will enable and empower healthcare professionals to deliver excellence of care, and to remain with patients and carers as 'companions on the journey'.

Keri Thomas
Shrewsbury
January 2003

About this book

Death belongs to life as birth does.
The walk is in the raising of the foot as in the laying of it down.

Rabindranath Tagore, *Stray Birds*

Care of the dying at home matters to us as people and as professionals

Amidst the diversity of the human condition there is one thing we know we all have in common; that one day we will die. And for most of us, given a choice, we'd prefer to remain at home for the majority of the time, and to die at home if possible, given adequate support. Added to this, there is a consistent trend in all areas of healthcare towards increasing community care and reducing expensive hospital bed occupation in this country; but currently far fewer are able to die at home than would wish to do so and there are too many inappropriate and possibly preventable admissions to hospitals and, occasionally, hospices.

Cancer is now the biggest killer in the UK. About two in five of us will get cancer at some point in our lives and one in four of us will die of it.[1] Adding heart disease to this total will cover the majority of all deaths; most of us will be affected by these conditions, either ourselves or within our families. So there are three reasons why community palliative care is a vitally important subject:

1 At some stage in our lives, we are likely to be personally affected as individuals – this can happen to anyone, whether medical or not, to ourselves or our families and friends.
2 Secondly, most within primary care feel strongly that this is an inherently important issue which we pride ourselves on getting right. As community professionals we are able to build on the unique relationship with our patients, developed over time, and can use our privileged position to ensure the highest quality of care is given on a personal basis; these are people not just patients, usually living amongst our patients, and the impact of care we provide in primary care will be debated amongst those we live with in the community – we may bump into patients' relatives at the school gate, at the supermarket and frequently through other patients of the practice. So there are many incentives to do well for the dying, and the ripples can be far reaching.
3 Finally there are some looming imperatives on the horizon in the form of clinical governance agendas, primary care cancer standards, BMA contract awards, etc. At present there are many who have developed this work out of interest and commitment to better care; sometime soon it is likely there will be some mandatory targets for all of us in primary care to reach. But before this becomes another 'must do' from on high, I appeal to the former desire of all healthcare professionals to continuously strive to improve care for the dying at home, as a basic ingredient of good primary care, and affirm the essential supportive role of 'being there' for our patients.

So in varied ways, we may all have a vested interest in community palliative care; it is an area that affects us as healthcare professionals and as people. The key questions are:

- What is the ideal model of care we would wish for ourselves and our families?
- How can we in primary care best respond to this challenge?

Although most of us in primary care have been caring well for the dying for many years, this is a rather neglected area of development which is now under the spotlight. Despite being seen as a somewhat Cinderella service, primary care is very heavily involved in this stage of care. It can, at minimum, take a few minutes and a quick tick of the right boxes to refer someone to hospital for investigations for a suspected malignancy, although of course it may be a far more complex process than this. But at the other end of the cancer journey we can be very extensively involved, maybe visiting daily and at weekends, becoming personally challenged in providing much more than just medical care. We may use ourselves as people even more than we use our prescription pads. We inherently understand the meaning of supportive care and often provide the mainstay of palliative care for our patients. We are spurred on now to raise our standards, inspired by the examples of the palliative care/hospice movement, to improve care even further: inspired to bring about the kind of care that we would wish for ourselves and our families – the 'doctor–family index'.

The aim of this book

The purpose of this book is to support, encourage and enable those in primary care to make improvements in the care provided for their patients with any end-stage illness. It aims to strengthen the role, confidence, system and skills of the primary healthcare teams (PHCTs) as they deliver 'generalist' palliative care or supportive care to their patients.

This book is also something of a journey, describing:

- *why* community care of those in the last months of life is important in the current context, responding to the challenges of the palliative care movement and based on patients' needs (Part 1)
- *how* we can begin, using the evidence from published literature, knowledge of change management and some key clinical information to help anticipate problems and reduce the chance of tripping up, with other available help in the Appendix and on the websites (Part 2)
- *what* practical steps can be introduced, such as the Gold Standards Framework (GSF) for Community Palliative Care, with information on the Macmillan Gold Standards Framework Programme, now extended across the UK (Part 3).

The main message is that caring for the dying at home is an important and integral aspect of primary care, which we generally do well, but in which we can, with help, do even better. It is an area close to our hearts and many see this as one of the most important things we do – and maybe as a barometer of all other aspects of care. Putting patients at the centre of care and drawing together the collective wisdom and experience of those involved in hands-on primary palliative care, informed by the evidence from the literature, we can make changes and raise standards, stronger together, to ensure we deliver the kind of care we would wish for ourselves or our families. We can improve our own enjoyment, support and job satisfaction and we can enable more to die well in the place of their choice.

> *Good palliative care is achievable. It is simply an application of normal primary care skills and approach. It doesn't involve major changes. It is appreciated by patients and families. It improves morale and team functioning and is very rewarding for all the team.*
> GP, Huddersfield, GSF Phase 1 and first GSF reference group

Hospital and hospice staff, managers, social workers, clergy, patients and carers may find much of this of interest, but the focus is mainly on improving care delivered by healthcare professionals in the community, specifically primary healthcare teams. I write as a GP who has worked extensively with hundreds of GPs and district nurses to deliver better care, so I seek to represent the whole primary healthcare team (PHCT) here.

This book is intended for two general audiences and to be used in two ways:

1 Parts 1 and 2: as a resource book for anyone with a general interest in, and a desire to improve, palliative care in the community, particularly those from PHCTs, i.e. GPs, district nurses (DNs), practice managers and Macmillan nurses, and other clinical nurse specialists, social workers, etc. The chapters on the role and developments in primary care, the current context of the health service, change management and the evidence base for developments in community palliative care such as the GSF programme will be of interest to any involved in this area. The needs-based care chapter summarises some available user views and sets the tone for further consideration.

The two useful clinical chapters, written by Dr Susan Salt, Consultant in Palliative Care, are specifically directed towards those in primary care, to help with the proactive management of patients with the major cancers. In the advanced planning of future care for our patients, a constant theme of this book, such information helps inform and alert us to the possible clinical problems that may be lurking around the corner. Palliative care is based on good general medicine, but there are several specific differences in drug usage and conditions which are seen more frequently in hospices than in primary care. These can sometimes catch us out and are summarised in the chapter on 'tripwires'.

I hope these pages will encourage and inspire you to look further into specialised texts, and allow you to reflect on your current practice in the light of some very pragmatic, rooted examples of good practice. Additional material can be accessed via the website, www.radcliffe-oxford.com/caring.

2 Part 3: as a handbook for those involved in the Macmillan Gold Standards Framework (GSF) Programme for Community Palliative Care, currently running in the UK. This is based on the *Handbook for Practices* used in the initial two phases of the programme. The programme is supported by a central support team running conferences, training, a website and project area facilitators who run local feedback meetings. The resource material in the other parts will be of interest in explaining the foundation of the Framework. Anyone interested in joining this programme, please contact us through Macmillan Cancer Relief – see below.

For further information and details relating to the Macmillan Gold Standards Framework (GSF) Programme for Community Palliative Care:

Email: gsf@macmillan.org.uk
Tel: 0207 840 7840
Fax: 0207 840 7841
Website: www.macmillan.org.uk (from Sept 2003)

Some details are currently available at www.modern.nhs.uk/cancer
www.pcclsupport.org.uk

These two audiences have different perspectives but may well overlap, causing this book to be of specific use as a guide for the GSF programme and of more general interest to others.

In deference to the habit of many doctors (myself included) of reading books from back to front and picking out the relevant sections that leap out of the page, and also because some pages may be used fairly independently as stand-alone portions, there is occasional repetition of a point across the three parts. For these two reasons I seek your forbearance and ask that you use the parts you find most helpful, whether relating to the GSF or of general community palliative care interest. If when you've read the first part and felt inspired to get on with it you want to jump straight to what to do about it in Part 3, please do.

Although fairly broad-based, there is always more to add and there are omissions I've had to make. This does not claim to be a comprehensive text, and there will still be areas that may rapidly become out of date. It is a collage of images of the current situation of 'generalist' palliative care in the community in this country, with some pointers and worked examples of possible ways forward for the future.

The Gold Standards Framework

The Gold Standards Framework (GSF) is further explained in Part 3. The framework is being supported and rolled out UK-wide by Macmillan Cancer Relief with other partners, notably the Cancer Services Collaborative of the NHS Modernisation Agency. The key features of GSF are:

- It is a practical tool to facilitate better coordination, communication and delivery of primary palliative care and improve the patient's experience of care. This includes:
  - *identifying* this group of patients
  - *assessing* and responding to their needs
  - better *planning* of care
  - with improved *communication* being the glue that binds it all together.
- It is characterised by having developed from grass-roots general practice upwards, rather than a 'top-down' dissociated directive, with much listening, debating and testing by those on the ground. It has to date been tested out in over 100 practices across the UK, involving about 5000 patients, varying in detail as it is adapted and modified to fit a variety of situations, but retaining the basic form.
- Three stages are suggested, to be used flexibly to establish the GSF in an area:
  - step 1 – background work, raising interest and C1 and C2 (*see* p. 186)
  - step 2 – adding on C3, C4 and C5 (*see* p. 186)
  - step 3 – finally C6 and C7 (*see* p. 186), and the development of practice protocols and six-monthly review/audit meetings
  - later extending to supportive care of other patients from diagnosis.
- We can demonstrate improvements by measuring specific global outcomes, which are increasingly important for clinical governance.
- Even more importantly, however, there are some intangible benefits which we find difficult to measure but which have been found to improve, such as better levels of care and support, better levels of communication, a greater sense of security and confidence in our patients and their carers and better staff satisfaction and teamwork, etc.
- It is patient centred in that it attempts to improve the assessment of needs and refocus on patients' and carers' priorities, both physical and psychosocial; this agenda-sharing with patients aims to promote more involvement in decision making and retention of control. Improving the sense of security at home is a key element.

- It is not a one-size-fits-all measure, and there will be variation in response to it, but its success lies in the will of the people to improve care of the dying, with some suggested tools and ideas to speed up the process; using borrowed piloted tools rather than continuous wheel reinvention. All can find something of benefit in it.
- It is a locally owned, people-based programme, with a central team providing support to local project facilitators who work with the coordinators from each practice.
- It is a dynamic momentum, evolving and responding to the reflections and needs of the primary care teams involved. It is constantly being evaluated and refined. Local ownership and sustainability are important.
- Once established for cancer patients it can be extended to those with non-malignant conditions and also to support patients at an earlier stage in the cancer journey, i.e. from diagnosis or from fast-track referral.
- It aims to make life easier for practices not harder, saving time instead of costing time in the final analysis – working more effectively. With central direction and resourcing, shared ideas and worked examples, practices enjoy being part of a momentum across the UK to improve community palliative care.
- It sits comfortably with other emerging themes such as clinical governance and legitimises our supportive role. It affirms the aspiration to be a 'companion on the journey'.

The GSF helps build confidence that 'being there' is important – it's not just about science, but it reinforces that we can make a positive contribution. Once established in cancer patients, the principles can be extended to help all cancer patients at any stage and those with any life-threatening condition.

HT, GP, Halton, GSF Phase 2

- At a time when many in primary care feel de-skilled, it reinforces the essential contribution that good community care can provide in an area that may otherwise not be addressed for any but the lucky few. It reinforces the effective doctor–nurse teamwork.

The Gold Standards Framework promotes and encourages that special and important triad of the doctor, the nurse and the patient.

GP, Aberdeen, GSF Phase 2

- It specifically focuses on and formalises improving support for carers.
- It builds on the natural enthusiasm of the majority in primary care to develop this area.
- In line with the current trend towards community and intermediate care, primary care commissioning, improving supportive care and responding to the lead given by the modern hospice movement, the time is right to formalise developments in community palliative care.

The GSF is like a crossword clue – when you see the answer it's really obvious. It's non-threatening, non-prescriptive and awareness-raising, with attention to real individual patient care.

EP, GP Facilitiator, Glasgow, GSF Phase 2

Many of the ideas, reflections and quotations put forward here have been derived from experiences from practices across the UK involved in the first two phases of the GSF programme. Hearing colleagues from one end of the country to another enthusing and enlivened about the subject is both convincing and heartening, and I personally have been greatly encouraged to continue with this work by the inspiration and enthusiasm of those taking part in the GSF programme. I am extremely grateful to all those involved and indebted to them for their pragmatic wisdom and constant encouragement.

The view from the nations

Increasingly since devolution, there are significant differences in approach and in organisational structures across the four nations of the UK. However, despite these variations, people are basically the same across all borders, and the care we wish to provide for our dying patients will be much the same. All the nations are responding enthusiastically to the GSF programme, Scotland and Northern Ireland particularly, with a large number of practices involved in Phase 2 and more planned in future. For example, there are plans for most practices in Scotland to be aware of, or implement, the GSF in the next three years.

It is too clumsy to itemise each different organisational structure for each nation in the text; this book is written from the experience initially in the English system, although it has been a great joy and privilege working with projects across the nations. Therefore, this general disclaimer asks you to read the equivalent regional term for each English one where appropriate and to adapt the language as needed. However, brief notes are given below regarding the significant differences in health service structures and a view of the response to the Framework.

The view from Scotland (with thanks to David Millar, Macmillan GP Advisor, Aberdeen)

Scotland lagged a little behind England in that the Scottish NHS Plan *Our National Health: a plan for action a plan for change* was published in December 2000 and the Cancer Plan *Cancer in Scotland: action for change* in July 2001. The latter, which was intended more as a strategy than a plan, did support the development of managed clinical networks (MCNs) but had very little to say about the role of primary care.

The 12 mainland health boards and three island health boards are the equivalent of English health authorities. There are 27 acute hospital trusts, 12 primary care trusts and one integrated trust. Local healthcare cooperatives (LHCCs) are the equivalent of primary care groups (PCGs), although the average population served is less (65 000–70 000) and they have no role in commissioning hospital services. There are three cancer networks covering the west, north and south-east of Scotland (regional cancer advisory groups) with differing structures and composition.

The Clinical Standards Board for Scotland (CSBS), which was set up in 1999, oversees the monitoring process within the NHS in Scotland and relies heavily on guidelines produced by the Scottish Intercollegiate Guidelines Network (SIGN). There are no specific primary care cancer standards, although all but one of the Scottish health boards have agreed to utilise the Royal College of General Practitioners (RCGP) Scotland Practice Accreditation (PA) as a quality assessment process to satisfy the requirements of clinical governance. Included in PA is the audit/significant event analysis of a number of cancer cases within each practice.

Palliative care at home is an important issue to us, particularly in rural areas of Scotland, far from any specialist input. The Scottish response to this Framework has been hugely enthusiastic, with 16 practices involved across three project areas in Phase 2, and extensive plans for the future across the whole country. We are keen to extend it to all cancer patients from diagnosis and to use it to develop the primary cancer care agenda in Scotland.

The view from Northern Ireland (with thanks to Brendan O'Hare, GP and Macmillan GP Facilitator, Castlederg)

In Northern Ireland we had a review of cancer services based on the Calman Hine Report. Stemming from this review, a cancer centre based in Belfast and five cancer units throughout the province were established to deliver a high quality of cancer care to the population. The number of palliative care consultants was increased and a network of Macmillan GP Facilitators was established to raise the profile and standard of cancer and palliative care at a primary care level.

Local Health and Social Care Groups (LHSCGs), our equivalent of primary care trusts (PCTs), are currently struggling with negotiations between the GPC and the Department of Health. GPs do not currently participate in these groups but hopefully will do in future, and our input can ensure that palliative care receives a high priority at a strategic level.

The Macmillan GP Facilitators have been tremendously successful in addressing deficiencies in palliative care provision in their various 'patches'. However, much work remains to be done and Gold Standards provide a framework to ensure that the highest possible standard of care is delivered to all patients in Northern Ireland. The Gold Standards Framework is actually a benchmark or common standard against which we can measure the effectiveness of our efforts.

In Phase 2 of the project there were three practices in Northern Ireland involved, but it has been embraced with enthusiasm by the Macmillan Northern Ireland GP Facilitator Group and the number involved will expand rapidly in future. It is anticipated that at least 20% of all practices will be involved in Phase 3 of the GSF, with more planned in future.

The view from Wales (with thanks to Kate Whitfield, GP and Macmillan GP Facilitator, Powys)

Wales differs from England in several ways.

1 *Structural differences.* At the time of writing there are five health authorities in Wales with 22 constituent local health groups (LHGs). As from April 2003, the five existing health authorities and the LHGs will be dissolved and 21 local health boards (LHBs) will be created with the same boundaries as the existing unitary health authorities. These LHBs will be directly accountable to the Welsh Assembly Government. There will be no equivalent to the English strategic health authorities. There are just three cancer networks covering huge geographical areas.

2 *Delivery of care.* Models of care have to be variable because most of the population is concentrated in a few urban areas, but the majority of the countryside is very sparsely populated with patients living great distances from district general hospitals and hospices. In these areas palliative care is often provided by GPs, using the community hospitals. Macmillan funded a number of GP Facilitator posts in Powys to develop palliative care in the community. Clearly, the Gold Standards Framework is very useful for raising standards in these situations.

3 *The Welsh Collaborative Care Pathway Project.* This project is being widely adopted by hospitals, hospices, GP practices and nursing homes across Wales, supported by the Welsh Assembly. This relates specifically to the care of those in the last days of life and is based on the Liverpool Integrated Care Pathway for the dying. The GSF programme

for those in the last months of life would therefore become a natural extension of this work.

An evolving Framework: people and paperwork

The GSF is an evolving programme, and this book is part of a dynamic movement, with templates and updates available on the website which link in with recent national developments; for example, the Supportive Care register sheets are updated in line with recommendations on cancer databases from the NHS Information Authority.

But more than this, the real benefit is the fact that you embark on the journey together as a practice team and group of motivated innovators. The papers are useful, but the people are more important. They are the powerhouse behind this programme, and to me the real strength and reason for the success of the Framework. The structures that bring people together set off a process that will inevitably lead to real rooted change. As Don Berwick, founder of The Institute of Healthcare Improvement, affirms, we need many things to improve care but most importantly we need the dynamic momentum of a group of motivated people moving on together.

> Most striking is the enthusiasm of the PHCT – the typical reply is 'We're really busy but this is something we all care about and we will make the time'. It is something about putting people back in touch with the reasons they came into healthcare.
>
> CCS, GP, Dorset

The real strength lies in living out the pages of the book in the most appropriate form. Practice is reflected on and the quality of end-of-life care provided is built up slowly and imperceptibly. New ideas and improvements in care will develop as teams take protected time to consider ways to do this. (It's helpful to share these ideas with others via the website, e-mail, conversations or at workshops.) Investing in people is the key, guided by a fresh look at an important but age-old subject. We only have one chance to get this right. We may struggle to succeed, but we owe it to our patients to try.

Aims of the Gold Standards Framework

1 *Patients* – that patients are enabled to live well in the last months of life and, finally, have a 'good death' (a) in their preferred place of choice (b) symptom-free (c) with a greater sense of security and support, with fewer crises and reduced fear or anxiety.

2 *Carers* – that carers feel supported, informed, involved, acknowledged, empowered and satisfied with care.

3 *Staff* – that staff grow in confidence, have a sense of teamwork, job satisfaction, with improved communication and co-working with specialists and hospital staff.

Reference

1 Office of National Statistics (1999) Registration of cancer diagnosed in 1993–96, England and Wales. *Health Stat Quart.* **4**: 59–70.

Acknowledgements

Gold Standards Reference Group

I would like to thank all those from Calderdale and Kirklees Health Authority who were involved in the original multidisciplinary reference group: Dr Mary Kiely, Dr Susan Salt, Jo Love, John Murgatroyd, Dr Chris Martland, Angela Robinson, Miranda Morris, Rosie Norbury, Anne Briers, Lorraine Macdonald, Christine Springthorpe, Margaret Spark, Joyce Swift, Julie Hoole, Cathy Inman, Helen Thornton, Dr Chris Houghton and Dr Birt Jindall. Thanks particularly to Dr Susan Salt for her invaluable clinical contributions in Chapters 7 and 8.

Pilot practices: Phase 1

Many thanks to all those participating pilot practices in Phase 1, especially the wonderful team of district nurse coordinators who I grew so fond of and who did such valiant work: Joyce Swift, Brenda Bowers, Katie Meredith, Chris Pyrah, Angela Robinson, June Wilkinson, Anne Calloqhan, Carol Atkin, Ann Fearnley, Audrey Keeshan and Dawn Gordon; and the very supportive lead GPs: Mark Davies, Peter Gorman, Kate McMichael, Richard Gatecliff, Chris Martland, Sheila Bennett, Lyn Mason, Mark Taylor, Mike Pacynko, Gill Bradley, Chris Houghton and Sue Cameron.

Calderdale and Kirklees Health Authority, West Yorkshire

I would like to thank my old health authority, to which I will be forever indebted, for giving me such a wonderful springboard for this work and providing me with such great encouragement and support, especially Dr Chris Veal, Philip Sands, Dr Graham Wardman, Elaine Fry, Claire Butler and the fantastic secretarial support from Alexis Duval and Helena Condon. Also Drs Hilary Felton, Liz Higgins and Rob Lane of the local hospices I worked in, and Lorraine Macdonald, Sarah Cost and other Macmillan nurses in the area.

Macmillan Cancer Relief and the Cancer Services Collaborative: Phase 2

Thanks to all those who helped get Phase 2 going, in particular Glyn Purland (Macmillan Project Director and a very good man to know); Marie Patchett, Claire Henry, Jodie Mazur and Sally Cook of the Cancer Services Collaborative (wonderfully energetic and encouraging stalwarts); Professor Helen Bevan and Jean Penny of the NHS Modernisation Agency for their enthusiasm; the Macmillan GP Advisors, Drs Jane Maher, David Millar, Greg Tanner, Gill Harding and Rosie Loftus; the GSF Steering Group, particularly Katie Booth, Jane Maher and Frankie Shutt, plus other advisors, Dr John Ellershaw, Dr Bill Noble, Judith McNeil, Tonia Dawson, Jane Bradburn, Alison Hirst, Kate Whitfield, Ros Johnstone and Katie Burall; and for the encouragement and contributions from all Macmillan GP Facilitators taking part, especially Euan Paterson, Brendan O'Hare, Charles Campion-Smith, Chris Woodyat,

Peter Kiehlman, Rosalie Dunn, Steve Fraser, Darin Seiger, Cathy Hubbert, Christine Moss, Kate Tully, Pam Selby and Cliff Richards. Also, the Yorkshire Cancer Network PCT cancer leads and nurse facilitators, Rosaleen Bawn and Sue Stearn. Particular thanks to Dr Hong Tseung, Jane Melvin and Dr David Lyon of the Halton project for their wonderful support of the GSF and contributions to this book.

Also, many thanks to those whose work has contributed enormously to this project: Paul Morris, MGPF, St Helens, Pat Turton of the Bristol Cancer Centre, Dr Tim Greenaway and Donna McLeggan of Manchester ACTS, Becky Miles of the National Cancer Alliance, Peter Kaye for his excellent and inspiring writings, Dr Michael Downing and team from the Victoria Hospice Society, Victoria, British Colombia, Canada for the wonderful home care work and handbook, Dr Robert Dunlop, Dr Max Watson, Reverend Roger Cressey, Chaplain at Pinderfields Hospital, Wakefield and Reverend Harry Edwards, Chaplain, Drs Wendy Jane Walton, Teresa Griffin and Jeremy Johnson of Shrewsbury, and many others. Thanks also to Gillian Nineham and Jamie Etherington of Radcliffe Medical Press for their encouragement and forebearance.

I am greatly indebted to Macmillan Cancer Relief and to many others not mentioned here, but especially to all patients, doctors, nurses, friends and family who have contributed in various ways to this work. I hope that this book is a testimony to the dedication and commitment of so many working in our NHS and voluntary sectors to maintain the kind of 'loving medicine' that is at the heart of good patient care.

Thanks also to those in the parish of St Chad's, Shrewsbury, my home church and where my husband is vicar, who have within a short space of time made us feel completely at home, supported and enriched by their friendship – and especially Ronnie Bowlby and Mary and Lawrence Lequesne for their support in writing this. I breathe in strength at St Chad's to keep me going all week – I couldn't do without it.

Finally and most of all, thanks to my fantastic husband, Mark, who has been most wonderfully supportive and long suffering, supplying me constantly with fresh rounds of coffee and much needed support and common sense, and tolerating this sixth gestation, and to my five stunningly gorgeous children, Megan, Ben, Bethany and seven-year-old twins Sophie and Imogen, for being so tolerant of a distracted mum. They have put up with a cardboard cut-out with only remnants of a brain remaining and have been a constant reminder of the life-affirming and love-fulfilling joy that is the reason I keep going.

I would also like to dedicate this to the memory of Andrew Rodger, my first husband, who died 20 years ago to the day (ironically, almost to the minute as I write!), who was and is an inspiration to me in this work, and to his father, The Right Reverend Patrick Rodger, who died only recently and sadly will not see in this life this edition of the book dedicated to his son ... but maybe he knows anyway.

Cover illustration: 'The Healing Touch'

I need to know that this body is my body. And I need to know everything that is happening to my body. But most of all I need to know that you know that within my body there is me.
Healing is brought about not just by medicine. It's not just treatment which cures you but all that encompasses the human touch.

'Healing Touch' is taken from the series of paintings and words 'The Emotional Cancer Journey' (along with three other illustrations: 'So Much Love' p. 1, 'Rest' p. 61 and 'Everything You Need to Know You Have Learnt on Your Journey' p. 173) that document Michele Angelo Petrone's experience of cancer.

Michele Angelo Petrone, a professional artist, was diagnosed with Hodgkin's Disease in 1994. The enormous response to this work, and the art workshops, lectures and educational work for patients, carers and health professionals has been formalised into the charity, the MAP Foundation (www.mapfoundation.org, email: info@mapfoundation.org).

Glossary

Cancer Network
Group of primary, secondary and tertiary cancer services covering several PCTs. There are 34 Cancer Networks in England.

DN
District nurse.

DS1500
A fast-track attendance allowance form completed when a patient's prognosis is about six months or less.

Generalist palliative care
Generalists (GPs, dentists) only some of whose work involves caring for palliative care patients.

GP
General practitioner.

GSF
Gold Standards Framework.

Macmillan nurse
Nurses specially trained in palliative care who work in an advisory capacity in the community, funded (initially) by Macmillan Cancer Relief (a UK charity).

PCT
Primary care trust in England. There are equivalent primary care organisations in Scotland (LHCCs), in Wales (LHGs/LHBs) and in Northern Ireland (LHSCGs).

PHCT
The primary healthcare team – GP, DN, practice managers, receptionists, practice nurses, health visitors and other community providers, based around a GP practice.

Primary care
GP, DN, general practice and other community-based services.

Secondary care
Hospital-based services.

Specialist palliative care
Trained palliative care personnel most of whose work involves palliative care patients.

Tertiary care
Specialised units in hospitals taking referrals from larger areas.

PART I

Palliative care at home: why is it important?

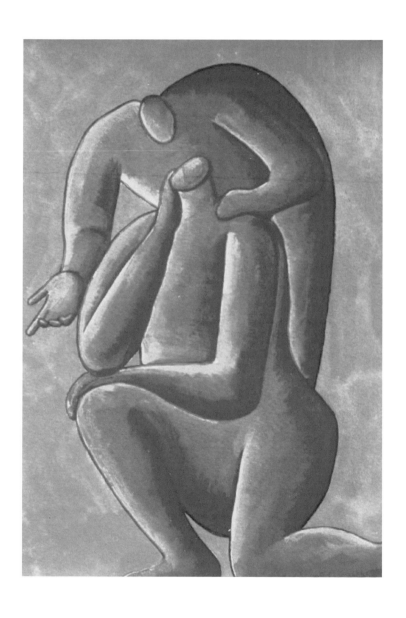

CHAPTER I

Introduction: companions on the journey

This chapter emphasises the importance of improving community palliative care and offers a framework to begin to do so. It includes:

1 Maps and journeys
2 Making changes: resolving the practice–theory gap
3 A matter of life and death: the inner and outer journeys
4 The head, hands and heart of community palliative care
5 A practical model of good practice
6 Seeking wisdom: learning from the dying.

Maps and journeys

In various ways, we're all involved in journeys. Over recent years, in common with many, my work has required me to travel across the country, in my case as Macmillan GP Advisor in Cancer and Palliative Care, to discuss ways of improving palliative care in the community. When setting off, for example for Leicester from my home in Shrewsbury, West Midlands, I first have to be clear about my destination – a clear goal. With train journeys it is important to know the final destination of a train to ensure you catch the right train to your station. With that in mind, I have to plan a means and a route. I could meander by car across country and make my way slowly to Leicester, and I would no doubt arrive eventually, but it would take me all day and I might give up in the process! However, if I consult a map, take a tried and tested route that other travellers have followed and use signposts to guide me, then my chances of arriving at my destination in time are greater.

I can gauge my progress by the road signs or stations passed. If I come across a hold up, I may take a temporary detour, adapting to new directions, and by chance discover a more delightful short-cut previously known only to seasoned travellers. Or, as happened recently, I may suddenly come upon a stunning field full of poppies, a celebration of diversity, that takes my breath away, lifts my spirits and sets me back on track in a deeper sense. In being lost, I became found anew. If several of us travel together and pool our collective experiences, then we may develop an even better route to the destination and have some fun in the process. So in work, as in life.

In aiming for a goal, such as the best quality of care for the dying, there are many routes, many detours and barriers, many signposts. Therefore a recommended route from a fellow traveller, or even a map, is a helpful start to our journey. Briefly 'helicoptering' ourselves out of the immediate situation provides us with the means of examining where we are, where we have come from and where we are heading, allowing us to renew a clear sense of direction and perspective.

The Gold Standards Framework is such a map, tried and tested to help practices take the first steps in developing improvements in community palliative care.

> *The GSF is an important and valuable 'map', especially in the present climate of increasing time constraints and increasing demands on current general practice. In the long run, it will make our job easier.*
>
> GP Facilitator, Halton, GSF Phase 2

Making changes: resolving the practice–theory gap

In many areas of life there is a practice–theory gap – a space between where we are and where we want to be. We may know what to do but somehow we just don't get around to doing it. Why not? There are many varied reasons for this, but one is the difficulty moving from first base, taking the first steps towards the goal. Don Berwick from the Institute of Healthcare Improvement, USA, which has supported and inspired the NHS Modernisation Agency's work in the UK, says that to implement real change within a system we need to have:

1 **Aims**
2 **Optimism**
3 **Measures**
4 **Creativity**, ideas, curiosity about other ways of doing things
5 **Group behaviour** – a collective synergy of ideas.[1]

Aims

We need to be clear about our aims or intended destination – our vision – and take time to crystallise these thoughts. In this case, we are attempting to improve generalist palliative care in the community, delivered by our primary healthcare teams. More specifically, we are trying to improve:

1 the care of patients, so that they are enabled to live well until they die, to have a 'good death' in their preferred place of choice, symptom-free, safe and secure, with fewer crises
2 carer support, so that they feel supported, involved, empowered and satisfied
3 staff confidence, teamwork, satisfaction, communication and co-working with specialists.

Optimism

It's good to be optimistic that we can make a difference and encourage constructive thought. How hard it is to build a house of cards and how easy to knock one down. When cynicism creeps in (a feature that seems to come with the stethoscope in medicine), we might reflect whether we alone could do any better?

The journalist, Libby Purves, commenting on a recent MORI report which suggested that the middle-aged are the new, whinging 'Meldrew' generation of cynical disparagers, affirms that: 'The history of humanity tells us that great reforms are made and great civilisations built out of optimism and energy and the willingness of individuals to work together without much immediate personal gratification, for a good purpose. Psychology ... tells us that the secret of happiness is making the best of what you have, and believing that you are contributing to something good.'[2] Refuse to allow others to drain your enthusiasm and optimism for constructive change, tempered by a degree of realism, and keep perspective. For every force for change there is always an opposite resistance.

In the current climate of 'change fatigue' and dispirited exhaustion in some, we need to retain a positive approach and affirm our ability to change things for the better. Is the *status quo* alright? Are we going to be part of the problem or part of the solution? Many resist change, sometimes indignant and resentful that change is with us always, sometimes quite justifiably as not every change is for the better: 'Every improvement is a change, but not every change is an improvement.'[3] Sometimes it is an unwillingness to adapt to a new way of working ('we've always done it this way'), and sometimes it may be because the current system appears to be working well enough, to them. But is it the best for all our patients all the time, and can we raise the quality of our service so best practice becomes routine care? Can we be sure of always delivering the kind of care for all patients that we would wish for ourselves?

Measures

We need to build in measures so we can demonstrate to ourselves and to others how far we've progressed from our starting point, and we can perhaps use our findings to call for better services from those who hold the purse strings. We can measure recurring problems in community palliative care, such as lack of carer support or district nursing, or problems accessing drugs and equipment out of hours, etc. We can then assess how often these factors cause crisis admissions to hospitals or prevent patients dying in their preferred place of choice, which enables us to develop better service provision for our patients. The measures are there to develop improved services, not to make us feel bad: 'measuring for improvement not for judgement.'[4]

We can measure *structure* matters such as numbers on the register, *process* matters such as how often we send a handover form to the out-of-hours service and *outcome* matters such as levels of satisfaction and numbers dying in their preferred place of choice. The focus is very pragmatically on the patient in front of us, and how we can improve the provision of care for them and for those who come after them (*see* Box 1.1 and www.radcliffe-oxford.com/caring).

Box 1.1 Suggested categories for measurement

1 **Is it acceptable to the practice?** (*structure*)
  time spent, workload, numbers using a register, etc.

2 **Does it change practice?** (*process*)
  are things being done now that were not done before, e.g. PHCT meetings, handover forms to out-of-hours provider, assessment tools, etc.?

3 **Does it make a difference to patients and carers?** (*outcome*)
  numbers dying in preferred place of choice, reduced crises, numbers of hospital bed days per patient, better symptom control, better information and sense of security, patient, carer and staff needs met and satisfaction improved, etc.

Curiosity and creative thinking

Curiosity about other routes may allow us to discover new directions, applicable for others. Sharing examples of good practice is fruitful; not all solutions are transferable but highlighting the problems we have in common can be constructive. Informed by a wide reading of the literature, brainstorming problems, lateral thinking, spreading real-life solutions across peer groups, modifying and adapting ideas from other areas of care, and taking the risk of trying out possible ideas on a small scale are all ways of creatively addressing change from the bottom up.

Group behaviour

Group behaviour as a team is a wonderful resource, sometimes untapped, to develop good practice. We have only recently discovered in primary care the value of working together in out-of-hours cooperatives and undertaking Significant Event Analysis as part of our reflective practice as a team. We rediscover the shared dynamic of undertaking the task together, of allowing protected time as a group to reflect and rethink priorities, goals and means of getting there. In the process we are supporting each other, sharing burdens, building teamwork and improving our enjoyment of the daily jobs we do. This synergy of ideas, where one plus one equals three,[5] allows groups to become very creative, where rooted but real change can occur, 'owned' by those undertaking it – the best ideas are the ones thought up by the people involved.

> *I felt so isolated in this work before. It's good to have the support and back-up of others.*
> Dorset GP, part-time partner of GP Facilitator of GSF Phase 2 practice

Many practices are using their 'in-house' protected learning times to debate such issues. Having a specified time to raise these identified palliative care patients to the forefront of our thinking, discuss collectively their problems, care and planning needs and share ideas and solutions, leads to a greater concerted wisdom. Some will find holding meetings difficult, but improvements can still be made and six-monthly practice review meetings are a valuable reflective tool (*see* Chapter 12, C1). Just as many hospital staff find that the introduction of multidisciplinary team meetings for all cancer patients has radically improved patient care (and many see it as one of the key developments in reducing cancer mortality[6]), so we in primary care might follow suit and organise structures to prioritise our most needy patients.

> *A positive outcome was the fact that when I went to see my partner's patient out of hours, I was able to say: 'Dr A. has told me about you and I understand that X and Y are your main difficulties.' Patients really appreciate the continuity of care and the fact that we have cared enough to discuss them as a team.*
> MH, Northern Ireland GP, GSF Phase 2

A matter of life and death: the inner and outer journeys

There are many parallel journeys. Here we are considering the goal of improving community palliative care and the suggestion given is to use the map of the Gold Standards Framework. There are other routes of course, and other means of achieving the goal.

There are other journeys too. We are all on our own journeys, caught in the same 'time capsule', where the end-point will be the same for all of us. We live in the context of our death.

> *Death is one of the attributes you were created with; death is part of you. Your life's continual task is to build your death. One should be ever booted and spurred and ready to depart.*
> Montaigne

For some of our patients entering the final stages of their lives, this journey's end can seem terrifying or welcoming, but usually both. The sudden biting of the reality that this journey is going to have an end. This may come the day the diagnosis of cancer or another serious illness is given, or it may not come at all. We may glibly call it denial, but others call it living in hope, and we have to tread gently here. There are many shifts in personal identity here – our views of ourselves – from being a person who lives for ever to being a dying patient, and many points of vulnerability where support may be needed most (*see* Figure 4.3, p. 55). This is, of course, much harder in the premature dying of a younger person, than in the culmination of a full life of an older person.

There are both outer and inner journeys: the outward conveyor belt of hospital investigations, appointments, treatments and medications, and the inner transitions towards a different view of ourselves, our lives and our priorities – a new perspective. Both the outer and inner journeys are important and need to be recognised. Being a witness to these transitions is a great privilege and a great teacher, an honour we never tire of.

As many have observed over the years, most notably Dame Cicely Saunders in her pioneering work with the dying, the quality and dignity of the dying is something very special, and is a constant pointer for us who accompany them as we busy ourselves with the fretfulness of daily living, to something beyond this tangible existence before us. We are particularly privileged to accompany patients on this journey.

Elisabeth Kubler-Ross, an American psychiatrist and author of the ground-breaking book *On Death and Dying*, was one of the first to describe these final stages of the inner journey. She later related how much she learnt from dying patients as she took time to listen to their deeper thoughts:

> *Later someone would ask what all these dying patients had taught me about death. First I thought about giving them a very clinical explanation, but then I would have misrepresented myself. My dying patients taught me so much more than what it was like to be dying. They shared lessons about what they could have done, and what they should have done, and what they didn't do until it was too late, until they were too weak or too sick, until they were widows or widowers. They looked back at their lives and taught me all the things that were really meaningful, not about dying ... but about living.*[7]

'Companions on the journey'

For our patients and their loved ones, we in primary care may become companions on the journey. It is one of our greatest callings and one of our greatest challenges.

> *The essential concept is that the doctor or practice team will stay firmly with the patient and relatives at their time of need and not desert them.*[8]
>
> TB, retired oncologist who cared for his dying wife

As they travel along their journeys, how can we best meet patients at their point of need? How can we promote a sense of security around them and their families? And how can we look after ourselves as people, thinly disguised as healthcare professionals, as we attempt to support them on their way? Can we rise to the challenge of quality care for all those dying at home?

> *Good palliative care is appreciated by our patients and their families, and is at the core of good primary care, and in many ways is probably the best thing we do.*
>
> GM, Northern Ireland GP – a statement on the wall at the local GP cooperative

The 'head, hands and heart' of community palliative care

In researching this area over many years, looking through the current writings and debating at workshops and practice visits, I have come to the view that there are three main areas for improvement of services for palliative care patients (*see* Figure 1.1):

1   clinical competence, e.g. assessment and diagnostic skills, knowledge of what to do, which treatments to use, when to refer, symptom control, etc.

the 'what to do' – *the head*

2   the organisation – the way processes are involved, the systems (e.g. communication and information transfer), accessing other support, coordination and continuity (e.g. out of hours), primary healthcare team workload issues and managed system of care, social (e.g. benefits)

the 'how to do it' – *the hands*

3   the human dimension of care – to improve the patient's experience of care, compassion, dignity, patient and carer autonomy/choice, the intangible dimension of human relationships, the spiritual inner journey – 'loving medicine'

'why' we do it all – *the heart*.

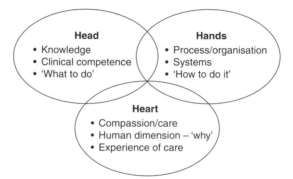

Figure 1.1: Head, hands and heart of community palliative care.

It has been the experience of many Macmillan GP facilitators and others when examining this area that the main gaps in community palliative care are often related to the organisational aspects of care – the 'hands'. We need the 'head' knowledge – clinical effectiveness and competence is vital – but if in doubt we may know where to seek help or advice, such as a friendly textbook or specialist palliative care doctor (*see* Chapters 16 and 17). But it is in the organisation or system of care, which has perhaps inadvertently developed over time ('we always do it this way'), that there can be most problems. This may lead to unanticipated problems causing insecurity in our patients, inadequate support and inappropriate crisis admissions. By addressing the system of primary palliative care we are most likely to improve the multifaceted dimensions of care provided.[9]

This area is addressed largely in the GSF. By improving the system and the priorities of quality, patient-centred care of the seriously ill in our practices, real changes can be made, and we can put more of the 'heart' back into our day-to-day practice. Small things can make a huge difference. The informing of the cooperative doctor, the passing visit to show support, the phone call after receiving bad news, the enquiry about the spouse's feelings, describing what to do if a bleed should happen, the intuitive feeling that a break is needed and respite being organised: it is the attention to detail, informed by regularly consulting the 'map', that is so much appreciated.

Support for staff

In supporting practices as they improve the 'hands' and then the 'heart' issues – the experience of care – we have to question the level of support for our staff as well as for our patients. As healthcare professionals, we may struggle at times to cope with the realities of this interface between life and death. We are challenged clinically, but also at a deep level of our own humanity. This may be on a backdrop of declining morale,[10] or unhappiness for other professional or personal reasons and so could, in some cases, become the 'last straw'. The sentiments of those already undertaking the Gold Standards Framework impart something of the personal satisfaction, support and encouragement people have felt as they work together, using the GSF as a springboard to better care and more fulfilling teamwork. Use of significant event analysis and other reflective practice helps develop a shared understanding of each person's contribution and builds morale. Looking after our staff and improving enjoyment of our work are such vital elements.

There is a high incidence of burn out and clinical depression in healthcare professionals (*see* Chapter 17, C6), especially around issues that affect us as people, beyond our roles. What are we doing to care for our professional carers when they feel burdened by the task or guilt that there is little they can do? Many studies, most notably David Jeffrey's examination of GPs' views in *Cancer: from cure to care*[11] and the Commission for Health Improvement's (CHI) report of GP and district nurse (DN) focus groups across the country,[12] reveal the depth of feelings amongst those in primary care, the guilt when struggling and the overall ever-present commitment of staff. This is an area that many feel is the best of primary care and yields great job satisfaction, and yet there is a personal cost. Building in support for our staff, enabling practice teams to fulfil their ambition of best quality palliative care and encouragement to enjoy the satisfaction of a job well done are noble virtues to which this work aspires.

Empowerment and sustainability

These words, though often reeled off in 'management-speak', hold part of the key to success of a new development. What is the difference between this being a sustained, embedded improvement that lasts, or a flash in the pan, a good but short-lived idea that melts like a snowflake after the initial enthusiasm? If it chimes with long-held beliefs and ideas of those within the team, now empowered to translate them into reality, if it helps to release the potential for creative ideas that develop into owned systems maintained with pride, and if tangible benefits to patients and to staff can be felt, then sustained improvements will be made. The reasons for continuing the work will outweigh the drawbacks that will come with staff changes, workload struggles and other real-life issues in the health service. If patients feel a greater sense of security at home, staff take an even greater pride in their work, or one nurse feels it has triggered better care and eased bottlenecks, then it has been effective.

Sustaining change requires changing hearts and minds, building in ongoing learning and measurements, mainstreaming of ideas that fit with other values and visions and then celebrating success, renewing and setting the bar higher (*see* helpful Improvement Leaders' Guides on the NHS Modern website).[13]

A practical model of good practice

Putting theory into practice is harder than it looks. How can practices begin to improve care with a simple stepwise plan? The GSF handbook in Part 3 describes in detail seven key tasks, the seven Cs, which build together in stages and inter-relate to form a comprehensive whole, rather like pieces of a jigsaw puzzle coming together to reveal the whole picture.

Essentially three processes take place which form the model of good practice (*see* Figure 1.2 and Box 1.2):

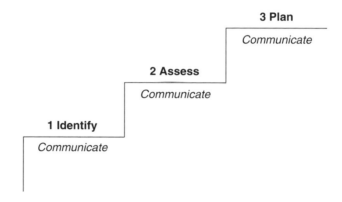

Figure 1.2: Three practical steps to better primary palliative care.

1 specific *identification* of patients in the last months of life
2 improving the *assessment of their needs*, both physical and psychosocial
3 building in *planning* of anticipated problems and future care.

Improved *communication* between all involved, and specifically improved listening to patients and carers, should occur at each level.

> There have been many improvements, but if I was to pick out one particularly since starting this GSF project in our practice it would be that now we leave a supply of the anticipated drugs in the home of those palliative care patients we have identified on the register. Having assessed their particular problems and likely needs, the drugs are all ready in the home in case they are needed out of hours by the visiting doctor (who also has information on them in a handover form). There have been no crisis calls for drugs and no 50-mile round trips chasing chemists at weekends since we started doing this.
>
> DN coordinator, Shropshire, GSF Phase 2

So by picking out this group of patients for special treatment and taking time to listen and fully assess their needs (physical, emotional, spiritual and practical), we can plan better for the predicted future course of events and anticipate possible problems. As we go through this process, by building up stage by stage the seven key tasks suggested (C1–7), perhaps

---

Box 1.2 Model of good practice for primary palliative care

This consists of a primary healthcare team who will:

1 **IDENTIFY** palliative care patients as a special group (*pick out this group of patients*)
   - a *register* of eligible patients using certain criteria, e.g. last six months of life from DS1500*
   - *communicate* information within the team, e.g. at a PHCT meeting
   - *record* and communicate about these patients using register sheets as prompts and audit tools
   - identify *carers* and their own needs

2 **ASSESS** and respond to patient and carer need (*patient-centred care responding to needs*)
   - physical problems (symptom control)
   - holistic/psychosocial needs (emotional, social, spiritual and practical)
   - discuss these needs with patients and carers and prioritise according to patient's agenda
   - plan regular reassessment and respond to need, at appropriate level of intervention
   - support offered, e.g. initiated weekly contact, asking about carer, etc.
   - symptom control given
   - referral to specialist palliative care where needed, triggered by criteria, e.g. eligibility criteria, Problems and Concerns Assessment Tool (PACA) scale
   - *communicate* better with patients, carers and staff

3 **PLAN** care (*change from reactive to proactive in advanced planning for likely problems*)
   - nominate specific coordinator in practice
   - *communicate* with team members and those outside the team
   - carer support anticipated, e.g. respite care, night sitter
   - carer education, empowerment and co-working
   - preferred place of care/death discussed and noted
   - drugs needed in home provided
   - equipment needed in home provided
   - out-of-hours handover form sent
   - information given to patient/carer, including crisis care
   - terminal phase planned according to protocol
   - teamwork and staff support developed
   - plan of proactive support – revisits/further contacts initiated

NB. Improved *communication* is a thread running through each area.
*DS1500 is a DSS attendance allowance code for rapid access when patients are considered to be terminally ill, i.e. last six months of life.

---

imperceptibly there will be an improvement in the quality of our care and a greater professionalism about our service. Patients will remain as symptom-free as possible but the purpose is also to enfold them and their carers with a sense of security and support, to enable them to progress on their journey (*see* Chapter 4).

When my wife, Joy, was diagnosed with cancer of the liver, our excellent GP said three things: first, we can do a great deal to control pain these days; second, we must see that the quality of life will be as good as it can be; third, we must see that she dies at home. With the help of our Macmillan nurse all these points were met. At every stage of the next 14 months our GP, district nurse and Macmillan nurse were on hand to suggest, reassure and predict, helping not only Joy but me and our children. Their assistance in dark days was priceless.

MC, widower and carer, Shrewsbury

Seeking wisdom: learning from the dying

The much loved lines from TS Eliot help to set the right course:

Where is the life that we have lost in living?
Where is the knowledge we have lost in information?
Where is the wisdom we have lost in knowledge?

TS Eliot, *Four Quartets*

We live in an era of ever-increasing data and information, but very little knowledge and even less wisdom. The study of 'informatics' looks at this inter-relationship (*see* Figure 1.3). Increasingly, with evidence-based clinical governance issues hitting us, we may be in danger of missing the wood for the trees.

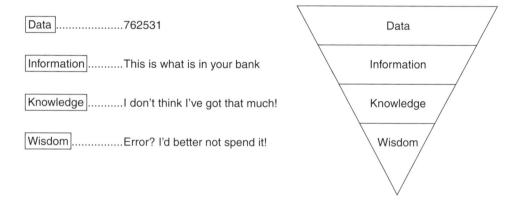

Figure 1.3: Example of informatics: relationship between data, information, knowledge and wisdom.

Perhaps within general practice we are better placed than many to maintain that vision of wisdom in a data-obsessed world, and to represent this to our patients. We are often asked to interpret or translate the information given to patients from hospitals; the common question asked is 'What would you do?' It takes great skill to move from bald figures towards an interpretation that contains some humanity and wisdom for the patient in front of us. It is the ability to see through the noisy facts and figures to the silent wisdom or 'truth' revealed within, which we must nurture. Not the truth that relates to us (not 'If I were you ...') but to the patient in the context of their lives, about which we may know some things but not everything.

Bill Gates, the IT multimillionaire, was asked once, in the context of the ever-increasing digitalised information available to us all at the touch of a button, 'What is the role of the human being in the digital age?', to which he answered 'The role of the human being in the digital age is to be a human being'.[14]

In considering the needs of our future doctors, with all the access to data, information and knowledge available to them, the skill is to be able to translate that humanity to patients in real human terms, to learn the language of wisdom. We need to nurture wisdom and encourage that ability to translate it into our daily practice and contact with patients.

Wisdom is concerned not so much with knowing the right answers, but in asking the right questions. What is wisdom? It is that mysterious mixture of truth intertwined with love – you cannot have one without the other.[15]

Having made the case for seeking a wider wisdom than is merely found in the pages of the medical journals, what can these pages tell us that will help us to develop improvements in primary palliative care? Chapter 5 'Evidence-based care' addresses some of the questions, seeking the recurring barriers or problem areas as a brief distillation of the wisdom available in the current literature that relates to the organisation of community palliative care.

Box 1.2 is a summarised model of good practice in primary palliative care, with practical pointers towards improvement, detailed further in Part 2 of this book. This is one means of developing the potential of primary care and affirming the fact, sometimes unacknowledged, that supporting patients is one of the most valuable functions we can perform.

The district nurses who have taken part are all very keen because they feel, although they are giving up their time, this makes their job easier in the end. Relationships between DNs and GPs are much better. Everyone is so busy they can tend to go off and do their own thing. This way, sitting down together to discuss patients, brings them together and makes so much of a difference.

PCT Manager, Halton, GSF Phase 2

My hope is that some of the ideas presented here will be of benefit to anyone involved in caring for the seriously ill or dying, in particular those in primary care, and that using this book, whether as part of the GSF programme or not, you will be enabled to discover more of your own path as you accompany your patients on the final stage of their journeys.

If we give more 'loving medicine' to these important patients by improving their care, whilst opening ourselves to the messages of those approaching death, we will receive a greater wisdom of how to live our lives now, a deeper understanding of 'the life we have lost in living'. As Elisabeth Kubler-Ross puts it.[16]

By listening to dying patients, all of us learned what we should've done differently in the past and what we could do better in the future.... The lessons each individual taught us boiled down to the same message:
Live so that you don't look back and regret that you've wasted your life.
Live so you don't regret the things you have done or wish that you had acted differently.
Live life honestly and fully.
Live.

References

1 Berwick D (2002) Introduction to NHS Modernisation Agency Associates Day, March 2002. London.

2 Purves L (2002) For goodness sake stop whinging [Comment]. *The Times*, August 27th, 2002.

3 Goldratt E (1990) *The Theory of Constraints*. North River Press, Great Barrington, MA.

4 NHS Modernisation Agency (2002) *Improvement Leaders' Guide on Measurements for Improvements*. DoH, London.

5 Covey S (1997) *The Seven Habits of Highly Effective People*. Simon and Schuster, London.

6 NHS Executive (2000) *Manual of Cancer Services Standards*. DoH, London.

7 Kubler-Ross E (1997) *The Wheel of Life*, p. 168. Bantam Books, London. Also see Kubler-Ross E (1973) *On Death and Dying*. Tavistock Publications, London.

8 Brewin T (2001) Deserted [Personal View]. *BMJ*. **322**: 117.

9 Berwick D and Nolan T (1998) Understanding medical systems. *Ann Intern Med*. **128**: 293–8.

10 Edwards N, Kornacki M J and Silversin J (2002) Unhappy doctors: what are the causes and what can be done? *BMJ*. **324**: 835–8.

11 Jeffreys D (2000) *Cancer: from cure to care*. Radcliffe Medical Press, Oxford.

12 Robinson A (2001) Commission for Health Improvement and Audit Commission Report on Cancer Services, December 2001.

13 NHS Modernisation Agency (2002) Sustainability and spread. www.modern.nhs.uk/improvementguides/sustainability

14 Professor Muir Grey, at the launch of the National Electronic Library of Health, London, October 2000.

15 Thomas M (2002) Personal Communication.

16 Kubler-Ross E (1997) *The Wheel of Life*. Bantam Books, London.

CHAPTER 2

A modern way of dying

This chapter examines our attitudes to death and dying and explores the invaluable contribution made by specialist palliative care. It includes:

1 Death and dying: a modern way of dying
2 The palliative care movement
3 Integrated care pathways: care in the last days of life
4 Working together: dovetailing care.

Death and dying

Death and taxes: the only certain things in life

Are you ready to die? If not, then you might begin some preparation. Every BMJ *reader will die this century, and death is constantly beside us.*[1]

At the beginning of the new century the leader in the *British Medical Journal* began with these words, having allowed us only a few days to recover from the millennium festivities. It continued by affirming that death should no longer be seen as failure, but rather as an important part of life and be brought back centre stage. The Age Concern 'Debate of the Age' argued that: 'We believe it is time to break the taboo and to take back control of an area (death) which has been medicalised, professionalised and sanitised to such an extent that it is now alien to most people's daily lives.'[2]

Death comes to us all – we know this as an immutable fact. Yet we live as if we are immortal, as if 'by the time we're old they will have invented a cure for dying'.[3] As Heath comments: 'The welcome success of scientific medicine carries other dangers. The chief of these is the implication, the false promise, that science offers a cure for every ill and the indefinite postponement of death. Death, which is inevitable, and often unpredictable, arbitrary and unjust, is seen more and more as a simple failure of medicine and doctors. Medicine cannot promise immortality and yet we, in Western society, begin to convince ourselves that it might.'[4] And as Skrabanek puts it: 'Since life itself is a universally fatal sexually transmitted disease, living it to the full demands a balance between reasonable and unreasonable risk.'[5]

Although from the outset achievement of a 'good death' was a goal of the palliative care movement (*see* Box 2.1), some would argue that the 'medicalisation of dying' has meant that some elements of the ideal of palliative care have possibly been diluted.[6] In primary care, we spend the majority of our time and energies caring for those with psychosocial problems, the acutely ill, some with self-limiting conditions, for the 'worried well' and for those who are coming to terms with illness and with the possibility of dying, as well as those in the last stage of life. Supporting those living with dying is a key element of general practice. If the

---

Box 2.1 Elements of a 'good death' in modern Western culture[6]

- Pain-free death
- Open acknowledgement of the imminence of death
- Death at home, surrounded by family and friends
- An 'aware' death, in which personal conflicts and unfinished business are resolved
- Death as personal growth
- Death according to personal preference and in a manner that resonates with the person's individuality

---

new definition of *supportive care* is essentially to help the patient and their family cope,[7] then this is an area in which we may have valuable experience and certainly plenty of opportunity to do so.

Have you ever pictured yourself as you approach death and considered the scene – you or a member of your close family? Can you envisage where you would like to be in your final months and days, with whom, and what you would be doing? Many of us would be attempting to cram in a little more of life's experiences, fulfilling dreams, smoothing troubled waters, easing our passing but living life to the full right up to the end. It is about living until you die. We all go this way once only. We have one chance to get it right – for ourselves and for our patients.

> *Dying is a very important part of living – it's a very important time of life for the patient and their families. It's vital that they get the care that they deserve.*
>
> District nurse, Yorkshire[7]

> *You only get a chance to die once, so you've got to give it your best. We've got to provide the service for people to die in the best way they can.*
>
> District nurse, Wales[8]

People are beginning to discuss 'death plans' in the same way as they do birth plans (there are many analogies with the world of obstetrics) and finding that a sense of control and choice play a vital part and that small details really matter.[9] The Age Concern 'Debate of the Age', listing the 12 principles of a good death, mentions control and choice at least seven times (*see* Chapter 4, Box 4.1).[4] This highlights the need for people to maintain some control in a world gone mad, turned upside down by a diagnosis of an end-stage illness. Maintaining some control is more important for some than others, but helps retain 'a little bit of me' amidst this depersonalising, devastating medicalisation of a natural process – refocusing on the person not the patient. As Rabbi Julia Neuberger put it: 'If the locus of dying is the home then people are more likely to retain control.'[10]

A modern way of dying

Until the last few generations we had little time to choose our mode of dying – most died of catastrophic infections, accidents, diseases that were found at advanced stages, on the battlefield, in childhood or childbirth. Those who were chronically ill took to their beds and stayed there. In terms of healthcare provision, we have never been here before. We have more warning of our dying now, but we seem still to be caught by surprise by its inevitability.

We react against it, waving before us the shield of modern scientific advances to quell the deathly dragon in our attempts 'to beat it'. Just note the language of the tabloids after the death of a celebrity: 'he finally lost the battle against cancer', 'she bravely fought her illness but finally gave in'.

Many live so much longer now – longer and at times sicker. Cancer is becoming another chronic disease in a trend towards increasing longevity. Recent Office of National Statistics (ONS) figures for England[11] show that quantity and quality of life do not go together; poor health is marring longer life for millions of older people, and this is particularly notable in Northern England. Although life expectancy is an average of 77.5 years (from 73.4 years for men in the North West to 81 years for women in the South West of England), they are likely to suffer an average of 9.2 years of ill health in their late years (from 5.7 years for men in the South East to 12.3 years for women in Northern and Yorkshire areas). So ill health may be the norm for many from their mid-sixties onwards.

The medicalisation of dying

In our very human struggle with the inevitable, and in our search for the elixir of eternal life, we may look down the sterile linoed corridors of hospitals for hope. We can tend to over-medicalise and over-institutionalise the journey towards dying. Illich was the first to warn of the dangers of the medical establishment becoming a major threat to health.[12] Some now warn that increasing medical inputs will at some point become counter-productive and produce more harm than good. So where is that point and how will we know when we face it?

> Death, pain and sickness are part of being human. All cultures have developed means to help people cope with all three. Indeed, health can even be defined as being successful in coping with these realities. Modern medicine has unfortunately destroyed these cultural and individual attempts to defeat death, pain and sickness. It has sapped the will of the people to suffer reality.[13]

We always hope and suspect a cure is round the corner. As doctors we still fret that we may be missing something, causing us at times to err towards over-investigating and intervening, with the ever present concern of litigation never far from our thoughts. Even the speciality of palliative care, 'a speciality that opens up a space somewhere between the hope of cure and the acceptance of death',[16] can tend towards over-intervention and medicalisation of dying. There may be covert intimations of the financial burden of the elderly, that the medicalisation of old age may hide cost-cutting requirements; but it is dying in hospital – not an ageing population – that costs money.[14]

Dying in hospital or at home

Many patients, especially those undergoing curative treatment, may die in hospital during an admission for further investigation or treatment – this is usually appropriate and inevitable. However, it is the crisis 'inappropriate' admissions we must try to avoid. Dying in hospital can be the best place, but despite all best efforts it can sometimes be inadequately managed and less than dignified. Patients moved to side wards to avoid the acute frenzy of busy hospital life may be poorly supervised with inadequate symptom control and their carers made to feel in the way and a nuisance. Almost a quarter of hospital bed days are taken up by patients in the last year of life.[15] Dying patients may be seen as 'bed-blockers', yet there may be difficulties or resistance in moving them elsewhere, often from nervous carers who feel unable to cope at home. There can be a de-humanising of dying. On busy hospital wards, focusing on cure and discharge, it is the failure of medical technologies to coexist appropriately with dignified dying that can cause such social isolation and inadequate care.[16] Some cited examples of dying patients left abandoned in side rooms with ECG monitors to notify staff of their death, or the over-enthusiastic resuscitation bringing patients back from the brink, only for them to die later in an undignified way with tubes in every orifice, seen as a 'failure' of medical competence.

> But tragically the worst cases – those people in the last stages of illness, those who were in the process of dying – were given the worst treatment. They were put in the rooms furthest from the nursing stations. They were forced to lie under bright lights they could not turn off. They were denied visitors except during prescribed hours. They were left alone to die as if death might be contagious.[17]

In the first half of the twentieth century most deaths in the UK occurred at home, but by the 1960s this had dropped to one-third and its current level is about a quarter of cancer patients but a fifth of all deaths.[18] Hospital deaths are inevitable for some and appropriate for others, but there is still the indicting figure of 50% of cancer patients and 66% of those with other conditions dying in hospitals. In an age when we can provide so much in our centres of excellence, shouldn't we be looking to extend this beyond the boundaries of our hospitals and into our homes? And why does the home situation break down so often, requiring hospitalisation of those in the terminal phase? Is the main reason that we have lost confidence in our ability to cope in the community and we are inadequately resourced and empowered to provide it? Home can be the best and worst place to die.[19] Isn't it about time we came of age and developed our palliative care services in the community to such an extent that there would be no need to recourse to crisis hospital admissions as a last resort?

Increased longevity, demographic changes, fragmentation of the family unit, fewer women staying at home, a reduction in the number of children per family – all contribute to the need to institutionalise care at the end of life. But is there a clue we have been missing in this death-denying culture of ours? Does the white-coated, jousting physician, bearing all the drugs and mind-boggling glinting armoury of modern science, represent our last hope of beating off the dark figure approaching us with the sickle? How much is denial and how much is wisdom in our choices of how to manage the patient in front of us?

> One GP tells the salutary story of a patient who changed his thinking. He visited a young man with colorectal carcinoma, undergoing aggressive chemotherapy, who was bleeding from every orifice, desperately ill, and admitted him to hospital where he died a few days later. When he later visited his widow, she berated him, asking him why had he allowed him to die like that – and he asked himself the same question on the long journey home. He later instituted the first primary care oncology nurse in the country, acting as advocate and coordinator for cancer patients, in an effort to prevent such a sad situation recurring. This scheme continues, funded by Macmillan Cancer Relief.[20]

In the UK, we lead the world in the field of palliative care, since the inception of the modern hospice movement by Dame Cicely Saunders. But we cannot be complacent. There is still a lottery of differing qualities of care out there, and it can be hit or miss as to the care we may receive. The recent National Patients' Survey, collating the views of 65 000 NHS cancer patients in England, confirmed the marked inequities in the quality and appropriateness of care received by patients with different cancers, despite 86% of patients having total faith in their doctors.[21]

The US experience

In the USA, the over-medicalisation can be even more marked. In one New York hospital, in a group of elderly patients with advanced cancer or dementia, 47% received invasive non-palliative treatments during their final few days and 11% of cancer patients and 55% of dementia patients died with feeding tubes still in place.[22]

Dr Joanne Lynn, a US geriatrician, has led the development of a US collaborative in improving end-of-life care and is co-director of the Institute for Healthcare Improvement Breakthrough series. She asks how can we accept the situation of the disparate standards of end-of-life care. Why is it that if you ask anyone about the death of a family member you may hear a sad tale of pain, confusion and a mismatch of services offered and received, or you may hear of sustaining respectful care and support, but the final thought is 'Weren't we lucky!'.

Why lucky? We don't think we're lucky if an aeroplane lands safely or when we wake up after surgery because many people are doing their job well in a managed system designed to help people do their jobs effectively. Yet we accept it as our lot that our final days will be comfortable only if we're lucky.

> *How did we come to do so poorly on care at the end of life? A fundamental reason is we have simply never been here before. We face problems our grandparents would envy – the problems that come from growing quite old and dying rather slowly.... So what will we need when we have to live with an eventually fatal chronic disease? More than anything else we need reliability – we need a care system we can count on.* To make excellent care routine we must learn to do routinely what we already know must be done ... *All it takes is innovation, learning, reorganisation and commitment. People should not expect end-of-life care to be miserable and meaningless ... we should get good care for our expense – without having to hope for good luck.*[23]

Surely we should be able to anticipate good care in the final days of our lives in the same way that we count on safe plane landings and good anaesthetics. Not everyone flies and not all of us go under the knife, but we're all travelling on a journey that will eventually lead to our death. So we're all in this together: without having to hope for good luck, we all wish for a 'good death' when the time comes.

The palliative care movement

A shift from cure-for-all to care-for-all

Family doctors in the UK have been caring for the dying at home since the nineteenth century days of the apothecaries. The history of the speciality of the general practitioner is interesting. A trade demarcation dispute allowed the physicians and surgeons to gain control of the great hospitals whilst the generalist apothecaries initiated the sole gate-keeping role of referrals of the patients to them. This pivotal position of British general practice has been a much emulated success across the world. Specialist care is vastly more expensive than generalist care, and cost-effectiveness is assured by controlling access via a generalist who is able to treat the majority of all illness episodes presented.[24]

However, since the early 1950s concerns about improving care at the end of life have been developing both in institutions and at home. A home death was no guarantee of dignity or a good death, and hospital deaths were a sign of failure. The response was the emergence of the palliative care movement. Dame Cicely Saunders, the outstanding innovator and founder of the modern hospice movement, led the way in 1967 at St Christopher's Hospice, Sydenham, which still plays a major role across the world in the continued development of the speciality. Within a decade the principles of hospice care were being practised across all settings – in the newly founded hospices, on the intimidating hospital wards and stretching out into the community.

The growth of the palliative care movement in this country answered to some extent the calls for euthanasia, so vociferous in other parts of the world. Gone were the days of the Brompton Cocktail, and the speciality began to have a far-reaching educational role, influencing care for patients with all end-stage illnesses. Palliative medicine was later recognised as a separate medical speciality by the Royal College of Physicians in 1987, with the ensuing accredited training schemes.

Macmillan Cancer Relief, the UK cancer charity, has been striving to improve care and represent the patient's voice for over 80 years, both in hospitals and in the community.[25] The rise of Macmillan nurses in the early 1990s continued to spread the message that effective palliative care for all was possible and necessary. Since then Macmillan has increasingly focused on primary palliative care, developing the role of Macmillan GP facilitators across the UK and helping to establish the speciality of palliative care physicians and supporting oncologists, other therapists, pharmacists, etc. The donation of patient grants, improved social care and the building of palliative care centres and information units are all part of Macmillan's vision. Along with Marie Curie hospices and other organisations in the voluntary sector, their contribution to patient care has been significant in this country.

It is hard to overstate the importance of the palliative care movement in radically changing the perceptions and practices of caring for the dying over the entire world. The wonderful advances in symptom control, holistic care and people-centred medicine are matched by an increasingly well-researched and evidence-based scientific approach, which enhances all our thinking. Hospice care, having started in this country, has become a worldwide movement, radically changing the way in which death and dying are approached. Some regard it as one of the greatest social innovations of the past 100 years.

The challenge for those of us in generalist care now is to take what we have learnt in the centres of excellence, the hospices and specialist palliative care units across the world, and apply this to the area of generalist palliative care in the community. To use 'hospice care' as a verb and take the lessons learnt out into the home. Rather than undermining the work of hospices and specialist units, in fact it affirms them, using them more appropriately to back up generalist care in the community.

The palliative care movement has helped shift the cure-for-all mentality towards a more care-for-all understanding, which is being developed further with the current thinking around the term 'supportive care'. In the community there is generally no longer talk of a takeover of care, but of dovetailing better the generalist and specialist care for patients by working more closely and more fruitfully together. In improving palliative care in specialist settings over recent years, standards have been raised but so have heckles. Some GPs felt they were being de-skilled and their patients, often known to them for years, were being taken over by strangers without the balance of cooperative shared care being achieved. That was one of the reasons for the popularity of community hospitals. There may still be some tensions around between hospice and other specialist staff, Macmillan nurses and their primary care colleagues, but increasingly as the speciality has become established we are working better together in our patients' best interests. We need each other and we need to find the best way of working together – there is plenty of work for us all!

Many palliative care units have developed 'hospice at home' or other outreach services, extending out into the community. Some units in rural areas have 'virtual' hospices with hospice staff to care for patients at home with minimal in-patient back-up;[27] some in inner cities such as London tend to take over all care once patients are diagnosed. But in the majority of areas there is a developing relationship of shared care and complementing skills.

Box 2.2 Definitions of palliative care

Palliative care:

- affirms life and regards dying as a normal process
- neither hastens nor postpones death
- provides relief from pain and other symptoms
- integrates the psychological and spiritual aspects of patient care
- offers a support system to help patients live as actively as possible until their death
- offers a support system to help the family cope during the patient's illness and in their own bereavement.

Palliative care is care that focuses on quality of life (including symptom control), takes a whole-person approach, encompasses both patient and those that matter to them, respects the patient's autonomy and choice and emphasises open and sensitive communication.

The World Health Organization's definition of palliative care is:

> *The active total care of patients whose disease is not responsive to curative treatment. Control of pain, of other symptoms and of psychological, social and spiritual problems is paramount. The goal of palliative care is the best quality of life for patients and their families ... palliative care ... offers a support system to help patients live as actively as possible until death ... offers a support system to help the family cope during the patient's illness and in their bereavement.*[26]

The current funding crisis of the voluntary sector

Much of the drive to improve palliative care comes from locally fundraised hospices and other charitable sectors. The voluntary and charitable sectors provide most of the hospice and specialist palliative care, including around 75% of in-patient hospice units (152 of the 208 units in Britain), with an estimated 56 000 admissions to hospices each year and 28 000 new patients attending day care each year.[28,29] There are currently 3029 hospice beds, with 334 home care teams and 243 day care units. The NHS manages 56 acute palliative care units, providing 6000 beds. Nineteen per cent of all cancer deaths occur in specialist palliative care units.

However there is currently a crisis in the funding of voluntary hospices, with some now beginning to close beds and turn patients away. Chronic state underfunding combined with increasing staff inspection and development costs over the past five years means that many voluntary hospices are having to dig deeply into their reserves to meet running costs. More than half our hospices are reported to be running at a deficit. Only a small proportion of promised state funding has as yet reached hospices. Although government funding has risen by 14% in cash terms, growing costs have pushed up expenditure by 23%, with total running costs estimated at £300 million per year. Only 28% of that is from the state purse as opposed to 37% five years previously. New government funding is now available for palliative care, but is it enough?

If current trends continue, many smaller hospices will have to close some of their beds. We in the community need the back-up of hospice beds as well as the expertise of those in specialist palliative care, and patients appreciate the services of day care and respite amongst many others. In England, with primary care trusts (PCTs) soon to be managing the budget, will the commissioning of local services change in future?[30]

> *At first I didn't want to go because I thought a hospice is where you go to die. But what I actually found when I got there is that it's somewhere you can come to life.*
>   BC, breast cancer patient at Overgate Hospice, Elland, Halifax[31]

Despite improving generalist palliative care with, for example, the GSF programme, there will always be a need for the invaluable contribution made by hospices in care of the dying. Having led the world with charitably-funded, pioneering hospice work, we must ensure that good palliative care remains available to all patients in whatever setting via the NHS and the inequities of voluntary-run and state-funded provision are ironed out. We need to 'mainstream' these compassionate people-centred developments into the standard NHS care, so the best examples of care become our standard practice.

Integrated care pathways: care in the last days of life

Increasingly we are being asked to demonstrate clinical effectiveness in the current climate of clinical governance, with tangible measures of the outcome of our care. For example, the Quality Peer Review (QPR) Project, developed in Yorkshire, promotes peer review of neighbouring hospices to push standards up against certain agreed benchmarks.[32]

Integrated care pathways (ICPs) are now a very popular American import into the UK, used extensively across all areas of medical care, but particularly in the hospital setting.[33,34] They provide a clear description of the ideal model of care and the processes and outcomes required to get there – another kind of map. In succinct outcome terms they provide guidelines and appropriate supporting documentation is included for reference. The ICP becomes central to the patient's care and is completed by all healthcare professionals involved with the patient. Thus they replace all other documentation.

Despite the particular challenges in attempting to develop hard outcome measures in palliative care, an ICP has been developed for care of the dying in the last days of life.[35] The excellent Beacon-awarded Liverpool Integrated Care Pathway, devised by Dr John Ellershaw and his team in Liverpool, is a very well developed tool, piloted firstly in hospitals and later in the community, nursing home and hospice settings. It focuses on the last days of life, using standards which if not adhered to become 'variances' and lead to an account or action. For example, one standard would be that patients should be pain free and if they are not this is noted, an action triggered and reassessments made. This aims to improve generalist palliative care provided by those less used to caring for the dying, and has been shown to radically improve care across many settings.

This work overlaps considerably with the GSF programme, focusing as it does on the last months of life in the community and including care of the last days of life. The quality of care for patients in the dying phase will follow on from the care already developed using the previous plan. So C7, the terminal phase, is a natural extension of the other six standards. But there are a few details specific to the care in the dying phase that are also worth looking at routinely, such as stopping non-essential treatments, the use of syringe drivers/subcutaneous drugs, the routine prescribing of drugs as required PRN, checking relatives know what to do after a death, etc.

We are extremely grateful to John Ellershaw and the Liverpool team who have combined forces with us for this work, contributing enormously to the improvement in the Framework.

Many practices are initially undertaking one of the two programmes which then leads on to the other in time.[36] They have also greatly improved the C3 symptom control section, introducing the validated tool of the PACA assessment scale.

The Wales Collaborative Care Pathway Project[37] has adapted this model and is currently implementing it across the whole of Wales, with training, support, website, newsletter and telephone helpline. Central collection and analysis of data have established a baseline measure, facilitated local and national benchmarking and indicated future directions for research and development.

Working together: dovetailing care

Generalist and specialist care

There is increasing debate about the terms 'specialist' and 'generalist' in palliative care as in other areas, although there is little conflict about the value of both. The 'specialist' develops expertise within the complexity of a defined clinical area, and the 'generalist' (in general practice) focuses on the complexity of the patient's medical, psychological and social contexts.[38,39] Generalist care is provided by those healthcare professionals who see patients with end-of-life conditions amongst patients with other conditions, such as on hospital wards, in nursing homes or in GP practices. There can be some confusion about the overlapping roles of specialists and generalists, such as the functioning of district nurses and Macmillan nurses in the community. The development of 'eligibility criteria' for referral to specialist palliative care services[40] has clarified this in some areas and helped improve the timeliness and appropriateness of referrals to specialist services (*see* Box 10.1, p. 164). The use of an integrated care pathway such as the Liverpool ICP for the Dying (detailed above)[35] also empowers and raises standards for generalist care. The National Service Framework for Older People (*see* www.radcliffe-oxford.com/caring) also broadens the generalist palliative care remit to include all older patients approaching the last stages of life, and the NSF for CHD likewise specifically integrates palliative care practices.

It has been estimated that between 25% and 65% of patients may need specialist palliative care advice on symptom control.[41] With the principles of palliative care now extending to such conditions as end-stage heart failure[42] and chronic obstructive pulmonary disease (COPD), there are many more patients out there than any specialist service could deal with; GPs and district nurses must exercise basic generic palliative care for all patients that require it and use discretion in referring appropriately and at the right time for further specialist help. It is sometimes a fine tightrope to tread.

Requirements of generalist palliative care

Recent discussions led by the National Council of Hospice and Specialist Palliative Care Services about definitions, standards and performance indicators in specialist palliative care and supportive care have led to a consultation on the minimum standards that are felt to be required by any generic workers involved in generalist palliative care. Although still in early draft form, it is felt that the patient and family's usual professional carer should be able to:

- assess the palliative care needs of each patient and their families across the domains of physical, psychological, social and spiritual need
- meet those needs within the limits of their knowledge, skills and competence
- know when to seek advice from and refer to specialist palliative care services.

In order to meet these requirements the health and social workforce will need appropriate training and guidance in basic symptom management, assessing the palliative care needs of patients and families, communication skills and when to refer to specialist palliative care services.[43]

What do GPs want from palliative care services?

GPs are generally appreciative of specialist palliative care services, although they vary in their use of them.[44] Shipman *et al.* explored GPs' use of and attitude towards specialist palliative care services across a range of urban and rural locations.[45] Predictably they found a spectrum of usage, from seldom using such services to handing over care or responsibility entirely (mainly in inner city areas), with the majority using the service as a resource. Some used specialists as part of an extended team, perhaps the ideal scenario, but this depended on good personal working relationships, teamwork and better communication. Availability of services was obviously a factor, but usage varied also according to patients' needs. The challenge for specialist services will be to develop strategies and resources to respond to such variations in demand. There has also been a clear message from GPs that more help and more education in palliative care for non-cancer patients is a high priority, as they suffer equally distressing symptoms often with second-class support.[39,46]

A recent systematic review confirmed that GPs deliver the majority of palliative care to patients in the last year of life, and generally do this in a sound and effective way, especially when they have appropriate specialist support and facilities.[47]

Dovetailing care

We obviously need each other and patients will benefit from good, respectful working relationships between generalists and specialists. Putting patients at the centre of the circle and focusing on this issue from the primary care viewpoint, the aim here is to improve generalist palliative care to interlink better with specialist services and complement each other. By affirming primary care in its role of caring for the dying, and enabling us to fulfil our potential in this area and do what we do best, we can overcome any residual territorialism, we can be stronger together and dovetail with those valuable colleagues who specialise in this vital area of medicine. This is one of the goals of the Gold Standards Framework.

References

1 Smith R (2000) A good death. *BMJ.* **320**: 129–30.

2 'Debate of the Age' Health and Care Study Group (1999) *The Future of Health and Care of Older People: the best is yet to come.* Age Concern, London.

3 Hornby N (2000) *Fever Pitch.* Penguin Books, London.

4 Heath I *The Mystery of General Practice.* The John Fry Trust Fellowship, Royal College of General Practitioners' website www.rcgp.org.uk

5 Skrabanek P and McCormick J (1992) *Follies and Fallacies in Medicine.* Tarragon Press, Chippenham.

6 Clark D (2002) Between hope and acceptance: the medicalisation of dying. *BMJ.* **324**: 905–7.

7 National Council for Hospice and Specialist Palliative Care Services (2002) *Working Definition of Supportive Care.* NCHSPC, London, May 2002.

8 Richardson A (2001) *Cancer and Primary Care: the role of GPs and Community Nurses in Caring for People with Cancer.* CHI and Audit Commission Report, supporting paper 5.

9 Ferguson J (2002) Death Plans. *Information Exchange.* London.

10 Rabbi Julia Neuberger, at the APM Congress, Warwick, 2000.

11 ONS Health Statistics, Quarterly Report. *The Times,* May 24th 2002.

12 Illich I (1976) *Limits to Medicine.* Marion Boyars, London.

13 Moynihan R and Smith R (2002) Too much medicine? *BMJ.* **324**: 859–60.

14 Ebrahim S (2002) The medicalisation of old age. *BMJ.* **324**: 862–3.

15 Higginson I (1999) Evidence-based palliative care. *BMJ.* **319**: 462–3.

16 Seymour J E (2001) *Critical Moments: death and dying in intensive care.* Open University Press, Milton Keynes.

17 Kubler-Ross E (1997) *The Wheel of Life,* p. 124. Bantam Books, London.

18 Higginson I, Astin P and Dolan S (1998) Where do cancer patients die? Ten-year trends in the place of death of cancer patients in England. *Pall Med.* **12**: 353–63.

19 Parkes C M (1985) Home, hospital or hospice? *Lancet.* **1**: 155–7.

20 Macmillan Primary Care Oncology Nurses, www.macmillan.org.uk. Contact adawson@macmillan.org.uk

21 More details of the National Patients' Survey on www.doh.gov.uk/nhspatients/cancersurvey

22 Ahronheim J C, Morrison R S *et al.* (1996) Treatment of the dying in the acute care hospitals: advanced dementia and metastatic cancer. *Arch Intern Med.* **156**: 2094–100.

23 Dr Joanne Lynn, Institute of Healthcare Improvement. Collaborative on improving end-of-life care. 'Accelerating Change Today', October 2000. National Coalition on Health Care, www.nchc.org and Institute of Healthcare Improvement, www.ihi.org

24 Fry J and Horder J (1994) *Primary Healthcare in an International Context.* Nuffield Province Hospitals Trust, London.

25 www.macmillan.org.uk

26 World Health Organization (1990) *Cancer Pain Relief and Palliative Care.* Technical Report Series 804. WHO, Geneva.

27 Bibby A (1999) *Hospice Without Walls.* Calouste Gulbenkian Foundation, London.

28 Eve A, Smith A M and Tebbit P (1997) Hospice and palliative care in the UK 1994–95. *Pall Med.* **11**: 31–43.

29 Garry A (2002) Palliative care. In M Baker (ed) *Modernising Cancer Services.* Radcliffe Medical Press, Oxford.

30 See National Association of Primary Care booklet on the commissioning of palliative care services by PCTs. In press.

31 Freen A (2002) Funding Shortfall Forces Hospices to Refuse the Dying. *The Times,* August 28th, 2002.

32 For more details of QPR, contact Liz Barker on Liz.Barker@nycris.leedsth.nhs.uk

33 Overill S (1998) A practical guide to care pathways. *J Integrated Care.* **2**: 93–8.

34 Campbell H, Hotchkiss R, Bradshaw N *et al.* (1998) Integrated care pathways. *BMJ.* **316**: 133.

35 Ellershaw J *et al.* (1997) Developing an integrated care pathway for the dying patient. *Eur J Pall Care.* **4**(6): 203–7.

36 More details of the Liverpool Integrated Care Pathway available from Marie Curie Hospice, Woolton, Liverpool L25 8QA or jellershaw@mariecurie.org.uk

37 More details available from wccpp.manager@nww-tr.wales.nhs.uk

38 Heath I, Evans P and Weel C (2000) The specialist of the discipline of general practice. *BMJ.* **320**: 326–7.

39 Carnell D (2000) Specialists and generalists. *BMJ.* **320**: 388.

40 Bennett M, Adams J, Alison D *et al.* (2000) Leeds Eligibility Criteria for specialist palliative care services. *Pall Med.* **14**(2): 157–8.

41 Higginson I (1997) Prevalence and Incidence. In: A Stevens and J Raftery (eds) *Palliative and Terminal Care: health care needs assessment.* Radcliffe Medical Press, Oxford.

42 Seamark D A, Ryan M, Smallwood N and Gilbert J (2002) Deaths from heart failure in general practice: implications for palliative care. *Pall Med.* **16**: 495–8.

43 Tebbit P (2002) *Definitions of Supportive and Palliative Care: a consultation paper.* National Council for Hospice and Specialist Palliative Care Services, London.

44 Higginson I (1999) Palliative care services in the community: what do family doctors want? *J Pall Care.* **15**: 21–5.

45 Shipman C, Addington-Hall J, Barclay S *et al.* (2002) How and why do GPs use specialist palliative care services? *Pall Med.* **16**: 241–6.

46 Addington-Hall J, Fakhoury W and McCarthy M (1998) Specialist palliative care in non-malignant disease. *Pall Med.* **12**: 417–27.

47 Mitchell GK (2002) How well do general practitioners deliver palliative care? A systematic review. *Pall Med.* **16**: 457–64.

CHAPTER 3

Living and dying at home

Mission Impossible? Palliative care at home embraces what is most noble in medicine: sometimes curing, always relieving, supporting right to the end.[1]

This chapter examines the current state of primary palliative care, arguing that primary healthcare teams should be the 'conductors' of the orchestra and that now is the time to develop and enhance this crucial aspect of primary care. It includes:

1 Living and dying at home: improving home care is important
2 Promoting security
3 The role of the primary healthcare team
4 Primary care developments
5 The primary care-led NHS: our opportunity for action.

Living and dying at home: improving home care is important

Home care

Home holds a special place in our affections. Home is both a state and a place; we say we 'feel at home' somewhere, 'home is where the heart is', an ethereal spiritual quality from which we draw strength to face the external world, and yet we make these homes amidst the physical structures that surround us.

> *And when we were still far off you met us in your son and brought us home.*
>
> Anglican Service Book

Home represents life and living, and the surroundings of our homes will encourage us to live whilst dying. We feel comfortable with the familiar, surrounded by symbols of our lives, youthful photos of times past, mementoes of treasured times. Those of us privileged to visit people in their homes are witness to a special kind of sharing; we see *people* in their homes, not *patients*.

We should not rush to separate people from their homes, especially for those approaching a natural conclusion of their lives. The final departure from home, if it should come, should not be hurried to allow a sombre, decent farewell. A crisis admission is in many ways a real catastrophe and many long to return, even briefly, to catch up with their emotions. Spilling, a GP interested in care for the dying, writes:

> *The decision to move a terminally ill patient from home should be taken in the knowledge that in addition to loss of familiarity and freedom, an element of hope will be lost.*[2]

Despite accusations that death is the last taboo, it still makes good television. In most of the current soap operas and series over recent years there has been a description of a character dying, often at home, and there have been several real-life documentaries following the lives of dying people, accurately reflecting the inequities of care in the real world.

The preferred place of death

Most people, when asked where they would like to die, express the preference for a home death and yet only a minority achieve this (26%).[3] However, even for those who die in a hospice, nursing home or hospital, most of the final year of life will be spent at home under the care of the primary healthcare team.[4] Many patients particularly value the psychosocial support provided by GPs, DNs and Macmillan nurses.[5] Primary palliative care is important, no matter where the final place of death is. As Thorpe so succinctly put it in his two paradoxes:[6]

First paradox
1   Most dying people would prefer to remain at home but most of them die in institutions.
Second paradox
2   Most of the final year of life is spent at home but most people are admitted to hospital to die.

Improving home care is important, no matter where death eventually occurs. Yet those final days are important too: a 'good death' involves taking into account the patient's preferred place of care. Too rarely are patients asked where they would wish to be cared for at the end. We know that when it is asked, it is more likely to be fulfilled.[7] By sensitively approaching this question, we are more likely to raise the patient's agenda higher and enable them to retain more control of the situation. It is very difficult to ask this question – it requires sensitive discussion and it is not always possible to note it. Possible ways of opening the conversation might be by asking: 'If your condition worsens/when the time comes, have you thought about where you'd like to be cared for?' It's very helpful to note the answer and date it. If the person eventually dies in a place other than the stated place of choice, it's useful to note why, e.g. carer couldn't cope, difficult symptoms, etc., which will contribute to the overall picture and may be used to institute improvements. Informing relatives of the likely process at the end, discussing decisions such as where and how, and bringing up the uncomfortable question of whether to treat or resuscitate – all this prepares the family, avoids crises and enables a more gentle letting go.

> *I was terrified at first when they said they would discharge him home – I didn't think I could cope. But in looking after Peter dying at home, I felt I was fulfilling his wishes and we were a real family – this really helps me now. Our GPs and district nurses were really caring and professional and kept pace with us at each step – we felt so grateful to them. Although it was so sad, it was also in some ways a very good and satisfying experience, etched for ever on our minds. The children and I are so glad that we were able to look after him at home, where he wanted to be, with the help of our marvellous team.*
>
> Maureen, wife of Peter, cancer patient who died at home

It might be easy to interpret the evidence in the literature as focusing only on the home death rates. This is a relatively easy measurement and has been used as a proxy outcome measure in several studies. Many feel this is not the whole story nor is it our whole aim in improving community palliative care. It would be good to increase the home death rate eventually, moving it closer towards the estimated number who would prefer to die at home. However, this is not the overriding factor and it needs to be emphasised that the goal should not be altering numbers dying at home but ensuring a 'good death', where possible in the patient's preferred place of care.

Hospices have led the way in care of the dying and for many patients, especially those connected with day care or receiving respite care, the local hospice will be the preferred final resting place. If so, this could possibly be planned in advance, though increasingly demand for hospice beds is outstripping supply. Some voice the concern however that we may be raising expectations, and hospice admissions are not always possible at the time they are required.

Box 3.1 Why improve community palliative care?

Community palliative care needs to be improved for the following reasons:

- Sicker patients are living longer and mainly in the community.
- There has been a shift into community care – less hospital/hospice care is available.
- Hospital is more likely if patient is poor, elderly or has no carers.
- The home death rate is low (26%), yet home is preferred by most.
- 90% of the final year is spent at home.
- Gaps are apparent in community care, e.g. symptom control, nursing support.
- Specialist palliative care raised standards but is changing – the average length of stay in a hospice is two weeks and 50% are discharged.
- 96% of hospice patients have cancer, which accounts for 25% of all deaths.
- Patients with non-malignant conditions may have inequity of access and levels of support.
- Better care increases family and staff satisfaction – GPs and DNs are keen to improve and see this as intrinsic primary care.
- GPs and DNs can make a real difference for some of our most vulnerable patients.
- NHS Cancer Plan, Supportive Care Strategy, National Patient Survey and other documents highlight that patients' experience of care is variable: 'The care of all dying patients must improve to the level of the best.'[8]
- The user voice is becoming stronger and better heard: 'Need for good communication, clear information, best possible symptom control, psychological support – being treated with humanity, dignity and respect.'[8]
- National directives such as the NHS Cancer Plan as a National Service framework, British Medical Association/General Practitioner Committee proposed new contract for GPs,[9] New Opportunity Funds bids, Out of Hours Department of Health Review,[10] Department of Health DN training grants, etc.

The impact on hospitals: reducing inappropriate admissions

The quality of palliative care we provide in the community has a significant impact on secondary and tertiary hospital services and hospices. Reducing inappropriate admissions, especially in a crisis, is a key priority for all. Not only is this best for patients, but it also makes best use of our expensive hospital services. Wastage is intrinsic in most healthcare systems. Some feel that for us in the UK it is the overusage of hospital admissions that is our greatest misuse of resources.[11]

Areas of inequity in community palliative care

Currently there are several areas of inequity within primary palliative care:

1 The current inequity in provision of palliative care in the community – variations in knowledge, organisation of care, levels of communication and in provision of services such as district nurse availability, night sitters, etc.
2 The lack of specialist palliative care services in some regions – several areas do not have a palliative care consultant yet and some are unable to extend their service into the community. (The GSF or equivalent may be even more necessary in these areas.)
3 The variation in standards of primary palliative care provided within regions in the UK, between different general practices and even within a single general practice partnership, where one GP may be more interested than another, leads to inequities in the quality of care received.[12] With the initiatives in England of Department of Health (DoH) funding for district nurse education in palliative care, some of the disparities in knowledge levels of nurses may be reduced, but this is currently also very variable.

Promoting security

In many ways a critical factor in the care of the dying at home is whether patients and carers are surrounded by a sense of security – the knowledge of what might happen, who to contact and what to do if it does and the reassurance of the 'seamless' continuity of care that the home team can provide (*see* Chapter 4, p. 45). One of the reasons patients and their carers wish to be admitted to hospital or a hospice is that they feel 'safer' there. How can we engender that feeling of safety in the community? Dunlop, a former hospice Medical Director, feels that: 'Even when symptoms are minimal, there is a feeling of constant anxiety for patients and family; a vulnerability and helplessness, a burden of responsibility, a fear of future problems and difficulties interpreting the patient's condition. Professionals may sometimes make these problems worse.'[13] Yet when asked, especially when well, most would choose to stay at home. If we could create that same sense of security in the home, would there be fewer panic cries for help and breakdown of home care leading to admissions?

Although inadequate symptom control is a significant cause of admission, many such symptoms are dealt with in the community elsewhere. Some argue therefore that the greatest cause of admission is breakdown of the ability to cope at home by patients and their carers. If we strengthen this confidence in the patient and carers' ability to cope, promoting a sense of security at home, fewer crisis calls will arise and more will remain at home longer or die at home, if that is their wish.

In some ways there are three groups of patients (*see* Figure 3.1):

1 **Institution preference.** Those who would always wish for an Institutionalised death. They may be attached to a hospital or hospice because of previous links (e.g. hospice day care, breast clinical nurse specialist/links with an oncology ward, etc.). This group of patients may have prolonged illness trajectories and much hospital/hospice contact; however they may alternatively have shortened illnesses and have heightened defences or denial, suddenly deteriorate and be unprepared for a worsening of their condition.

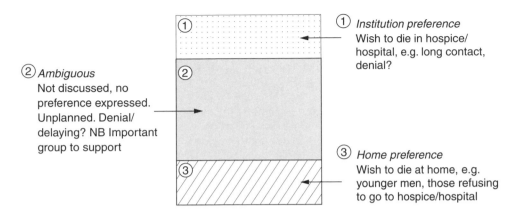

② *Ambiguous*
Not discussed, no
preference expressed.
Unplanned. Denial/
delaying? NB Important
group to support

① *Institution preference*
Wish to die in hospice/
hospital, e.g. long contact,
denial?

③ *Home preference*
Wish to die at home, e.g.
younger men, those refusing
to go to hospice/hospital

Figure 3.1: Categories of patients and preferences for place of death.

2 **Ambiguous.** Those who fall in the middle of these groups, where a preference has been hard to discuss or not expressed, or no preparations made. It is this group of patients to whom we should particularly direct our energies for good community care and anticipation of concerns and needs. Hinton suggested that many late admissions to a hospice were related to initial attitudes of denial, conscious fighting of the disease and unrealistic expectations.[14]

3 **Home preference.** Those who would never want admission to a hospice or hospital, perhaps because of stigma, other experiences or preconceptions. These may typically be younger men wishing to remain at home with their families or older people who have never been to hospital.

When a crisis admission does occur, perhaps this raises the question 'what could we have done in the community that could have prevented this?' Of course not everything is preventable, but with good planning, communication and proactive care, many issues can be addressed before they reach crisis proportions. We must not allow ourselves to feel guilty about a 'crisis' hospital/hospice admission – there will always be many unpreventable reasons for admission – but we should question in order to prevent recurrence.

This view of 'seamless care', much quoted since first used in the Calman Hine report,[15] has been criticised heavily. In many ways the reality is that there are seams, as in any garment, but we must strive to ensure they are only on the inside and hardly visible to the patients and their families. There is much we can do to allow easy movement across these seams or boundaries of care.

Caring for carers (*see also* Chapter 11)

Community palliative care is important for our patients with an end-stage illness. This may be even more true for those caring for dying patients, for whom the ordeal may be almost too much to bear – some would say at times an even harder journey than for the patient. GPs and district nurses play a particularly crucial role in their care, looking after them before, during and after bereavement.

It is formally recognised that, for many carers, the most important initial point of contact is with their GP or another member of the primary healthcare team ... It is clearly regarded that GPs have a key role in supporting carers and influencing service providers in their local community.[16]

For those of us as professionals caring for the dying, in hospices, the community, nursing homes, etc., we also need to allow care for ourselves, to nurture team support, debriefing and a celebration when things go well. This is an area which is close to our hearts and affects our self-esteem as professionals; it carries a burden with it of guilt and self-criticism alongside the satisfaction of a job well done. When things go wrong, we must protect ourselves not with defensive anecdote and alcohol, but with realistic team support and the opportunity to share feelings of inadequacy and a sense of improving care – bringing good outcomes from bad scenarios. Usually great time and personal effort goes into the delivery of care and we need the chance to acknowledge this, promote teamwork and also celebrate its success (*see* 'traffic lights' significant event analysis, pp. 92–5 and p. 235).

The role of the PHCT
The speciality of the generalist

GPs, it has been said, specialise in their patients. It is the speciality of the generalist, putting people first and diseases second. Family physicians 'are committed to the person rather than to a particular body of knowledge, group of diseases or special technique and seek to understand the context of the illness'.[17] We act as 'an interpreter and guardian at the interface between illness and disease and as witnesses to the human experience of, and search for meaning in, both illness and disease'.[18]

It is said that in hospitals, diseases stay the same and patients come and go, but in primary care, patients stay the same but diseases come and go. Others claim that specialists know more and more about less and less, whilst generalists know less and less about more and more! It can be hard being a generalist.

In primary care we offer something special to our dying patients: continuity of care, the 'being there',[17] the ability to act as a guide in this new and frightening territory, the care for the carers, the promise of being 'companions on the journey'. District nurses play a crucial and sometimes unsung role in the management, co-ordination and delivery of palliative care, and their care makes an important and much valued contribution to patients in their homes. Extra training in palliative care is available, e.g. the recent DoH £2 million grant for DN training in England, and they are often the most motivated and enthusiastic agents of change in their areas.

A recent important systematic review of palliative care delivered by GPs confirmed that GPs value this work and they feel comfortable working with specialists.[19] The contributions from GPs that patients particularly appreciate are their ability to listen, allowing ventilation of feelings, being accessible and basic symptom control. The review concluded that GPs can and do provide sound and effective palliative care, but recommends programmes of joint working with specialists. This important role of listening and accessibility is one that needs to be affirmed and enabled, in the ever-increasing demands placed on general practice today.

Caring for the dying presents us with considerable challenges of coordinating care, effective communication, clinical assessment and acumen. These are challenges not just to our clinical skills (head knowledge) but to the organisational abilities within our practices (hands/systems) (*see* Figure 1.1, p. 8).

Iona Heath reminds us: 'Where we cannot cure we must be available to help the patient make some kind of sense of their suffering ... The GP, often seeing patients through 20 or 30 years of illness and disease, both major and minor, as well as a series of significant life events, is in a unique position to help the patient make some sense of what is happening to them. The key skill here is *to listen* and in so doing to allow the patient to find their own pattern and explanation. The doctor witnesses the suffering, the struggle and the fortitude of the patient and the relationship is one of solidarity.'[16]

The conductor of the orchestra

So how can we play our part in primary care to get this right? How can we maintain the human touch whilst still orchestrating the right notes to be played at the right time?

We need to help develop systems in our routine care that will enhance our companionship and smooth the journey for those nearing the end of life. We must develop teamwork so that together we present our patients, and perhaps even more importantly, their carers, with the kind of supportive care that will sustain them as they travel this way. There are some of us who have been this way before – in primary care we are in an ideal position to help patients, as they travel this way for the first time, sharing the wisdom we have gleaned from experience. The small details that can make all the difference such as anticipating future needs, talking sensitively about the dying process, forewarning and reassuring, and helping our patients approach dying with more confidence. 'Being there' is very important.

> As death draws close we visit frequently, even though there is no specific task for us to perform or problem to solve. Together with the district nurses we shepherd our patients through this intensely emotional and often frightening time. Simply by being there, we acknowledge the gravitas of the events taking place, bearing witness to courage, to love seen within families and between friends.[20]

Without this pivotal role of primary care for our patients they can feel deserted, lost, without a guide in a foreign territory. There may be others who pick up the baton, for those patients fortunate enough to be under the care of a good hospice service or well-organised hospital department, but the chances are that they may fall between all available stools and feel abandoned by the system that is there to support them.

> Some GPs continued to visit regularly and gave regular support. Some visited only occasionally – often stiffly, awkwardly and with no promise to call again. Many never visited. Both nurses and relatives would have liked a regular, friendly, weekly call, but it never came.
>
> The essential concept is that the doctor, or at least the practice, will stay firmly with the patient and relative at their time of need and not desert them ...
>
> When a patient is dying at home ... it makes a big difference if the doctor continues to call regularly ... otherwise they are likely to feel abandoned and deserted when they least expect it ... The promise of a regular visit gives a special kind of support unlike any other.[21]

In Rachel Clark's *A Long Walk Home*, an evocative and moving account of her treatments and experiences whilst she was living with and dying from cancer, she describes her experiences of being lost in the system of care.[22] The loss of important scans, cancelling of vital appointments and the general confusion of where to go next are themes that will be familiar to us all as professionals and users of the health service. As Williams comments: 'When cancer is diagnosed patients are linked into several different professionals and agencies – multidisciplinary working is essential in cancer and palliative care. But somebody needs to conduct the orchestra. In the UK the obvious person to carry out this role is the general practitioner, yet GPs are often unintentionally sidelined. Many GPs may feel they have little to offer, especially when things change so quickly and letters arrive so slowly. Patients consumed by hospital appointments may not see the relevance or have the energy to make yet another appointment with the GP.'[23]

Yet if the GP or the PHCT does not conduct the orchestra, who will? Patients are more likely to become lost, abandoned and deserted at this most bewildering of times when they need to muster all their emotional energy to cope with the demands of their changing perspective. It is a vital and important role. Many primary care teams respond by having a dedicated nurse or other member of the team to offer this coordination and support. (This is the role of the nominated practice coordinator of the GSF (*see* Chapter 13). This has been extended by some to include patients from diagnosis.)[24] It can therefore be argued that the conductor of the orchestra should be the PHCT, notably the GP and District Nurse. It is a challenging but immensely rewarding task, which we in primary care must reaffirm and embrace, as life becomes increasingly complex and de-humanised for our patients.

Just one concern amongst many in general practice?

Cancer patients, though relatively few in number, will represent a considerable proportion of practice time for GPs and district nurses due to their increasing morbidity as their illness progresses. If you add to this the burden of other non-malignant conditions, e.g. COPD, end-stage heart disease, etc., the community palliative care workload can be considerable (*see* Box 3.2).[25]

Box 3.2 An average GP practice

For every GP (average list size 2000 patients) there will be:

- about 20 patient deaths from all causes per year
- approximately 30–40 patients with cancer at any one time
- nine new patients with cancer per year
- five patients with cancer die per year
- 26% cancer patients die at home
- 12% cancer patients die in nursing homes
- i.e. a total of 38% patients die under the care of the PHCT
- out-of-hours services provided by a local cooperative and/or deputising agency.

There are some hurdles to the ideal of seamless, patient-focused, competent and compassionate care:

- constraints on time – a big factor as workload demands on GPs and DNs increase (particularly for single-handed practices) as some GPs, not uncommonly, may still see over 50 patients in a day
- difficulties with communications across the boundaries of care (and in the 'hand-offs' between them)
- difficulties maintaining continuity of care between different professionals within a team or during the out-of-hours periods
- difficulties knowing what is available and how to access it – thinking creatively in trying to address a person's needs
- difficulties dealing with rarely seen, challenging clinical conditions
- coordination – somehow not letting things slip through the net
- problems in fully assessing and treating patients' symptoms.

How can we better coordinate what we have? This is probably a task that will never be fully completed, but my hope is that the GSF will contribute towards a solution.

In primary care we see many different kinds of problems in much greater numbers than just palliative care or cancer patients, so why prioritise them? Increasingly, we are being asked to pick out certain groups and organise their care on a pathway, having 'mapped the patient journey'. We may collect our hypertensives, asthmatics and diabetics in specific clinics, and since the advent of the National Service Frameworks have had registers, databases protocols and meetings for heart disease patients.

The World Health Organization (WHO) has developed some global measures to represent the burden of disease in a population which take into account the years of life lost due to premature mortality (YLL) and the years of life lived with disability (YLD), summarised into a specific index: the Disability Adjusted Life Year (DALY). This has been used to indicate that despite GPs not seeing many cancer patients per year, the 'burden of disease' of cancer patients is second only to heart disease in primary care.[26] The DALY could be used to inform policy and monitor the effect of certain changes over time.

So, the care of cancer patients and others with end-stage illnesses in primary care is important and does occupy a significant amount of our time.

Prioritising dying patients in primary care: a barometer of care

In the current climate of general practice, it may be easy to feel that we're sinking in a sea of overwhelming needs from patients below, whilst simultaneously being rained upon by a continuous stream of dictates and 'must-do's' from on high. This causes all of us to question why we are doing it at all, to perhaps try to get away with the minimum for survival or to 'de-compensate' and give up altogether (the inference of high retirement and drop-out rates). It's obviously important to protect ourselves and our family life outside medicine. We must do this to survive. But there are also other aids to survival such as prioritising the work, to 'think team' and to develop workable systems within our practice that make life easier, not harder.

Traditionally, general practice has always been described as care provided from 'cradle to grave'. In primary palliative care we know we only have one chance to get it right – we all go this way once only. Many GPs and district nurses have an instinctive feel that amongst all the needs and demands placed upon us, those in the last stages of life should take precedence over others – we must prioritise so that we're able to see the woods for the trees again.

I would argue that of all the demands on us, the two defining criteria could be:

- the needs of the most seriously ill in our practice, and
- those for whom we can make the most difference.

Despite GPs' crowded schedules and demands on time, there is real evidence of a genuine desire to prioritise care of the seriously ill patients in the community.[19] In terms of job satisfaction, it is thought to be one of the top three most satisfying parts of the job (good births, good deaths and getting the right diagnosis), and many are drawn to the holistic and very human nature of palliative care in general practice.

Overall those in primary care strive hard in this area and achieve a good standard of care, although this may be variable. This is often at the expense of considerable extra time and effort, sometimes outside normal working hours, which is much appreciated by patients and carers; many GPs and also DNs still give their home phone numbers to dying patients, which is very commendable, but not practicable in every case as standard procedure.[27] The preferred model for sustainable care in future is that of sharing care within the team and with the out-of-hours service, building a bridge over these gaps in services so that all can still have real time off from work and patients are still well covered at all times (*see* Chapters 12, 15 and 16).[28]

Many consider caring for cancer patients and those with palliative care needs as top of their agenda, as a 'barometer' of other aspects of care. Of all the people we see in general practice, from those with self-limiting conditions, chronic diseases, psychosocial problems and so on, who better deserves our greatest efforts than those with a serious life-threatening illness? If there is a genuine emergency call for a myocardial infarction, for example, we will drop everything, blue lights flash and we will rightly prioritise them because they may be near to death. But there is another group of patients for whom there is no blue flashing light, who are also near to death – do we prioritise them amidst all the demands of the working day? Is there more we could do for those in the last year, months or days of life? I would argue that often there is, but that it is partly a matter of organisation, of an improved system of care, to improve the service we provide for these most needy and most deserving of our patients.

There is a great emphasis from the Government at present on improving community care and 'intermediate' care and preventing inappropriate hospital admissions. National Service Frameworks, the National Cancer Plan and plans for revalidation and accreditation of practice, etc. are with us and there may be less option soon, with more 'top-down' directives. However, using these 'bottom-up changes', we will be moving in the right direction.

Primary care developments

Macmillan GP Facilitators

For about 10 years Macmillan Cancer Relief have been investing in making real grass-roots changes in community cancer and palliative care. They set up the innovative posts of Macmillan GP Facilitators in Palliative Care in the early 1990s[29] and currently there are about 70 MGPFs across the UK. This book, the Gold Standards Framework and other pieces of work all developed from the protected time given to me in my capacity as Macmillan GP Facilitator at Calderdale and Kirklees Health Authority, West Yorkshire and draws from the collective experience of many MGPFs across the country – for which I'm very grateful.

MGPFs are practising GPs with an interest in palliative care. Their remit is largely to develop educational activities and to be catalysts of change in their own areas, by peer to peer support and instigating local strategic developments.[30] More recently Macmillan have been helping to support the role of Primary Care Organisation Cancer Lead in England, which is having a significant impact in developing real strategic changes, linked with the Cancer Networks and the Cancer Services Collaborative. Macmillan have part-funded this work in Phase 2, and are running the Macmillan GSF Programme to roll out the GSF across the UK – more information is available at www.radcliffe-oxford.com/caring and from Macmillan Cancer Relief.[31]

Standards and accreditation for cancer and palliative care

There are currently several different groups across the UK, mainly involving Macmillan-sponsored projects, which are working on the development of appraisal and standard setting for primary cancer care, such as the North West Macmillan Cancer Standards Project.[32] Work is ongoing as this book goes to press; this will be collated and primary care cancer standards may develop across the UK. The new GPC/BMA contract, if agreed, will have standards and achievement awards attached, as mentioned previously, which will relate to palliative care, as well as heart disease, etc. This is an area undergoing rapid development, but it may mean that practices will at least feel better resourced when they attempt to raise the quality of their care, such as in undertaking the GSF or other similar initiatives. Many practices in England have accessed funding for this work from their PCT, New Opportunity Fund grants, their Cancer Networks, etc.

The Shipman debate and its consequences

Dame Janet Baker's interim report on the Shipman Inquiry has significant implications for us all. As a well-liked and trusted GP in Hyde, near Manchester, Harold Shipman was found to have been responsible for the murder of at least 215 of his patients over a period of several years, with another 45 deaths for which he may have been responsible.[33] This has an impact on everyone, especially in considering the care of the dying at home and the use of strong opioids. Shipman began his series of murders by killing his terminally ill patients first, and after a lull, often restarted with them again. He seems to have become addicted to the sinister thrill of determining the course of other peoples' lives.

There will undoubtedly be implications for community palliative care. It has been joked that the home death rate for the Shipman practice was admirably high. However, the full impact of the report of his terrible atrocities is yet to be felt, but there will be developments and they will probably impinge on the work described here. In future there may be increased hurdles concerning, for example, the leaving of drugs in the home, and there will undoubtedly be tighter regulations on drug usage. The mind of a 'death-addicted, power-hungry murderer' disguised as a friendly GP will no doubt have significant consequences. We must ensure however that they do not have repercussions that will detrimentally affect patient care and leave many more in pain at home for lack of access to adequate analgesics. Living in the post-Shipman era, those of us with an interest in this field must be even more vigilant and rigorous in our monitoring (e.g. accuracy of recording), but also in our advocacy for our patients.

Out-of-hours palliative care[34] (*see* Chapter 15)

The long periods in the week outside normal working hours (up to 70% of the week) can be a living nightmare for patients with serious illnesses. There is great variation across the UK in the provision for palliative care patients, leading to vast chasms of inadequate care in some areas. There is often:

- little communication about these patients to out-of-hours providers, and
- greatly reduced access to support such as district nursing, specialist advice, carer support, equipment or drugs.

The commonest reasons for admission are a breakdown in support for carers, plus problems with symptom control and communication. There is evidence that there are more problems with the elderly, poor and those with no carers, along with other predictive factors (*see* p. 70). Other confounding issues are the increased mediation of NHS Direct or its equivalent as a first telephone triage for all out-of-hours calls, demographic changes leading to more people being alone or far from their families and the changing roles of hospices and rising need for community hospital or nursing home beds as places of intermediate care.

Patient control and issues of real choice are discarded in crisis situations. In an obstetric analogy, when asked in the cool light of day about birth plans most pregnant women request everything to be as natural and homespun as possible, but once in the agony of labour many (myself included) will cry out for any analgesic going and the ideals of autonomy are quickly discarded for removal of this pain. Likewise, patients in pain at home have already lost some control and real effective choice when their symptoms are not well relieved.

We need to ensure measures are in place before this situation occurs, using good *anticipated care*, and that patients, their families and the visiting on-call services know what to do and how to do it. Many leave a standard few drugs in the homes of those in the terminal stages, such as:

- diamorphine or equivalent
- hyoscine for secretions
- midazolam for agitation
- haloperidol/cyclizine/levomopromazine for sickness.

This entails an important change of mindset *from reactive to proactive* to be able to anticipate problems ahead and plan for them. The next step is to send information to the out-of-hours provider, e.g. using a *handover form*. Many are *developing a protocol* for out-of-hours palliative care to change the service as a whole, along with their GP cooperatives (with the help of the National Association of GP Cooperatives; NAGPC), deputising service and specialist palliative care service.

With improved access to drugs and better coordination of care, many developments such as the Western Health Board Review in Northern Ireland[35] and the PENDOC cooperative and health authority protocol in West Yorkshire[36] are rapidly making major improvements for patients out-of-hours. A few changes make a vast difference, especially in a crisis. In the West Yorkshire protocol mentioned, we were able to show real changes in the level of satisfaction of care from the district nurses and GPs as well as from carers. This is an area that is fast developing but urgently requires examination and improvement, and real change is possible.

The primary care-led NHS: our opportunity for action

The world of healthcare is changing around us. Nigel Edwards of the NHS Confederation argues that there is a new compact between doctors and society; the individual orientation that doctors were trained for does not fit with the demands of current healthcare systems. Medicine has been based on a model in which doctors are trained to deal with individuals, not organisations; to take personal responsibility rather than delegate; and to do their best for each patient rather than make trade-offs in a resource-constrained environment.[37] There is now greater accountability, an emphasis on greater availability, more collective working with other doctors and staff, a growing blame culture and a greater emphasis on 'consumerism', with consequent evaluation by patient-centred measures.

The older image of the respected family doctor caring personally for individual patients continues in some ways, perhaps quintessentially in care of the dying, but is supplemented with the other images of the manager of community resources, the organiser of services, the screener and preventer, the promoter of evidence-based guidelines and so on. Perhaps one of the particular attractions of primary palliative care is that it reflects more purely the traditional model of holistic care for our patients, which was the aspiration of many of us entering medical school.

The structures of our health service are changing too. Alan Milburn, MP and Secretary of State for Health, at the announcement of increased funding for the NHS, affirmed the vision of the 'primary care-led NHS' saying:

> Instead of all public capital being allocated by the Department of Health from Whitehall ... it will particularly focus on strategic shifts in configuration to more community- and primary care-based services. As regards revenue funding, locally run primary care trusts will hold over 75% of the growing NHS budget.[38]

The 314 or so primary care trusts across England will determine the provision of services, including the commissioning of the NHS subsidy for local hospices in response to locally determined needs, in discussion with social services. The equivalent bodies in the other nations, although not all having commissioning powers, are becoming increasingly influential; the focus remains on primary care. The opportunity to improve community care is with us now as never before.

Excellent as the secondary and tertiary hospital services are, with their death-defying heroics and increasing survival rates, one consequence of our investment of faith and hope in our medical institutions is that we may have been distracted from care in the community and 'taken our eye off the ball'. Now sicker people are living longer at home, are we unsure of the best way to offer support to them in primary care? When offered over-aggressive potential cures, how many families might wish in retrospect that their loved one had given up on treatment and enjoyed their remaining days without all the be-dripped, toxic medical paraphernalia.

Are we only focusing on the quantity of life, at the expense of quality of life? Are we focusing on cure for all at the expense of care for all? Have we forgotten the principle of curing sometimes, caring always? Is it time for primary care to rediscover its essential mission and reassert the importance of supportive care? Surely, in this new age of the 'primary care-led NHS', this is our opportunity to reaffirm the patient-centred supportive role of primary care for our most seriously ill patients above all else. Will there ever be a better time than now?

In society's championing of institutionalised dying, we may have forgotten the value of the time-honoured care and support offered to those as we walk with them on this journey. The palliative care movement has to some extent redressed this balance, sparked off by the inspiring example of hospices and palliative care teams across the world. But for those of us in primary care looking after patients in their own homes and communities, there can be a mismatch between the kind of service we feel we'd like to give our most needy patients and the day-to-day reality of overstretched busy primary care.

Real life is messy. Are we giving our seriously ill or dying patients in the community the kind of care that we would like to receive ourselves or are we relying on good luck? And is this the moment to take up the baton again in primary care and rediscover our mission impossible of 'sometimes curing, always relieving, supporting right to the end'?[1] In England at least, PCTs will be increasingly involved in the commissioning of palliative care services and overseeing hospices and other voluntary sector organisations. A useful booklet by the National Association of Primary Care details some of the challenges now facing us in developing community palliative care services.[39]

The time is ripe for change. There is much activity at present in the area of community palliative care in the UK, and an increasing momentum of improvements and developments both nationally and locally. The Gold Standards Framework for community palliative care, detailed in Part 3, is seen as part of the current exponential developments.

In care of the dying we only have one chance to get it right. We are seeking solutions, not dwelling on the problems. By thrashing out the issues together in a constructive way we will find ways through the problems.

Director of Public Health, Northern Ireland

References

1 Gomas J M (1993) Palliative care at home: a reality or mission impossible? *Pall Med.* **7**: 45–59.

2 Spilling R (1986) *Terminal Care at Home.* Oxford General Practice Series. Oxford University Press.

3 Higginson I, Astin P and Dolan S (1998) Where do cancer patients die? Ten-year trends in the place of death of cancer patients in England. *Pall Med.* **12**(5): 353–63.

4 Cartwright A (1990) *The Role of the General Practitioner in Caring for People in the Last Year of Life.* King's Fund, London.

5 Grande G E, Todd C J, Barclay S I G *et al.* (1996) What terminally ill patients value in the support provided by GPs, DNs and Macmillan nurses. *Int J Pall Nurs.* **2**: 138–43.

6 Thorpe G (1993) Enabling more dying people to remain at home. *BMJ.* **307**: 915–18.

7 Karlson S and Addington-Hall J (1998) How do patients who die at home differ from those who die elsewhere? *Pall Med.* **12**(4): 279–86.

8 NHS Cancer Plan, September 2000.

9 General Practitioner Committee (2002) *Your Contract Your Future.* British Medical Association, London, April 2002.

10 Department of Health (2000) *Raising Standards for Patients: new partnerships in out-of-hours care.* [Independent review.] DoH, London.

11 Berwick D, President and CEO of the Institute for Healthcare Improvement, NHS Modernisation Agency Associate Conference, London, 2002.

12 National Patient Survey (2002) www.doh.gov.uk/nhspatients/cancersurvey

13 Dunlop R (2002) Eliciting attributions and promoting security. [Personal communication.]

14 Hinton J (1998) Which patients with terminal cancer are admitted from home care? *Pall Med.* **12**(1): 51–3.

15 NHS Executive (1995) *Commissioning Cancer Services: report of the Expert Advisory Group on Cancer.* NHS Executive, Leeds.

16 Simon C (2001) Informal carers and the primary care team. *Br J Gen Pract.* **51**: 920–3.

17 McWhinney L (1997) *A Textbook of Family Medicine.* Oxford University Press.

18 Heath I *The Mystery of General Practice.* The John Fry Trust Fellowship, Royal College of General Practitioners' website www.rcgp.org.uk

19 Mitchell G K (2002) How well do general practitioners deliver palliative care? A systematic review. *Pall Med.* **16**: 457–64.

20 Lee E (2002) Learning from death. *Br J Gen Pract.* **52**: 267–8.

21 Brewin T (2001) Deserted. *BMJ.* **322**: 117. [Personal view of a retired consultant oncologist.]

22 Clark R, Jefferies N, Hasler J *et al.* (2002) *A Long Walk Home.* Radcliffe Medical Press, Oxford.

23 Williams M L (2002) Book review of *A Long Walk Home. BMJ.* **325**: 446.

24 For more details, contact adawson@macmillan.org.uk and jane.melvin@gp-n81019.nhs.uk

25 Addington-Hall J and Higginson I (2001) *Palliative Care for Non-cancer Patients.* Oxford University Press.

26 The DALY and its use in policy decision making for PCTs – Ian Wilkinson, Centre for Health-care Development, Manchester. Personal communication, 2002.

27 Shipman C, Addington-Hall J, Barclay S *et al.* (2002) Providing palliative care in primary care: how satisfied are GPs and district nurses with current out-of-hours arrangements? *Br J Gen Pract.* **50**: 477–8.

28 Thomas K (2000) *Out-of-hours Palliative Care in the Community.* Macmillan Cancer Relief, London. [Available free from Macmillan suppliers on 01344 350310 or www.macmillan.org.uk]

29 Macmillan Cancer Relief and Royal College of General Practitioners' General Practice Primary Care Facilitator Project 1992–94. Report and Executive Summary.

30 Thomas K and Millar D (2001) Catalysts of change. *Pall Care Today.* **9**(4): 54–6.

31 www.macmillan.org.uk

32 More information from the NorthWest website, www.nwrcocancer.org.uk

33 *The Times,* July 20th, 2002.

34 For more details see the Macmillan Out-of-hours Palliative Care Report (*see* Reference 27).

35 O'Hare B J (2002) Review of Community Out-of-hours Palliative Care Arrangements in Sperrin and Lakeland Area, Northern Ireland, May 2002.

36 King N (2002) Report of Calderdale and Kirklees Out-of-hours Palliative Care Protocol. Huddersfield University. In press. [More details available on the website.]

37 Edwards N, Kornacki M J and Silversin J (2002) Unhappy doctors: what are the causes and what can be done? *BMJ.* **324**: 835–8.

38 Alan Milburn, parliamentary speech, April 2002. www.modern.nhs.uk

39 National Association of Primary Care (2002) *Commissioning and Providing Palliative Care Services in the Community: the next challenge for primary care?* NAPC, London. www.napc.co.uk

CHAPTER 4

Needs-based care

> This chapter includes:
>
> 1 Generic needs: the basic human condition
> 2 What do our patients need: the findings of user groups and surveys
> 3 Addressing these needs.

This chapter explores the fundamental needs of our patients, which form the basis of the kind of service care we should be providing. From generic needs common to the human condition, to the current findings of some patient and user groups specific for cancer and palliative care, has developed a proposed model for understanding how best to respond to these varying levels of need. Dying is a natural process, with existential, relationship and spiritual implications, and the impact we have as healthcare professionals is only one part of a deeper process of witnessing to this human journey.

People live in a variety of ways and die in a variety of ways; our needs will vary at different times and will differ between people. If there is one thing perhaps that our dying patients in the community require of us more than anything else, once they are released from the restrictions of troublesome physical symptoms, it is that we help to provide them with *a sense of security and support at home* – that they really do have 'companions on the journey'. We want them to feel safe in the knowledge of what might happen, what to do if it does and the reassurance that there will always be someone to help if needed. The gift of support that we offer can be one of the most appreciated yet one of the most neglected of our skills in primary care. Obviously there is far more to the art of dying peacefully than we as healthcare professionals may be involved with – in many ways we are onlookers as the story unfolds at different levels – but we have a definite part to play, and if we can play it well so much good may ensue. We cannot fulfil every need ourselves, but in helping patients become free of symptoms and feel secure and supported, they will be enabled to travel the rest of the journey themselves, seeking loving relationships, exploring matters of self esteem, worth and dignity and leading to some kind of sense of meaning, self-realisation and spiritual peace.

Generic needs: the basic human condition

Maslow's hierarchy of needs

We all have needs, whether acknowledged or not. Maslow in 1943[1] proposed that we are all motivated by our wish to continually satisfy needs. He commented that there are at least five sets of goals which he called basic needs (*see* Figure 4.1). These are:

1 physiological (food, sleep, warmth, health)

2   safety (security, protection from threats)
3   social (belonging, association, acceptance, friendship, love)
4   esteem (self-respect, reputation, status, recognition)
5   self-actualisation (personal growth, accomplishment, creativity, achievement of potential).

Maslow described a hierarchy of needs to show that at any moment we concentrate mainly on one, the lowest of the unsatisfied needs. We do not bother much about our social status if we are starving. Once the most immediate need is fairly well satisfied we are impelled to move on to the next. Patients recently diagnosed with cancer find themselves returned with a bump to the bottom of Maslow's hierarchy, to the level of the physiological needs for survival.[2]

There is an increasing emphasis on the benefits of psychosocial interventions in the support of patients with cancer, to meet needs beyond the purely physical.[3] There is some evidence that the psychological effects of relaxation and guided imagery include improved mood and quality of life, and importantly enhanced coping.[4] By meeting deeper needs, patients are better able to cope. Some are fortunate enough to have the benefit of specific psychological support, such as that provided by psycho-oncology departments or hospice counsellors, but the vast majority currently will not. How do we in primary care respond appropriately to the varying needs of our patients? How also do we protect ourselves from these needs becoming overwhelming?

In focusing on patient need, the goal or desired *outcome* is to meet those needs as far as is possible, using certain suggested activities or *processes* and tools or *structures*. As healthcare professionals, we focus particularly on meeting the first two levels of need, i.e. physiological and safety, that of maintaining comfort, being symptom free and promoting a sense of security and support, although we may also be contributing to other levels of need in helping people towards a deeper inner peacefulness.

The need for relationship: our emotional needs

We are made in relationship with each other – the presence of relationships in some ways defines us all. At a time of facing serious illness or death, many take stock of their lives, of the important relationships around them and of those that need restoring in some ways. The man on his death bed never wishes he'd spent more time at the office – the perspective of relationships becomes more important.

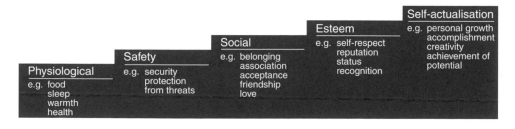

Figure 4.1: Maslow's hierarchy of need.

We all have emotional needs as well as physical ones. The ten most frequently experienced psychological needs, common to us all, have been suggested: these include our needs for *attention, affection, encouragement, approval, acceptance, appreciation, respect, security, comfort and support*.[5] We need all of these at various times, but in different degrees in different people.

If we were tired we'd sleep, or thirsty we'd drink, and yet we find it harder to acknowledge our emotional needs, built as they are on intangible relationships. We find fulfilment of these needs in relationships, both with each other and in a spiritual way, with God however perceived, or with something 'other' than ourselves. Where these needs are not fulfilled, other sources may be sought or other behaviour ensues, for example lack of attention towards a toddler leads to attention-seeking behaviour such as tantrums. Where we attempt as healthcare professionals to meet some of our patients' needs specifically, we are giving more than medicine. Many find that it is at this level that they also receive most in return from patients.

Comfort, security and support

In particular, dying patients may have a need for the latter three psychological needs – comfort, security and support. If we can articulate these in some shape or form, they are greatly appreciated. So by imparting the knowledge of what might happen and what to do if it does, we help to unpack the fears that underlie the words or symptoms, revealing their attribution and allaying concerns. The words of comfort and reassurance, the quiet 'being there', building up this sense of security for patients and carers at home, comfort from physical and emotional traumas and the support of someone acting as companion on the journey – these are important aspects to share with our patients.

Isolation

The power of isolation as a mortality risk factor and the healing powers of close ties are confirmed in numerous studies. Elderly people who suffer heart attacks but have two or more people giving them emotional support are more than twice as likely to survive longer than a year after an attack than are those with no such support.[6] So add the power of silence and aloneness to the list of emotional risk factors, and close emotional ties to the list of protective factors: 'Having people to turn to and talk with, people who could offer solace, help, and suggestions, protected them from the deadly impact of life's rigours and trauma.'[7] What implications does this have for our patients, especially the growing number of the isolated elderly?

The need for supportive relationships amongst staff: teamwork

The development of good working relationships enables us to be more fruitful and to feel better about our work. Stress and burn-out are a reality within the demanding roles of healthcare professionals (*see* Chapter 17) We need to watch the way we use ourselves – using the drug 'doctor' as Balint put it[8] – and the way we meet each others' emotional needs. Something imperceptibly special can happen as we work closely together as a team and as we reflect at meetings, building respect and appreciation for each others' contributions. In encouraging and affirming each other, we build teams and strengthen the resources we offer our patients.

Spiritual needs (*see* also Chapter 14 and www.radcliffe-oxford.com/caring)

Most people now distinguish between the inner *spiritual* needs we all have, and the outer *religious* manifestations of our beliefs, the tangible demonstrations of sacraments and religious ceremonies that will vary according to different cultures and religious systems.[9] Much sensitivity is required in seeking to address religious and cultural traditions and further advice may be needed from local religious leaders, particularly in relation to the increasing multi-ethnic society we live in.[10,11]

Many find it hard to recognise or verbalise spiritual issues – they say they are 'not religious' or may embody them mainly in terms of close 'horizontal' relationships rather than any acknowledged 'vertical' dimension. Spiritual care is based on the assumption that all people are spiritual beings, capable of transcending the here and now. Wright comments that: 'Fundamentally, spiritual care seeks to affirm the value of each and every person based on non-judgemental love.'[12]

But *spiritual distress* is as real as any overt pathology. The experience of 'death distress' amongst people with life-threatening conditions is associated with the psychosocial–spiritual dimensions of the patient's life. Attention to these may buffer the negative effects of death distress.[13] In dealing with these underlying issues – the 'icebergs' hidden under the surface (*see* Chapter 17, p. 249) – many of which relate to intangible spiritual issues, fears and concerns can be allayed with subsequent reduction of the 'total pain' and often a consequent reduction in the need for analgesia and the dosages required. In contrast, the peace reflecting an inner harmony of spirit, developed with insight and reflection, can be a tangible reality, as witnessed by many who have worked with dying patients. Not everyone may achieve this, but where it is attained something special and very awe-inspiring occurs.

Spiritual needs are inherently intangible and difficult to assess. They may easily be ignored, and yet in some ways the inner peacefulness of the spirit heads up the hierarchy of needs. If we do ignore the spiritual distress that some endure, then we are not caring for our patients adequately. Dame Cicely Saunders was the first to describe the reality of 'spiritual pain' and much has since been written on the subject.

Patients may well benefit from referral (with permission) to colleagues for further help, e.g. the local clergy or religious leaders. However, some spiritual care may be provided by any involved in patient care: 'Spiritual care responds to both religious and humanistic needs by meeting the requirements of faith and the desire for an accompanying person to "be there", to listen and to love.'[13]

In being there for our patients, listening and loving, and in maintaining the human touch, we can be of help to them as they unravel their inner thoughts, fears and impulses and in addressing their deepest spiritual needs.

What do our patients need?: the findings of user groups and surveys

Much work is developing to answer this question and to inform strategic policy decisions. There is no single answer, but a few examples are given below of the results of surveys and user groups in examining the needs of patients, here specifically cancer patients. The user voice is developing and becoming more integrated into mainstream strategic planning and the work of agencies such as Cancerlink,[14] Cancerbacup,[15] the National Cancer Alliance,[16] Patient Advisor and Liaison Service (PALS) and the new magazine for people affected by cancer, ICAN,[17] strengthens this. Cancerlink became part of Macmillan Cancer Relief in June 2001 and helps provide emotional support and information to over 750 cancer support and self-help groups nationwide, and training and consultancy in setting up groups. It also supports the Cancer Voices national project, working with individuals and groups affected by cancer who wish to use their experiences to shape the future of cancer services and research. Cancerbacup helps people affected by cancer by telephone or postal advice from qualified cancer nurses providing information, emotional support and advice, and the production of a large range of useful factsheets and booklets. It is also involved in conducting some surveys, such as in the recent 'Freedom from Pain' campaign.

Key vulnerability times and potential identity shifts on the cancer journey (with thanks to Pat Turton of Bristol Cancer Help Centre)

Figure 4.2[18] shows a fascinating alternative cancer journey which identifies the key stages of vulnerability for patients: waiting for investigations, at diagnosis, at end of treatment, at secondary diagnosis, when widespread metastases are confirmed and as the dying phase is entered. It also reveals the key stages of potential identity shifts, when people move from being a person with cancer towards being a dying cancer patient.

This helps to identify the key times and triggers for us to be able to offer support for our patients. Initiating support at these times is greatly appreciated, for example if a member of the practice team contacts the patient when they receive the diagnosis from the hospital, as an open offer of support, this may or may not be taken up but is so valued by patients and their families.

There are many new initiatives which are attempting to meet this need for support, such as primary care oncology nurses[19] or district nurses within a team taking on the role of supporting patients from diagnosis or referral. (It is hoped that the 'extended' GSF model will later include this.)

The impact of the illness on patients is one of:

- SHOCK – 'like a sledgehammer'
- LOSS – of confidence, control, certainty, continuity of care
- FEAR – of recurrence, of knowing more, of death and dying, of hospitals, tests and doctors
- and confusion, isolation, resentment, guilt, disillusion, etc.[20]

In affirming, strengthening and developing this supportive relationship between the patient and their family and the primary care team, especially as they move towards times of vulnerability or change of image, the rewards will be considerable for both.

The very first piece of information I tried to find out was how long I'd got left to live and that proved to be one of the hardest things. In fact nobody ever gave me that information.... The only person who did finally say to me that he would give his opinion was my local GP.

Male cancer patient

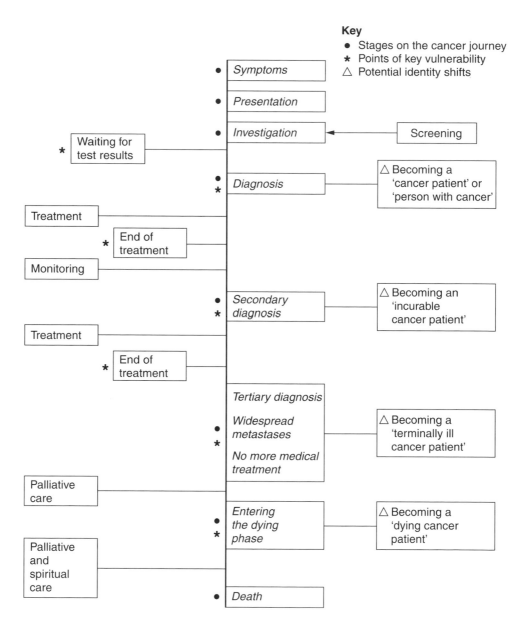

Figure 4.2: Stages on the cancer journey with points of key vulnerability and potential identity shifts. (Reprinted with kind permission of the Bristol Cancer Help Centre.)

Patients' 'top ten' requests from GPs

The National Cancer Alliance, led by Becky Miles, issued a list of suggested top ten requests to GPs from their cancer patients.[21] These included:

- GP willingness to take symptoms seriously and act fast to refer to a specialist
- diagnostic tests and diagnosis to be completed as quickly as possible
- doctors to be approachable and treat patients with respect, 'like being a human being'
- 'almost immediate' hospital appointment when GP refers
- chance to discuss treatment options and be given full information, especially about side-effects
- doctors who are willing to listen and explain (more than once if necessary)
- doctors who seem unhurried, or who pass patients to another appropriate health professional who does have time
- continuity of care
- communications training for doctors
- GP to make greater use of telephone for making hospital appointments

User groups in strategic planning

In 1996, the NHS Executive's Patient Partnership Strategy acknowledged the 'consumer' role and emphasised user involvement as key to the new NHS. The NHS Cancer Plan,[22] following the lead of The NHS Plan[23] before it, claims to 'put the patient at the centre of cancer care'. But with the cry of 'patient-centredness' always ringing in our ears, how can we claim to be patient centred if we don't ask patients? This is at two levels:

1 *Listening to patients.* We need improved skills and tools to enable structured listening to our individual patients for whose care we are responsible. Hence, teaching in communication skills which also focuses on open questions and listening, patient diaries, structured questions, weekly review sheets from patients and carers, etc. Communication must be two-way.

2 *Integrating the user view.* When organising services and developing systems, user involvement is increasingly being incorporated. Although initially daunting, there is now a growing band of well-trained 'expert patients' who are able to collect and express the user view. The Macmillan Cancer Voices Project of Cancerlink, the National Cancer Alliance and many other initiatives have been influential in strengthening the patient voice, which now is much more than tokenism in the world of modern NHS cancer care. Cancer networks have formal user groups and some take part in peer reviews. The NHS Reform and Health Care Professionals Bill is currently awaiting royal assent in England. This gives primary care trust patient forums considerably more power and along with the new Commission for Patient and Public Involvement in Health, they will be allowed greater independence and influence in future.[24]

Increasingly, however, patients and doctors are discovering the mutual benefit of working together, for both can suffer as a result of the inadequacies of a system. Partnership with patients should be seen as an enabling process that is essential to good standards of care, not as a threat to authority.[25]

The GSF has involved patients groups from an early stage and has been greatly enriched by co-working with Macmillan Cancerlink and other user groups, including that of the Cancer Services Collaborative, and we plan further developments in this area in future. A key element of the assessment tools used has been the structured listening to patients and their carers, who might otherwise be ignored. The Home Packs contain Weekly Review sheets with sections for expressing what has gone well, what not so well and what improvements can be made. These present a readily accessible means of structuring the listening to patient and carer views, leading to appropriate action.

The NHS Cancer Plan and the Supportive Care Strategy

The NHS Cancer Plan for England states the needs of patients are:

- rapid access to best possible treatment
- being treated with dignity and respect
- views being taken into account
- good communication, information and best possible symptom control.

A willingness to listen and explain is considered by patients to be one of the essential attributes of a health professional (along with sensitivity, approachability, respect and honesty).[26]

Improving patients' experience of care is one of the four key aims of the Cancer Plan so supportive and palliative care services are vital. Currently networks in England provide the framework for planning services and engaging commissioners at a high level.[27] The Supportive Care Strategy is being developed as part of the NHS Cancer Plan, to be produced towards the end of 2002 with further work in 2003.

The simplistic working definition of supportive care is 'care that helps patients and their families cope'. This strategy is an attempt to meet some of the needs discussed here, particularly regarding service provision at network, primary care organisation and other geographic areas. By building in minimum standards of service that should be made available to patients in the community and in hospitals, based on current available evidence, there is the hope that all patients will be able to access a more equitable level of care than is the case at present (*see* also Chapter 6).

Cancer Services Collaborative Patient Experience and User Group

There is currently much work underway on integrating the user views into our strategic and policy decision making, particularly with the Supportive Care Strategy (*see* Chapter 5). One such group, the Patient Experience and User Group of the Cancer Services Collaborative, has produced early thoughts reflecting patients' experiences as they travel through the cancer journey, mainly focusing on the early stages of diagnosis and treatment involving hospital care. This highlights the need for patients to receive clear information, their concerns to be taken seriously, good information flows between professionals across the boundaries of care, improvements in the systems of care and less of a deafening silence at crucial times during their journey (*see also* the summary of patients' views at www.modern.nhs.uk/cancer and www.radcliffe-oxford.com/caring).

What do patients and carers want from the services? Cancerlink's survey

As part of the process of developing the Supportive Care Strategy for Cancer Patients in England, Cancerlink undertook a questionnaire survey and held meetings of expert patients and carers. Results from these exercises highlighted the following domains as the key components of good supportive care for patients and carers:

1 *Being treated as a human being.* People want to be treated as individuals, and with dignity and respect.
2 *Empowerment.* The ability to have their voice heard, to be valued for their knowledge and skills, and to exercise real choice about treatments and services are central to patients' and carers' wishes.
3 *Information.* Patients and carers should receive all the information they want about their condition and possible treatment. It should be given in an honest, timely and sensitive manner.
4 *Having choice.* Patients and carers want to know what options are available to them from the NHS, voluntary and private sectors, including access to self-help and support groups and complementary therapy services.
5 *Continuity of care.* Good communication and coordination of services between health and social care professionals working across the NHS and social sectors is essential.
6 *Equal access.* People want access to services of similar quality wherever they are delivered.
7 *Meeting physical needs.* Physical symptoms must be managed to a degree acceptable to patients.
8 *Meeting psychological needs.* Patients and carers need emotional support from professionals who are prepared to listen to them and are capable of understanding their concerns.
9 *Meeting social needs.* Support for the family, advice on financial and employment issues and provision of transport are necessary.
10 *Meeting spiritual needs.* Patients and carers should have support to help them explore the spiritual issues important to them.

Recurring themes: control, information and support

Three important areas of need recur often (*see* Chapter 5):

1 the need for some retention of *control*
2 the need for *information*
3 and the need for *a supportive relationship and a sense of security.*

The need for control

This was highlighted in the Age Concern 'Debate of the Age's 12 Principles of a Good Death',[28] in which at least seven principles are based on control and autonomy (*see* Box 4.1). By working closely with our patients, listening to their real concerns, keeping them informed and offering various options and choices, we can improve their sense of retaining control and autonomy.

Box 4.1   12 principles of good death[28]

- To be able to retain control of what happens.
- To have control over pain relief and other symptom control.
- To have choice and control over where death occurs (at home or elsewhere).
- To have access to hospice care in any location, not only in hospital.
- To have control over who is present and who shares the end.
- To be able to issue advance directives which ensure wishes are respected.
- To know when death is coming, and to understand what can be expected.
- To be afforded dignity and privacy.
- To have access to information and expertise of whatever kind is necessary.
- To have access to any spiritual or emotional support required.
- To have time to say goodbye, and control over other aspects of timing.
- To be able to leave when it is time to go, and not to have life prolonged pointlessly.

The need for information and good communication[29]

Involving patients in decisions about their treatments or care improves health outcomes.[30,31] But how are they informed and how do we involve patients more in decision making?

Cancer can be frightening. When faced with the word 'cancer' most people's minds go blank. We can only take in a limited amount of information at any one time, whilst another part of our brain heads off into the stratosphere with all kinds of questions and permutations – both earth-shattering, heavy-duty questions of life and death alongside the more mundane questions of practical real life. One patient described how, when told she had cancer, the two thoughts in her mind were: 'Will I die tomorrow?' and 'Where is the bucket if I need to vomit?'

In some ways there are two parallel journeys here. The *outer journey* is represented by the numerous hospital appointments, scans, blood tests, brief conversations imparting serious information and so on. This is mirrored by the *inner journey* of the gradual evolution of a healthy person who implicitly thought they'd live for ever (as we all do) becoming a 'patient' with a diagnosis of cancer, who may well be cured, but who also lives with this 'sword of Damacles' – the possibility of recurrence – hanging over them for the rest of their lives. And most, of course, do become incurable and have to adapt internally to the fact that they will one day die of their disease. No-one is the same again after a diagnosis of cancer.

With the evidence that retaining some control is a key factor in patient and carer satisfaction[28] and that this is in part enabled by good information – 'information is power' – how then can cancer patients become better informed? Leslie Fallowfield, Professor of Psycho-oncology at the University of Sussex, clarifies the difference between bald information and real empowered control: 'The desire for information is not the same as a desire to participate in decision making. Patients cannot participate in decision making to their desired extent unless they have the right types of information, given in ways optimal for their own level of understanding.'[32]

There are many sources of information, both general and specific to the type of cancer or treatment. But one key element in all this is having patients' own questions answered by the relevant people involved in their care. Unfortunately, under stress the mind goes blank, only a minimum of the information given is retained and there is also the old problem that 'you don't know what you don't know!' Patients and carers need detailed information to become shared decision makers and help create customised care. Informed choice can lead to a greater involvement in decision making and a better sense of control.

In the recent Commission for Health Improvement/Audit Commission report on cancer services, 'NHS Cancer Care in England and Wales',[33] a detailed checklist of about 30–50 questions for patients was suggested, related directly to the 'hallmarks of a good service', i.e. what should happen during the three stages of diagnosis, treatment and care and palliative care. An excellent leaflet, 'Questions for Patients to Ask', was produced and copies are available free from Cancerbacup on 0808 800 1234.

Other checklists have been produced. www.radcliffe-oxford.com/caring contains a checklist of suggested questions to ask GPs and district nurses as well as hospital staff. These could be adapted and altered to suit each patient's needs. They could also be copied, with answers noted for future reference or to show other members of the family. The aim is to enable patients and their carers to be encouraged and supported in asking the right questions, in order to remain fully informed and active in decision making. Other examples are the 'Home Packs' used in the Gold Standards Framework project, with templates of phone numbers, care plans, etc. and feedback forms from patients/carers.

The concern from some of inappropriately raising patients' expectations must be balanced by the recognition of the vulnerability of patients at this time and their need for information. If those affected by cancer can become well informed at the most vulnerable stages along the journey, with adequate personalised information about their condition, treatment and care, then we will be making some strides towards the ideal of more patient-centred care.

The need for supportive relationships

The benefits of personal, supportive relationships were discussed earlier. The support of loving family as carers is the mainstay for most people, and facilitating the resolution of any conflicts or unfinished business is important. Therefore ensuring family know that death is imminent is vital, to allow last death-bed affirmations and goodbyes. And this includes children, who may be inadvertently neglected, with a consequent lifetime's regret about things not said.

The great satisfaction in primary care of looking after patients during their final stage of life revolves in the development of this supportive therapeutic relationship.

> *I think that terminal care is probably if not the most important then certainly one of the most important things that GPs can become involved in. I do feel very strongly that there should be continuity of care with patients you've known in the past and have been involved with in the diagnosis. From feedback from patients and the relatives, I feel it's personal involvement that is often the most important thing, that there is one person there, who you can turn to continuously, who you learn to trust, who really takes control of the situation.*[34]
>
> GP, Gloucestershire

Patients appreciate the sense of security that is provided by having good information, well communicated to them in written as well as verbal form. A sense of planning and anticipation of needs is a vital key, both for carers and healthcare professionals, contributing to feelings of safety, security and support.

Addressing these needs

Needs/support matrix

So how can we assess the needs of our patients and their carers? What too are the needs of the professionals involved in their care (focusing mainly on the primary healthcare team here)?

The needs/support matrix (*see* Figure 4.3), always evolving, was originally developed to describe the needs of patients and their carers at various stages of the cancer journey, with the support available at the time. It is also useful in examining the ongoing needs or requirements of the primary healthcare team and support available to them. Figure 4.3 shows where the Gold Standards Framework fits in, initially concentrating on the palliative care phase but later extending up the cancer journey from first suspicion of symptoms and diagnosis.

The cancer journey has been described in linear form, divided into three phases:

1 'I have cancer' – screening or presentation to diagnosis
2 'Living with cancer' – diagnosis to treatment, rehabilitation, follow-up and in some cases cure
3 'Dying of cancer' – palliative care (this may be from diagnosis in some cases, e.g. lung cancer to terminal care [towards last two weeks of life] and bereavement).

There will obviously be gaps and overlaps and the journey will vary with each patient, but this gives a workable framework when attempting to coordinate and improve the system of care.

Structure and relationship: the 'outer' and the 'inner'

The needs of our patients may be met at two levels:

1 the *structure of service provision* in the area, with access to 24-hour nursing services, out-of-hours palliative care provision, access to drugs and equipment, access to specialist advice, speedy and accurate communications and information transfers, better coordination of care, etc.
2 the *relationships* with those caring for them – many needs are met at the more personal level of professional yet human relationships. For this we need good communication skills, availability of dedicated time, support for ourselves as staff to be able to care for our patients, specific support for the family/carers, etc.

The GSF: patient needs informing the model of care

In summary, how do we know how best to support our patients and where to direct our resources? Why do we suggest using tools to assess symptoms or handover forms and written information to increase the sense of security for patients at home? Table 4.1 correlates much of what has previously been described, providing suggested examples relating to the care of the dying at home. This relates to the human areas of need (after Maslow) and has been broken down into:

- patient *need*
- *outcome* – the patient's inner dimension of needs met – comfort, security and support
- *process* – the active means of achieving this, i.e. identify, assess, plan
- *structure* – the practical measure required to achieve this, e.g. use of registers, assessment tools, etc.

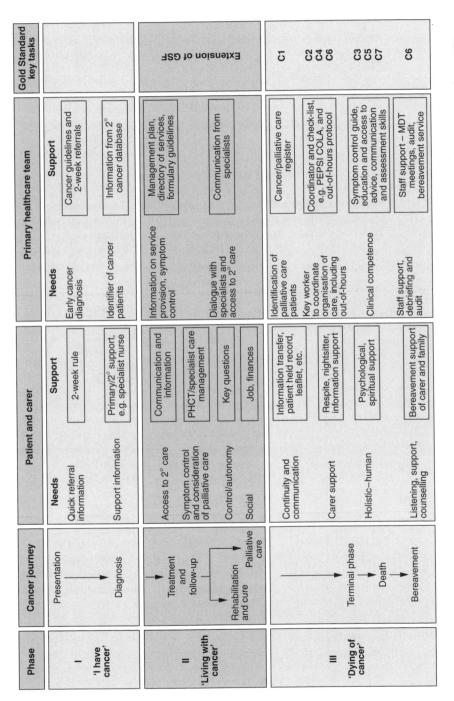

Figure 4.3: Needs/support matrix of the cancer journey: a map of an average cancer patient's journey, illustrating where GSF tasks address needs.

Table 4.1: Summary of suggested needs-based care

Hierarchy of need of patient (after Maslow) NEED	Patient feeling – 'inner' dimension OUTCOME	Provision – 'outer' determinant PROCESS	Practical measure – examples of suggested means or intervention STRUCTURE
1 *Physiological*	**Comfort:** Health Functioning body	Symptom relief – free of physical symptoms	• SC register – identification • Assessment – physical • Specialist advice • Out-of-hours palliative care • Access to 24-hr DNs
2 *Safety*	**Security and support:** Lack of fear and anxiety Protected from threats	Emotional support Information Continuity of care Practical support Anticipatory care Financial help	• Assessment – psychosocial/holistic • Information • Out-of-hours protocol • Access to key person • Equal access to resources and equipment • Specialist care register – identification and inform team • PHCT planning and coordination • Financial and benefits advice
3 *Social*	**Love:** Belonging Acceptance Harmonious relationships	Supportive, loving relationships Dealing with emotions	• Active listening • Communication skills • Information • Family dynamics and carer support
4 *Esteem*	**Dignity:** Self-respect Feeling good about themselves	Control Choice Confidentiality Respect Humane treatment Empowerment Being valued Truth and honesty	• Consultation • Information, e.g. Home Pack • Agenda – sharing • Patient review – sheets in Home Pack
5 *Self-actualisation*	**Spiritual peace:** Personal growth Inner calm	Acceptance Finding meaning Hope Wisdom Dealing with inner fears And all of the above	• Time – listened to • Prayer • Supportive relationship • Spiritual needs addressed • Religious support • And all the above

If we begin with the basic *needs* of the human condition, such as physiological body functioning, and then describe the condition that the patient is seeking if this need is to be fulfilled, e.g. healthy functioning body, free of physical symptoms, this could be described as the *outcome* we are trying to achieve. The *process* to achieve this may be to assess and treat any physical symptoms, and some helpful means of *structuring* this good symptom control, such as assessment tools, access to specialist advice, etc., are therefore of use.

> *We felt safer because the GSF project provides a system of care to make it less likely that people will slip through the net. It has formalised what we were trying to do in a very haphazard way before, a more watertight organised service which gives more patients better care and gives us more job satisfaction.*
>
> GP, Halifax, GSF Phase 1

> *We ring our GP at his suggestion every week and give him a progress report. Usually he comes round every Tuesday at 8.00 am and gives me a thorough going over. I could not have a better GP. He has done everything possible and has put himself out for me.*
>
> Cancer patient[35]

Spiritual peace and inner calm are the ultimate goals that will be achieved when most other pressing needs are met, i.e. patients are physically, emotionally and practically comfortable. Inevitably this may not be accomplished in all, for reasons that may be beyond our control. It is obviously so much harder with young premature deaths, especially in children and young adults, when the feeling of life being snatched away before the appropriate time can be quite overwhelming. Yet the goal of spiritual peace is perhaps the highest that we can aspire to, representing harmony in all other areas, and it is possible at any age. Some feel that we have the privilege of acting as medical companions on a journey that is largely a spiritual one.

Using these examples it is more apparent that we must not make the completion of forms or the holding of meetings an end in itself or a measure of success – they are the means (structures or processes) to achieve the end. Better assessment is there purely as a means to provide and respond in the most appropriate way.

So the aims of the GSF have been developed in a direct line with the assessment of patient, carer and staff needs (*see* Box 4.2). There are other possible goals but these appear to be the most significant ones with current knowledge available. They are reflected in the evaluation of GSF (*see* Chapter 19) with the global outcomes and specific measurables.

Box 4.2 The aims of the Gold Standards Framework

1 Patients are enabled to live well in the last stage of life and, finally, to have a 'good death':
   - symptom free
   - in their preferred place of choice with needs-based, customised care
   - with a sense of security and support, with fewer crises (or admissions).
2 Carers feel supported, informed, involved, acknowledged, empowered and satisfied with care.
3 Staff increase in confidence, with a sense of teamwork and job satisfaction, and with improved communication and co-working with specialists.

Needs-based care: the user view and the GSF

Patient and carer involvement has been intrinsic throughout the development of the Gold Standards Framework, so it is difficult to separate. The framework has been based on real life patient experience as described by members of the PHCTs involved in its development, with extensive literature searches for numerous articles and reports, e.g. from Cancerlink, Cancerbacup, CHI, NHS Executive, etc (*see* Chapter 5). It has also been under the scrutiny of the local Community Health Councils, local user groups across the UK, as well as listening closely to the Cancer Services Collaborative User Group and to individual patient voices. We believe that it is rooted in listening to patients and carers and also to primary healthcare staff, both GPs and nurses. We are developing even stronger links through the work of Cancerlink, as the user voice becomes better structured, and we look forward to developing this even further in future.

However, there is no one 'user' view, just as there is no one user – the underlying flexible approach is that we must respect individuality and adjust according to the needs of the patient. But there are some general common themes that need to be addressed, e.g. information, communication skills, round-the-clock cover, etc.

Primary care health professionals are dealing with hundreds of patients every week, so there is a need to structure better listening to *all* patients and to move on any remaining fixed, hierarchical professional mind-sets, as well as including patient representation at committee level, such as those trained by Cancer Voices. The voice of all patients must be heard, especially those weakened by illness, alongside those representing them on committees. Structuring listening and focusing on patient need, e.g. with the use of the PACA sheet and Weekly Review sheets of the Home Pack, is a step towards this.

However, I feel there should in fact be less 'us and them' between healthcare professionals and patients. We are all 'users' of the health service and have a vested interest in developing high-quality services – our professionalism is thinly veiled. Either as patients ourselves, or through members of our family or friends, all of us will have had personal experience of care, or in future will hope for the same quality of care that we wish to offer our patients. This is the 'doctor–family index' as quoted by Professor Mike Richards, the National Cancer Director – what kind of care would you wish for if it was you or a member of your family?

So, the ideal of 'needs-based care' put forward here, listens and responds appropriately not to our view of the world but to that of the patient. It is an ideal that is worth striving for.

> *Dad had lymphoedema of his leg and scrotum. I had enormous difficulty finding anyone to take notice of this and to know how to deal with it in spite of having regular assessments. These assessments must lead to the provision of appropriate action, care and relief.*
>
> JB, daughter of cancer patient

If we play our part in meeting the needs of our patients where we can, in enabling patients to feel comfortable and secure, allowing them to find love, a sense of dignity and self-respect amongst their supportive relationships, then they are more likely to die peacefully with loved ones around them who feel that a 'good death' has been achieved.

In basing our care on the needs of our patients and remaining alert to their changes, we are more rooted and informed of the significant developments required to provide good care. We are then, we hope, more likely to achieve this for more of our patients more of the time, and to feel satisfied that we are providing a good service for our patients.

References

1 Maslow A H (1943) A theory of human motivation. *Psychological Review*.

2 Rendell A (2000) *Management Theory and the Patient's Potential*. Information Exchange, London.

3 Shipman C, Levenson R and Gillam S (2002) *Psychosocial Support for Dying People: what can primary trusts do?* King's Fund, London.

4 Walker L (2002) *Surviving Cancer: does the fighting spirit matter?* Inaugural lecture, Professor of Psycho-oncology Dept., University of Hull, November 2000.

5 Ferguson D (1998) *The Great Commandment Principle*. Tyndale House, Illinois, USA.

6 Berkman L *et al.* (1992) Emotional support and survival after myocardial infarction. *Ann Intern Med*.

7 Goleman D (1996) *Emotional Intelligence*. Bloomsbury, London.

8 Balint M (1964) *The Doctor, His Patient and the Illness* (2e). Pitman, London.

9 Walter T (2002) Sprituality in palliative care: opportunity or burden? *Pall Med*. **16**: 133–9.

10 Neuberger J (1994) *Caring for Dying People of Different Faiths*. Mosby Palliative Care Series. Mosby, London.

11 Firth S (2001) *Wider Horizons: care of the dying in a multicultural society*. National Council for Hospice and Specialist Palliative Care Services, London.

12 Wright M C (2002) The essence of spiritual care: a phenomenological enquiry. *Pall Med*. **16**: 125–32.

13 Chibnall J T, Videen S, Duckro P *et al.* (2002) Psychosocial spiritual correlates of death distress in patients with life-threatening medical conditions. *Pall Med*. **16**: 331–8.

14 www.macmillan,co.uk or cancerlink@macmillan.org.uk Tel: 0800 808 0000

15 www.cancerbacup.org.uk

16 www.nationalcanceralliance.co.uk

17 www.ican4u.com

18 Reprinted with permission of the Bristol Cancer Help Centre www.bristolcancerhelp.org. From 'Meeting the Needs of People with Cancer for Support and Self-management'. The report of a collaborative research project by Bristol Cancer Help Centre and the University of Warwick, March 1999.

19 More details from www.macmillan.org.uk or from adawson@macmillan.org.uk

20 Turton P, Bristol Cancer Help Centre.

21 Miles B, National Cancer Alliance.

22 Department of Health (2000) *The NHS Cancer Plan*. DoH, London.

23 Department of Health (2000) *The NHS Plan*. DoH, London.

24 NHS Reform and Health Care Professions Bill, www.parliament.uk

25 Blennerhassett M (2002) What cancer patients need. In M Baker (ed) *Modernising Cancer Services*. Radcliffe Medical Press, Oxford.

26 Department of Health (2000) *The NHS Cancer Plan*, p. 63. DoH, London.

27 Richards M (2002) *Priorities in Developing the Supportive and Palliative Care Network Agenda.* Bristol, May 2002.

28 Debate of the Age Health and Care Study Group (1999) *The Future of Health and Care of Older People.* Age Concern, London.

29 Thomas K (2002) *What to Ask the Doctor.* ICAN Hayward Medical Press, London.

30 Towle A and Godolphin W (1999) Framework for teaching and learning informed shared decision making. *BMJ.* **319**: 766–71.

31 Charlton R *et al.* (1999) What do we mean by partnership in decision making about treatment? *BMJ.* **319**: 790–2.

32 Fallowfield L (2001) Participation of patients in decisions about treatments for cancer. *BMJ.* **323**: 1144.

33 Commission for Health Improvement and Audit Commission (2001) *NHS Cancer Care in England and Wales.* CHI and Audit Commission, London.

34 Jeffrey D (2000) *Cancer: from cure to care.* Radcliffe Medical Press, Oxford.

35 Meads J, Coe N and Davies D (2002) A qualitative evaluation of community palliative care: nurse specialists', patients' and carers' views. [Personal communication.] Avon, Somerset and Wiltshire Cancer Network User Group.

PART 2

Present knowledge and words of wisdom: how can we begin?

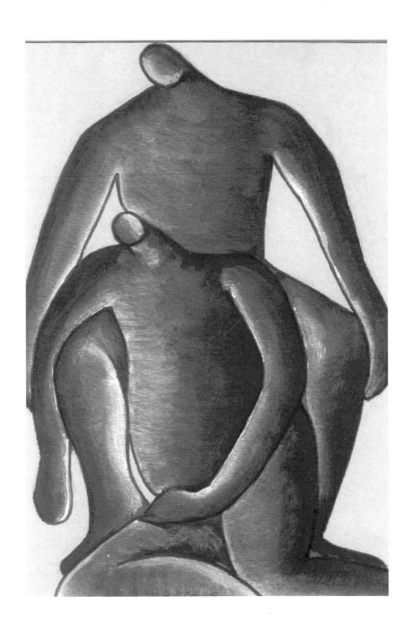

CHAPTER 5

Evidence-based care

This chapter includes:

1 Research-enhanced healthcare
2 Structure and relationships
3 Overview of the literature.

Research-enhanced healthcare

It is important to correlate as far as possible what we already know on a subject, to inform and to substantiate any future directions and develop clinical recommendations. *Bandolier* is an evidence-based journal which attempts to distil current learning from research and transfer it into practice. As the editor puts it: 'Doing better is what it all comes down to.'[1] Over recent years palliative care has built up an increasingly sound research portfolio[2] and primary care research has long been well established. We need to hear the wisdom gleaned from well-conducted research and be involved always with asking the right questions, using our rooted experience and questioning minds.

Evidence-based medicine (EBM) was promoted as a new approach to the practice of medicine in the early 1990s.[3] It has brought great benefits in many areas and has had a significant impact on improving quality care, not least through the consequent development of agreed evidence-based guidelines and with its financial consequences via the musings of NICE (National Institute for Clinical Excellence) and others, advising us on how best to spend our money. However, some are wondering if it is on occasions misused; originally it incorporated patients' preferences and choices and was seen as a sharpening of knowledge, not a replacement to thinking. One criticism directed at EBM now is that these and other important elements may become lost; as Haynes *et al.* put it: 'Evidence does not make the decisions, people do.'[4] The term 'research-enhanced healthcare' may be preferable, emphasising its complementary role in decision making (*see* Figure 5.1), and in integrating specific clinical circumstances with patients' views in the knowledge of current best practice according to the research.

The furious debates on this subject in the pages of the medical journals underline this tension, which is perhaps particularly relevant in primary care. The marriage of evidence-based medicine and clinical intuition is welcomed by many.[5] The debate centres in part around the fact that, as Polanyi put it: 'We know more than we can say.'[6] Wider acknowledgement of the role of tacit knowledge, intuition, creativity and the dialogues by which these processes are acquired and maintained is vital and some feel that EBM is going to have a diminishing shelf life if these broader areas are not integrated.[7]

However, the term 'evidence' is increasingly used in this current climate, promoted by such quality-improving organisations as NICE, CHI (Commission for Health Improvement) and the recommendations of NSFs (National Service Frameworks). In an effort to consistently use the appropriate treatments, it guides us in the clarification of what is already known about a subject and the position of new knowledge.

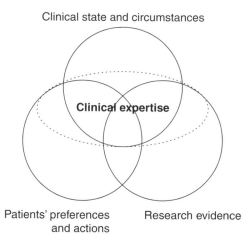

Figure 5.1: An updated model for evidence-based clinical decisions.

This may be entirely right when using a drug, or a standard treatment, but may not always take into account the 'people factors' of individual variation, clinical situations, multiple service provision and choice. The forceful, legal-sounding term of 'evidence' implies a real indisputable truth and transferability applicable to all scenarios. Of course this is not the case, especially when considering improving service provision in complex multifaceted settings such as healthcare scenarios, rather than the recommended use of one new drug or treatment. Top-down dictates from evidence-based systematic reviews only tell us so much – one facet of the truth. For those at the tail-end of such dictates there can be a sense of disempowerment, of hands tied and having no voice. This is true for health professionals as well as patients, even more so when attempting to improve system redesign, organisation or service provision. Just because something works in one situation does not guarantee its transferability to another. Developments from the bottom-up, rather than the transfer of a solution from one place to another, procure more ownership and empowerment and, in terms of service provision, more sustained improvements. (This is at the heart of the GSF programme – *see* Chapter 6.)

People factors

With the increasing inclusion of the 'user voice' to inform strategic decision making,[8] we are made more aware of the importance of including human factors and the danger at times of only listening to the 'evidence' from well-designed, validated clinical trials, important as they undoubtedly are. Sometimes we need to hear evidence from different sources – both the scientific and the more sociological are valid, both the quantitative and the qualitative research provide insights into truth and transferability.

There needs to be better ways of developing and measuring change, using what we do know but still moving the debate on. There needs to be clearer ways of acknowledging insight, perception and especially wisdom. There should be more recognition of the 'people factors', of the common-sense views of our 'friends in low places' as James Willis puts it in his dissection of our modern, apparently intelligent, systems:[9]

> *The new understanding is that life is not a simultaneous equation, however much logic tells us that it ought to be. It has no single solution, however intricate and beautiful we believe that*

solution to be. Our lives have opened into two parallel and utterly disparate paths. We are moving forward in two ways which cannot be formally reconciled. Structure and freedom, the fixed and the fuzzy, the professional and the amateur, the modern and the post modern, the specialist and the generalist, the game and the life …

Put humanity back at the centre of things, at the heart. We must not let society become too complex and too automatic for people to understand. We must keep it within our comprehension … It's about the fact that people are more important than systems. People are what life is about.

Amongst this search for truth, as real research essentially is, there may be times when we lose sight of the wider perspective, become obsessed with the detail, lose our map of the world. Just as if lost in a maze, we can't see the truth round the next corner or how near we are to the goal. Often good research can inspire and promote appropriate action, but how often does a carefully argued study tell you some aspect of common sense that your six-year-old daughter could have told you? Not that this is a belittling statement – children have that quality of searing profundity that cuts to the quick and shakes off the irrelevant barnacles of our thinking. We as adults, tortuously sophisticated, need to relearn their clarity of vision and their refining directness. As some have put it, there is sometimes EBO … 'evidence of the blindingly obvious'. The 'truth' in the end is often something quite simple.

However, we need the dispassionate academic approach and the development of good 'research-enhanced' evidence to inform our thinking, balance extremism and moderate skewed examples, and to guide us on the map in the right direction for future travel. We need to be constantly questioning and presenting null hypotheses. But more than this, we need to listen to wisdom from a variety of sources, most notably from wise people – and this will include a special kind of listening to our patients.

Structure and relationships

Amidst all the tangible structures around us, we are in danger of losing the real prize – people relationships. We must attempt always to make the structures work for us to enhance our relationships, not the other way round. We do not serve the computer, the guidelines, the forms and paperwork – they serve us! But we must make them work. So, for example, to deepen a friendship you invite someone to a 'structured' meal, and we have the wonderful structure of the mobile phone to keep family in touch; a simple document like a handover form becomes a vehicle to enhance the relationship between the patient and the doctor in the middle of the night or structuring a team meeting provides a time of shared support for staff and a moment to consider the real ordeal a patient and their family are undergoing. Use whatever structures are available, but only to enable better relationships and not as an end in themselves. It is the destination that matters and not the train. Form filling is there for a purpose. Consider the structures and the relationships and do not confuse the master with the servant!

There are some pointers to further wisdom that will help in clarifying why particular aspects have been developed. For example, many studies suggest that noting the preferred place of death or care enables more patients to attain their preference. Therefore if someone wishes to stay at home, by recording and communicating this fact home care can be better planned and managed, resources and carers permitting, and the patient's wishes are more likely to be fulfilled. So on the Supportive Care register front-sheet it is suggested that this be noted, dated and later audited, noting after a time maybe the reasons that it isn't being fulfilled, such as a lack of carer support, drugs access, etc. 'Evidence' or 'research-enhanced healthcare' must lead us to action. Structures must lead us to better relationships and improved care.

Overview of the literature

Townsend states that 'with a limited increase in community care, 50% more patients with cancer could be supported to die at home'.[43] This key assertion should motivate us to use existing evidence and research findings to improve community services, which is the message of the GSF and other initiatives. This framework is firmly evidence-based, using all current knowledge available to constructively present some answers to the questions posed. The challenge is to improve community care as Townsend affirms, to better support patients at home. But how do we do this?

Below is a brief interpretation of some of the collective wisdom obtained from a reading of some of the current literature, divided into subject areas that broadly relate to the seven sections of the GSF. Some are surveys, trials, even systematic reviews and others are expert opinions based on real experience. This is not a full literature analysis or systematic review, it is not comprehensive nor exhaustive and focuses mainly on brief points in primary palliative care, but it is broad and far reaching, and references are given for those interested in reading the original articles, some of which are stunningly helpful and perceptive. All have varying grades of 'evidence' – we must never underestimate the evidence of the wise experienced practitioner. The summary impressions are my own personal interpretations.

The broad categories used are:

1 General views on quality community palliative care provision
2 Role of the primary healthcare teams: GP and DN views
3 Preferred place of care or death
4 Communication and coordination issues: C1 and C2
5 Symptom control and education: C3 and C5
6 Out-of-hours palliative care: C4
7 Carers'/users' views: C6
8 Other care settings
9 Possible solutions, guidelines and protocols.

General views on quality and current needs in community palliative care provision

Summary Impression: there are consistent reasons for home care failing (lack of coordination, lack of teamwork/communication, carer breakdown, symptom control, etc.) and a need for specialists to work well together with generalists. Lack of district nursing support at night is an important issue.

- There are two paradoxes: firstly, most dying people would prefer to remain at home but most die in institutions, and secondly, most of the final year of life is spent at home but most people are admitted to hospital to die. Admissions are largely due to difficulties with carers rather than with patients – carer stress and breakdown is a more significant cause of admission than symptom control. To keep people at home we need:
  - adequate nursing care
  - night sitters
  - good symptom control
  - confident and committed GPs
  - access to specialist palliative care

- – effective coordination of care
- – financial support
- – terminal care education.[10]
- Admission to hospital does not necessarily imply improved care.[11]
- A systematic review of palliative care delivered by GPs confirmed that GPs valued this work, appreciated working well with specialists, and that GPs can and do provide adequate palliative care. However, better teamworking with specialists was recommended.[12]
- Audit of home-based palliative care in 1086 cancer patients in Grampian – key areas in palliative care at home are symptom control, improved teamwork, further education and training, communication, use of services, information provision.[13]
- Main areas of concern are communication, symptom control, staff support and facilities. Efforts to improve these lead to mixed results and time taken to develop guidelines is not always well spent.[14]
- GPs' views in a postal survey of 447 GPs on service priorities are: night district nursing, Marie Curie nurses, DN daytime, Macmillan nurses, palliative care consultants.[15]
- District nurse views of needs in Northern Ireland are Marie Curie nurses, twilight help, Macmillan nurses, respite care, hospice and 24-hour district nursing.[16]
- Postal survey of 167 GPs and 96 DNs on commissioning priorities found asking for hospice admission for both symptom control and terminal care, and Marie Curie nurses were the main priorities, also, home visits by medical specialists and hospital-at-home arrangements.[17]
- Inadequacies in DN and home help provision were perceived both to affect care and to discourage relatives from caring for dying patients.[18]
- More terminally ill patients were kept at home if there was more 24-hour district nursing availability.[19]
- In a large survey of 2074 bereaved carers in 20 health authorities which asked about care in the last year of life, a third needed help with activities of daily living and a third more care at night, 60% had DN help, 93% had GPs home visiting (one-third at night).[20]
- A systematic review confirmed the benefits arising from the introduction of specialist palliative care teams in the care of the dying in terms of health outcomes, compared with conventional services.[21]
- Sometimes the primary/specialist interface causes problems but specialist palliative care is usually regarded as helpful; those who are most negative are those who use it least.[22]

Role of the primary healthcare teams

Summary Impression: that palliative care is perceived to be an important and intrinsic part of the work of GPs and DNs, but there is some variability in the levels of care provided and need for support from specialists, community hospitals, etc. Some of the stresses are related to role domains and personal tensions with other healthcare professionals.

- In a large survey of GPs, most still regard care of patients with palliative care needs as an inherent and important part of their role.[23]
- Many argue that quality palliative care following the hospice example can be achieved by GPs. Key factors are teamwork, symptom control, time to anticipate problems and communication.[24]
- Physicians believe that advanced planning and good relationships are the major determinants of good decision making.[25]

- A particularly interesting study of 25 GPs confirmed again that care of the dying is viewed as a rewarding and satisfying part of their work. They see themselves as part of a team of carers, with themselves as the coordinators of such care, and with good relations with DNs though less good with hospitals and social services. They see a continuum in their relationship with patients, many of whom they have known for many years, and good honest communication at this point was seen to be essential. There were some problems of tensions with hospices and specialists in palliative care, care of non-malignant conditions and the role of the GP in the social construction of bereavement.[26]
- There have been radical changes in primary care: fewer GPs have personal lists, increased numbers of partners, more locums needed therefore less continuity, less visiting patients at home, increased public demand for a 24-hour rather than emergency service, changes in out-of-hours care with most using cooperatives or deputising services with poor transfer of information.[27] (NB. Many feel that palliative care patients may have suffered most in these changes.)
- Causes of stress for DNs in palliative care were poor family dynamics, a family wanting the nurse to be part of the unit, workloads, others expectations, family/patient denial of possibility of a cure. The DNs coped by developing support networks, talking about stress and sharing experiences in groups at work. This has important implications for employers.[28]
- Issues in home care provided by GPs: maintaining contact – giving explanations and support were reported to help as often as physical treatments and practical nursing. Weakness was a common symptom and led to more admissions than pain. Difficulties in relieving strain and fatigue in relatives also curtailed home care. Favourable comments about GPs were dependent on the frequency of their visits and the amount of support and time offered to patients and their families – DNs visited on average twice a week and GPs variably about once a fortnight (one-fifth having little or no involvement).[29]
- In a study in rural Wales most GPs saw palliative care as an important and rewarding part of their work and over half felt that they should be responsible for its coordination. They particularly welcomed the presence of community hospitals, allowing them to continue their involvement for those patients who did not die at home.[30]
- Job satisfaction was also high in interviews with DNs, stemming from the opportunity to provide holistic care, in contrast to work with other patients which is increasingly task orientated. The heavy involvement could be justified because it would be time limited, although the author notes that resource implications should be considered.[31]
- Survey of 203 family doctors over two years: referred on average 5.5 patients to in-patient specialist palliative care and 4.7 patients to specialist home teams. They wanted improved communication and liaison with palliative care services, input for patients with non-cancer illness and improved out-of-hours access.[32]
- DNs welcomed the chance to use all their nursing skills to help patients and their families and the opportunity to exercise some control over their work – emphasis of this work could illustrate DN activity for the purpose of strategic purchasing.[33]
- DNs in a Northern Ireland study feel they have a key role in coordinating palliative care and in supporting patients and families. The limiting factors are staffing, time constraints, limited resources, problems with equipment – these cause stress and require further help and training.[16]
- DNs play an important role in needs assessment and the development of a therapeutic relationship and are well placed to liaise well across the boundaries of care of primary and acute services.[34]

- The main problems expressed by a group of 53 DNs in care for the dying were to do with physical symptoms and work-related stresses of team relationships, but not many related to emotional problems.[35]
- A positive outcome had been achieved when patients retained control over their circumstances and died a peaceful death in their place of choice. Key factors in quality care provision were early referral of patients to DNs, family circumstances, the availability of time, the accessibility of services and equipment, and the relationship with other health-care professionals and informal carers.[36]
- On the whole, there was a high level of satisfaction with care from terminally ill patients and their carers of community-based services. Problem areas were perceptions of health professionals, especially in the domains of role, power and expertise, and some of the practical problems faced by some patients.[37]
- Ethno-specific needs of Bangladeshi patients in East London were explored and high-lighted socio-economic factors, recent migration and religious beliefs. Communication difficulties with patients and carers were common and there is reliance on children for translation. Fourteen patients died in London and 13 were buried in Bangladesh. The average age was young – 55 for males and 40 for females.[38]
- The main stresses for clinical nurse specialists in palliative care in the community were relationships with healthcare professionals (with relationships with GPs seeming to cause most difficulties), pressure of workload and the impact of sadness on the client group.[39]

Preferred place of care or death

Summary Impression: most people choose to remain at home to die but this is less likely to occur with some groups of patients, particularly the poor, the elderly, women, etc. Noting the preferred place of care/death makes this more likely to be fulfilled. Supporting carers is crucial and targeting services to meet community needs would increase the home death rate significantly.

- A post-bereavement survey of 229 people in inner London showed 21% died at home; 38% had expressed a preference of whom 73% had preferred home and 58% had achieved this. Key factors that increase the chance of achievement appear to be having access to equipment and stating a preference about place of death.[40]
- There is a clear preference among patients to die at home.[41]
- Home care in deprived areas may be particularly difficult to achieve: there is a wide variation in proportion of cancer deaths at home in different electoral wards of the UK. Of 1.3 million cancer deaths in 10 years, 27% died at home, 47% in hospital, 26% other. Home deaths were more common in areas of low deprivation (30%) and less common in more deprived areas (24%). Other social factors such as increasing age, Jarman index, ethnic variation and being female also lead to a low home death rate.[42]
- With a limited increase in community care 50% more patients with cancer could be supported to die at home, as they and their carers would prefer. In one study 84% of patients stated a preferred place of care: 58% preferred home (given existing circum-stances) and of those dying in hospital 67% had preferred home.[43]
- Most terminally ill patients would prefer to be at home despite satisfaction with hospice care.[44]
- An analysis of the 10-year trends in place of death of cancer patients showed that home deaths fell from 27% to 25.5%, with a slight increase to 26.5% in 1994, whilst

47.3% died in hospital in 1994. It was concluded that trends towards a reducing home death rate had halted, although this varied across regions, and the largest rise is in the increasing use of hospices.[45]

- An important target to improve home death rates is better support for carers. Unless factors associated with home death are identified and interventions targeted accordingly, further improvements may only help those already advantaged. Patients with carers are more likely to die at home and to access palliative support at home. Older patients are both less likely to die at home and to access home care. Women are less likely to die at home. There are suggestions that men are less efficient as carers so they need to be encouraged and enabled to take on the carer role. Therefore home deaths would increase if services were targeted towards poorer elderly patients, especially older females.[46]
- Home care is more likely if: younger patients, strong care systems, patients have expressed a preference, higher socio-economic group, longer trajectory of illness.[47]
- Reasons for hospital admission are continuous nursing care, symptom control, diagnostic test, elderly, public expectation.[48]
- Place of death is related to socio-economic groups with higher socio-economic groups dying in hospices and lower in hospitals.[49]
- Examining the factors related to admissions in 415 patients referred to St Christopher's home care service, it was found that the proportion requesting admission increased as care lengthened. Late admissions were more likely to be related to attitudes of denial, fighting the disease and optimism whereas earlier awareness of dying and stoicism in relatives favoured a home death. A growing preference for in-patient care usually preceded admission.[50]
- Preference for place of death is a clinical governance issue: figures of place of death of all patients should be compared with national figures and practices should be encouraged to present and discuss information as part of clinical governance.[51]
- In a USA study of elderly patients with cancer and non-cancer, making plans for pre-ferred place of death was common and was successful most of the time: 64% made plans for place of death and 91% of these were effected.[52]

Communication and coordination issues: C1 and C2

Summary Impression: Improving communication and coordination are seen as important in supporting patients better, though difficult to evaluate, but several factors have been shown to make an improvement, e.g. using registers, link workers, coordinated teams, etc.

- A matched controlled comparison looking at the effects of 'transmural' home care, which provides hospital back-up for community healthcare and increases the quality of life for carers (estimated one week after discharge and three months after death). Enhanced coordin-ation and cooperation between professionals and care-givers lead to improved supportive care for patients and carers compared with standard community care in the Netherlands.[53]
- A multiprofessional team approach with specialist palliative care input is beneficial and leads to improved satisfaction from patients with advanced cancer.[54]
- A small study of visits to terminally ill patients by five GPs following the establishment of a register, found that visits increased and tended to be planned; more patients also died at home and carers were more satisfied with the care given.[55]
- An informal study of the use of a register for palliative care patients and PHCT meetings in one practice showed a significant rise in the home death rate.[56]

- Use of a cancer 'link' nurse in primary care, linking between patients and professional services, led to fewer patient days in hospital, hospice or home visits and so was cost-efficient.[57]
- A palliative care intervention (coordination, consultant-led team) in Norway increased the home death rate from 15% to 26%, but time spent at home was unchanged.[58]

Symptom control and education: C3 and C5

Summary Impression: that symptom control, particularly pain management in the community, can be difficult and poorly achieved and that better assessment, use of guidelines and co-working with specialist palliative care can improve things. Education must be targeted and should include care of non-malignant conditions.

- Symptom control, especially pain management, in primary care can often be inadequate. There are several studies which show that difficulties in assessment, treatment and appropriate referral to specialist palliative care can be less than optimal. Better methods of symptom assessment and use of guidelines have been shown to improve such care.[59]
- A study of bereaved carers' views suggested that although satisfaction with GPs' care was high, symptom control may not be optimal. Particular concerns were the treatment of insomnia, loss of appetite as well as pain and shortness of breath.[60]
- The most severe problems were the effect of anxiety on carers and symptom control. The majority were extremely satisfied with their care from support teams and GPs/DNs but the negative comments referred to communication, coordination of services, attitude of doctor, delays in diagnosis and difficulty getting GPs to visit.[61]
- GPs want more targeted teaching and more help with non-malignant conditions.[32]
- There is increasing recognition that patients with non-malignant conditions suffer equally distressing symptoms and face similar emotional and social difficulties.[62]

Out-of-hours palliative care: C4

Summary Impression: that palliative care out-of-hours can be a major problem and that introducing changes in the transfer of information, nursing and other support, drugs access and advice from specialists can make a difference.

- Clear local policies and protocols for improvements in communication, carer support, adequate training and access to advice, and drugs and equipment access can improve out-of-hours palliative care in the community.[63]
- Inadequate out-of-hours palliative care is common across the UK since the changes in GP out-of-hours provision, leading to more patients being admitted to hospital where many will remain until their death. An example of a protocol is included.[64]
- There is a wide variation in out-of-hours palliative care service provision. GPs are less positive than specialists about the availability of out-of-hours specialist advice. There needs to be better primary–secondary dialogue, local needs assessments and adequate resourcing.[65]
- There is inadequate transfer of information to out-of-hours providers from those in primary care regarding patients with palliative care needs.[66]
- Few GPs hand over information to out-of-hours cooperatives. Although most GPs were satisfied with the out-of-hours arrangements (fewer DNs were), there were concerns about the quality of advice given, reluctance to visit and difficulties obtaining medication. There is a need for 24-hour availability of DNs, specialist palliative care advice and for protocols.[67]

- GPs welcomed help from specialist palliative care teams out-of-hours, especially telephone advice.[68]

Carers'/users' views: C6

Summary Impression: that carer breakdown is a crucial and sometimes unrecognised area of care and that carers have their own separate needs for support. This is a very important factor to address if any impact is to be made on home-based palliative care.

- Carer breakdown increases the chance of hospice referrals.[17,69]
- A postal questionnaire survey of carers indicated that information provision was deemed unsatisfactory for many carers and many were dissatisfied with care from hospital, GPs and DNs.[70]
- Another older survey found that admissions to hospital and hospice were more commonly due to carer breakdown/problems in providing care at home: in 22% of cases there was no lay carer and in 45% of cases the lay carer was unable to provide care.[71]
- Carers' needs should be assessed separately to balance the need for outside help with the preservation of independence, dignity and family aspects of life. Services should be introduced in ways that help patients to preserve independence, dignity and familiar aspects of life. The perception of accessibility of healthcare professionals may need to be reviewed.[46,72]
- Predictors of family care satisfaction were:
  - family care perceptions (greatest predictor)
  - family members' ages
  - family functioning – greatest need of support in those with poor functioning
  - length of time patients receive care.

  There is a need to sensitively explore the perceptions of care from the family to guide service provision.[73]
- Carers may have more concerns than patients, and they are usually neglected. There is little recognition of the significant unmet psychosocial needs of informal carers of cancer patients: to have a good relationship with the healthcare professional, receiving honest information, managing daily life, emotions, etc. 43% had significant unmet needs leading to poor health.[74]
- Most palliative care at home means heavy demands on family and friends: 84% reported above normal levels of psychological distress and 41% expressed high levels of strain relating to care giving. There was more strain in younger-aged carers and in females, and participants also reported life restrictions, emotional distress and limited support.[75]
- Friends and neighbours provide a small but significant source of support for the dying – the boundaries of friendship need to be negotiated. Friends may be left with complex, sometimes unrecognised, grieving processes.[76]
- Home care in Australia depends largely on the availability of a family care-giver. Family care-givers find significant meaning in their role but there are negative impacts on their health, schedules, anxiety and energy. They are involved in symptom control, take on all household tasks and they are asked to assess, monitor and deliver complex therapeutic interventions. There is a need to develop care-giver focused interventions.[77]
- In the USA there are about 20 million primary care-givers, supporting an estimated $190 billion industry. A qualitative study found that primary care-givers:
  - expressed that they did not immediately identify themselves as care-givers prior to initiating care

- found the shock and intensity of the tasks involved in care giving to be overwhelming
- believe they were ill prepared to meet the demands of the role
- desired help in managing.[78]

- Information is a key area in the carer's experience: there is a need to provide individualised care, answer questions and explore effects on couples and the complexity of the carer's needs. The nurse's role as sensitive mediator is important in this.[79]
- GPs' care in bereavement varies greatly – little is known about its quality or value or needs for intervention. GPs can feel too stretched to take a proactive role.[80]
- A survey of 500 senior GPs revealed that about a third routinely offered contact with a team member in bereavement. Practices with a special interest and those with a register were more likely to offer routine contact.[81]
- GPs may need training and support in bereavement. One study of GPs' attitudes to responding to death and bereavement revealed a strong sense of guilt about issues relating to death of their patients, based on a fear of making mistakes and lack of diagnostic precision. They felt they lacked training and tended to draw on their own experiences.[82]
- A bereavement protocol for general practice suggested that deaths should be recorded and a programme for review set up to make the GP practice accessible for grieving people.[83]

Other care settings

Summary Impression: that community hospitals and nursing homes are important and appreciated resources. Some standards, however, may not be adequate and may be unmonitored.

- Although widely agreed that nursing homes are appropriate settings for palliative care, there are concerns about the quality of care that can be given with mostly unqualified staff.[84]
- Community hospitals are an important resource for GPs seeking palliative care for their patients.[85]
- A study in Gwent, South Wales concluded that community hospitals may be the ideal setting in which to care for terminally ill patients who do not require specialist hospice beds.[86]

Possible solutions, guidelines and protocols

Summary Impression: many varied initiatives responding to perceived needs have had positive consequences. It is better to address these issues appropriately than to ignore them.

- The introduction of a patient assessment matrix within an audit framework led to a greater awareness within the PHCT of patients' preferred place of death and number of patients dying there.[87]
- A Dutch intervention to enhance coordination and cooperation of 'intra- and extramural' care led to a higher home death rate, with less re-hospitalisation.[53]
- An audit schedule (CAMPAS) was found to be suitable for monitoring palliative care standards in diverse primary care settings.[88]
- Nine key guidelines were developed for care of the dying in primary care in Devon. They included team meetings, symptom control, teaching carers, etc.[89]

- Setting and discussing multidisciplinary palliative care guidelines allows PHCTs to share ownership and develop initiatives within the practice. Key features are teamwork, coordinated management, early involvement of nursing staff and the identification of a key worker.[90]

References

1 July 30th (2002) edition of *Bandolier*, www.ebandolier.com

2 Higginson I J (1999) Evidence-based palliative care: there is some evidence and there needs to be more. [Editorial.] *BMJ.* **319**: 462–3.

3 Evidence-based Medicine Working Groups (1992) Evidence-based medicine: a new approach to teaching the practice of medicine. *JAMA.* **268**: 2420–5.

4 Haynes R B, Devereux P J and Guyatt G (2002) Physicians' and patients' choices in evidence-based practice. *BMJ.* **324**: 1350.

5 Greenhalgh T (2002) Intuition and evidence: uneasy bedfellows? *Br J Gen Pract.* **52**: 395–400.

6 Polanyi M (1996) *The Tacit Dimension*. Routledge, London.

7 Quinn M (2002) Intuition, creativity, dialogue, tacit knowledge and ... evidence? *Br J Gen Pract.* **52**: 588.

8 The Cancer Voices Programme and Cancerlink, www.macmillan.org.uk

9 Willis J (2002) *Friends in Low Places*. Radcliffe Medical Press, Oxford.

10 Thorpe G (1993) Enabling more dying people to remain at home. *BMJ.* **307**: 915–18.

11 Addington-Hall J M *et al.* (1991) Dying from cancer: the views of bereaved family and friends about the experiences of terminally ill patients. *Pall Med.* **5**: 207–14.

12 Mitchell G (2002) How well do general practitioners deliver palliative care? A systematic review. *Pall Med.* **16**: 457–64.

13 Millar D G, Carroll D, Grimshaw J *et al.* (1998) Palliative care at home: an audit of cancer deaths in the Grampion region. *Br J Gen Pract.* **48**: 1299–1302.

14 O'Henly A, Curzio J and Hunt J (1997) Palliative care services and settings: comparing care. *Int J Pall Nurs.* **3**(4): 227–31.

15 Hanratty B (2000) GP views on developments in palliative care services. *Pall Med.* **14**: 223–4.

16 McIlfatrick S and Curran C I (2000) District nurses' perceptions of palliative care services: part 2. *Int J Pall Nurs.* **6**(1): 32–8.

17 Barclay S, Todd C, McCabe J *et al.* (1999) Primary care group commissioning of services: the differing priorities of general practitioners and district nurses for palliative care services. *Br J Gen Pract.* **49**: 181–6.

18 Cartwright A (1991) Balance of care for the dying between hospitals and the community: perceptions of GPs, hospital consultants, community nurses and relatives. *Br J Gen Pract.* **41**: 271–4.

19 Pugh E M G (1996) An investigation of general practitioners' referrals to palliative care services. *Pall Med.* **10**: 251–7.

20 Addington-Hall J and McCarthy M (1995) Dying from cancer: results of a national population-based investigation. *Pall Med.* **9**: 295–305.

21 Heath J and Higginson I J (2002) Do specialist palliative care teams improve outcomes for cancer patients? A systematic literature review. *Pall Med.* **12**(5): 317–32.

22 Robbins M A, Jackson P and Prentice A (1996) Statutory and voluntary sector palliative care in the community setting: NHS professionals' perceptions of the interface. *Eur J Cancer Care* **5**: 96–102.

23 Pugh E M G (1996) An investigation of general practitioners' referrals to palliative care services. *Pall Med.* **10**: 251–7.

24 MacAdam D B (1983) Care of the dying: relevance of the hospice concept to general practice. *Aust Fam Phys.* **12**: 249–50.

25 Hanson L C, Earp J A *et al.* (1999) Community physicians who provide terminal care. *Arch Intern Med.* **159**(10): 1133–8.

26 Field D (1998) Special not different: general practitioners' accounts of their care of dying people. *Soc Sci Med.* **46**(9): 1111–20.

27 Barnett M (2002) The development of palliative care within primary care. In R Charlton (ed) *Primary Palliative Care: dying and bereavement in the community.* Radcliffe Medical Press, Oxford.

28 Wilkes L, Beale B *et al.* (1998) Community nurses' descriptions of stress when caring in the home. *Int J Pall Med.* **4**(1): 14–20.

29 Hinton J (1996) Services given and help perceived during home care for terminal cancer. *Pall Med.* **2**(10): 125–34.

30 Lloyd-Williams M, Wilkinson C and Lloyd-Williams F (2000) General practitioners in North Wales: current experiences in palliative care. *Eur J Cancer Care.* **9**: 138–43.

31 Griffiths J (1997) Holistic district nursing for the terminally ill. *Br J Comm Health Nurs.* **2**(9): 440–4.

32 Higginson I (1999) Palliative care services in the community: what do family doctors want? *J Pall Care.* **15**(2): 21–5.

33 Goodman C *et al.* (1998) Emphasising terminal care as district nursing work: a helpful strategy in a purchasing environment? *J Adv Nurs.* **28**(3): 491–8.

34 Daniels L (1999) Primary-led palliative care. *Br J Comm Nurs.* **4**: 108.

35 Dopp G and Dunn V (1993) Frequent and difficult problems perceived by nurses caring for the dying in the community, hospice and acute setting. *Pall Med.* **7**: 19–25.

36 Austin L, Luker K, Caress A *et al.* (2000) Palliative care: community nurses' perceptions of quality. *Qual Healthcare.* **9**(3): 151–8.

37 Jarrett N J, Payne S A, Wiles R A (1999) Terminally ill patients and lay carers' perceptions and experiences of community-based services. *J Adv Nurs.* **29**(2): 476–83.

38 Spruyt O (1999) Community-based palliative care for Bangladeshi patients in East London: accounts of bereaved carers. *Pall Med.* **13**(2): 119–29.

39 Newton J and Waters V (2001) Community palliative care clinical nurse specialists' descriptions of stress in their work. *J Pall Nurs.* **7**: 531–402.

40 Karlson S and Addington-Hall J (1998) How do patients who die at home differ from those who die elsewhere? *Pall Med.* **12**(4): 279–86.

41 Townsend J, Frank A *et al.* (1990) Terminal cancer care and patients' preferences for a place of death: a prospective study. *BMJ.* **301**: 415–17.

42 Higginson I J, Jarman B, Astin P *et al.* (1999) Do social factors affect where patients die: an analysis of 10 years of cancer deaths in England. *J Pub Health.* **21**(1): 22–8.

43 Townsend A *et al.* (1990) Terminal cancer care and patients' preferences for place of death: a prospective study. *BMJ.* **301**: 415–17.

44 Dunlop R J *et al.* (1989) Preferred vs. actual place of death: a hospital palliative care support team experience. *Pall Med.* **3**: 197–201.

45 Higginson I J, Astin P and Dolan S (1998) Where do cancer patients die? Ten-year trends in the place of death of cancer patients in England. *Pall Med.* **12**: 353–63.

46 Grande G E, Addington-Hall J M and Todd C J (1998) Place of death and access to home care services: are certain patient groups at a disadvantage? *Soc Sci Med.* **47**(5): 565–79.

47 Higginson I J and Sen Gupta G J A (2000) Place of care in advanced cancer: a qualitative systematic review of patient preferences. *J Pall Med.* **3**: 287–300.

48 Spilling R (1986) *Terminal Care at Home.* Oxford General Practice Series. Oxford University Press.

49 Sims A, Radford J, Doran K *et al.* (1997) Social class variation in place of cancer death. *Pall Med.* **11**(5): 369–73.

50 Hinton J (1994) Which patients with terminal cancer are admitted from home care? *Pall Med.* **8**: 197–210.

51 Holden J and Tatham D (2001) Place of death in 714 patients in a north-west general practice, 1992–2000: an indicator of quality? *J Clin Excellence.* **3**(1): 33–5.

52 Kaffengarger K P *et al.* (2000) Prevalence, effectiveness and predictors of planning the place of death among older persons followed in community-based, long-term care. *J Am Geriat Soc.* **48**(8): 943–8.

53 Smeenk F W M *et al.* (1998) Transmural care: a new approach in the care of terminal cancer patients: its effect on rehospitalisation and quality of life. *Patient Educ Counsell.* **35**(3): 189–99.

54 Hearn J and Higginson I J (1998) Do specialist palliative care teams improve outcomes for cancer patients: a systematic literature review. *Pall Med.* **12**: 317–32.

55 Buckley D (1996) Audit of palliative care in a general practice setting. *Pall Care Today.* 27–8.

56 Morris P Using a cancer register to aid communication and help patients die in their place of choice. [Personal communication.]

57 Raftery J, Addington-Hall J, MacDonald L D *et al.* (1996) A random controlled trial of the cost-effectiveness of a district coordinating service for terminally ill cancer patients. *Pall Med.* **10**: 151–61.

58 Jordhoy N S *et al.* (2000) A palliative care intervention and death at home: a cluster randomised trial. *Lancet.* **356**: 888–93.

59 Barclay S I (2000) The management of cancer pain in primary care. In: R Hillier, I Finlay, J Welsh and A Miles (eds) *The Effective Management of Cancer Pain.* Aesculapius Medical Press, London.

60 Hanratty B (2000) Palliative care provided by GPs: the carer's viewpoint. *Br J Gen Pract.* **50**: 653–4.

61 Higginson I J (1990) Palliative care: views of patients and their families. *BMJ.* **301**: 277–81.

62 Addington-Hall J M, Fakhoury W and McCarthy M (1998) Specialist palliative care in non-malignant disease. *Pall Med.* **12**: 417–27.

63 Thomas K (2000) *Out-of-hours palliative care in the community*. Macmillan Cancer Relief, London.

64 Thomas K (2000) Out-of-hours palliative care: bridging the gap. *Eur J Pall Care.* **7**(1): 22–5.

65 Munday D, Dale J and Barnett M (2002) Out-of-hours palliative care in UK: perspectives from general practice and specialist services. *J Roy Soc Med.* **95**(1): 28–30.

66 Barclay S I G, Rogers M and Todd C (1997) Communication between GPs and cooperatives is poor for terminally ill patients. *BMJ.* **315**: 1235–6.

67 Shipman C, Addington-Hall J, Barclay S *et al.* (2000) Providing palliative care in primary care: how satisfied are GPs and district nurses with current out-of-hours arrangements? *Br J Gen Pract.* **50**: 477–8.

68 Boyd K (1995) The role of the specialist home care team: views of GPs in South London. *Pall Med.* **9**: 138–44.

69 Seamark D A, Lawrence C and Gilbert J (1996) Characteristics of referrals to an in-patient hospice and a survey of general practitioners' perceptions of palliative care. *J Roy Soc Med.* **89**: 79.

70 Le Couturier J *et al.* (1999) Lay carers' satisfaction with community palliative care: results of a postal survey. South Tyneside MAAG Palliative Care Study Group. *Pall Med.* **13**(4): 275–83.

71 Herd E B (1990) Terminal care in a semi-rural area. *Br J Gen Pract.* **40**: 248–51.

72 Grande G E, Todd C J and Barclay S I G (1997) Support needs in the last year of life: patient and carer dilemmas. *Pall Med.* **11**: 202–8.

73 Medigovich K *et al.* (1999) Predictors of family satisfaction with an Australian palliative home care service: a test of discrepancy. *J Pall Care.* **15**(4): 48–56.

74 Soothill K *et al.* (2001) Informal carers of cancer patients: what are their unmet psychosocial needs? *Health Soc Care Comm.* **9**(6): 464–75.

75 Payne S, Smith P and Dean S (1999) Identifying the concerns of informal carers in palliative care. *Pall Med.* **3**(1): 37–44.

76 Young E, Seale C and Bury M (1998) 'It's not like family going is it?': negotiating friendship boundaries towards the end of life. *Mortality.* **3**(1): 27–42.

77 Aranda S K and Hayman-White K (2001) Home care-givers of the person with advanced cancer: an Australian perspective. *Cancer Nurse.* **24**(4): 300–7.

78 Lewis K L (1996) The invisible Americans: primary care-givers in the home setting. *Dissertations – Abstracts – International.* Sect B the Sciences and engineering. **56**(9-B): 4810.

79 Rose K E (1999) A qualitative analysis of the information needs of informal carers of terminally ill cancer patients. *J Clin Nurse.* **8**(1): 81–8.

80 Woof W R (1997) The future of bereavement care in British general practice. *Eur J Cancer Care.* **6**: 133–6.

81 Harris T and Kendrick T (1998) Bereavement care in general practice: a survey in South Thames health region. *Br J Gen Pract.* **48**: 1560–4.

82 Saunderson E M and Ridsdale L (1999) General practitioners' beliefs and attitudes about how to respond to death and bereavement: qualitative study. *BMJ.* **319**: 293–6.

83 Charlton R and Dolman E (1995) Bereavement protocol for primary care. *Br J Gen Pract.* **45**: 427–30.

84 Avis M and Jackson J G (1999) Evaluation of a project providing community palliative care support to nursing homes. *Health Soc Care.* **7**: 32–8.

85 Seamark D A, Williams S, Hall M *et al.* (1998) Palliative terminal cancer care in community hospitals and a hospice: a comparative study. *Br J Gen Pract.* **48**: 1312–36.

86 Llewellyn J, Evans N and Walsh H (1999) The role of community hospitals in the care of dying people. *Int J Pall Nurs.* **5**(5): 244–9.

87 Carroll D S (1998) An audit of place of death of cancer patients in a semi-rural Scottish practice. *Pall Med.* **12**: 51–3.

88 Rogers M, Barclay S I G and Todd C J (1998) Developing the Cambridge Palliative Care Audit Schedule (CAMPAS): a palliative care audit for primary healthcare teams. *Br J Gen Pract.* **48**: 1224–7.

89 Jones R (1992) Primary healthcare: what should we do for people dying at home with cancer? *Euro J Cancer Care.* **1**(4): 9–11.

90 Robinson L and Stacey L (1994) Palliative care in the community: setting practice guidelines for primary care teams. *Br J Gen Pract.* **44**: 461–4.

CHAPTER 6

Changes in a changing world

Knowing is not enough, we must apply
Willing is not enough, we must do.

Goethe

This chapter includes:

1   The world is changing
    - Policy context and clinical governance in England
    - The Supportive Care Strategy for England and Wales.
2   Change management
    - The head, hands and heart of improving community palliative care
    - Modernising services
    - Effecting change in primary care
    - Use of significant event analysis
    - Strategies for effective teamwork and productive meetings.

This chapter is in two parts: first, a brief overview of some of the recent national policy changes and their implications for primary care, and second, a discussion of change management and educational developments and how to attempt to cross the theory–practice gap to spread good practice.

The world is changing

The world of community palliative care is changing. Cancer is now the biggest killer in the UK, causing 25% of all deaths, and although the five-year survival rate is improving for many of the common cancers, the prevalence is likely to continue to rise.[1] Palliative care covers much more than cancer, although still the vast majority of patients in hospices have cancer. Along with the care for patients with other end-stage illnesses, currently there is a trend away from hospital and hospice care and into the community. With approximately 50% of patients discharged elsewhere from hospices and the average length of hospice stay being two weeks,[2] the roles of specialist and generalist palliative care are being redefined. There are more interventions and life-prolonging procedures available now, so the concept that the hospice once represented, as a safe place to die, is no longer as relevant as it once was. There is a rise in 'intermediate care' and means of preventing inappropriate admissions and keeping people at home longer, such as rapid response teams, continuing care funds, etc. More will be expected of us in the community in providing excellence of care for the dying at home, and yet currently some still regard this as a neglected 'Cinderella' service. Until, in particular, we have the availability of nursing cover 24 hours a day for patients at home in every part of the UK, it's hard to see how we can provide a full service for our patients.

Policy context and clinical governance in England

The issue of clinical governance is increasingly important, with evidence reviews, performance indicators and tangible outcome measures becoming part of standard practice. So in the context of improving palliative care at home, increasingly there will be a requirement to be accountable and to audit our care as much as is possible in this area. Initiatives such as the GSF programme incorporate some tangible outcomes measures that may soon become part of this process, if current trends continue – the 'must do's' rather than the 'add-on extras'. Although reluctant to have any more central diktats imposed on us, many in primary care feel that they wish to improve this area of care as a matter of professional pride and that such measures might be of use in indicating means of improving care (*see* www.radcliffe-oxford.com/caring).

The world of healthcare has been changing at an ever-increasing pace in recent years, to the extent that many are exhausted, cynical or at best dizzy with the number of turns of the merry-go-round. Several have seen a return of previously dismantled institutions under another name, such as primary care trusts replacing old district health authorities of a few years ago. However there are many new initiatives, such as the focus on clinical governance, evidence-based medicine, quality measures, intermediate care moving away from hospitals and supportive care, that have a subtle but significant bearing on our daily practice of medicine.

Box 6.1 contains a brief overview of some of the recent changes affecting primary palliative care in England, some of which also include other parts of the UK. The other countries of Scotland, Northern Ireland and Wales have many similar developments but are not specified here.

Box 6.1 The recent policy context of the NHS in England*

- ***Calman Hine Report 1995***
  - A framework for commissioning cancer services
  - a report to the Chief Medical Officers of England and Wales, it laid out the plan for the organisation of cancer services in future, including the development of accredited cancer centres and cancer units

- ***First Class Service 1997***
  - decentralisation; a new framework to deliver consistent, equitable services
  - national consistency measured against standards and informed by users' views

- ***NHS Plan 2000***
  - partnership, prevention, professions, performance, patient access, patient empowerment
  - Introduction of primary care groups and trusts, clinical governance, National Institute for Clinical Excellence, Commission for Health Improvement, etc. (*see* Figures 6.1 and 6.2)
  - National Service Frameworks developed

- ***National Institute for Clinical Excellence (NICE)***
  - standards/performance indicators and data sets

- ***User involvement – partnership groups***
  - Cancer services collaborative (CSC) patient experience project
  - Cancer Information Advisory Group
  - National Cancer Patient Survey

- *Palliative Care Survey 2000*
  - inequality of palliative care provision across the UK of in-patient palliative care beds, home care, nurses, etc.
  - uneven patchwork distribution not correlated with needs assessments
- *NHS Cancer Plan 2000*
  Aims:
  - to save more lives
  - to improve patients' experience of care
  - to tackle inequalities in health/cancer
  - to build for the future through education, research and workforce development

  1 *Faster treatments*
     - waiting is stressful
     - NHS Cancer Plan set out new targets, working with the Cancer Services Collaborative
     - two weeks between GP referral and specialist appointment
     - one month from diagnosis to treatment
     - effective communication, information and support
     - referral to first treatment – one month by 2008

  2 *Fairer, better treatments*
     - NICE appraisals, evidence-based COG guidelines
     - manual of cancer services standards – peer review and action plans for all hospital provision

  3 *Workforce provision*
     - 34 cancer networks developed across England
     - each primary care organisation (PCO) to have a cancer lead half day of protected time for strategic planning with Macmillan support programme backing

  4 *Improve patient experience*
     - Supportive Care Strategy, 2002–3
- *Shifting the Balance of Power 2001*
  - introduction of PCT commissioning
  - 75% of budget to be held by PCTs by 2005
- *CHI and Audit Commission 2001*
  - National Service Framework assessment
  - NHS cancer care in England and Wales
  - 'snapshot' of cancer services before introduction of NHS Cancer Plan
- *Out-of-Hours Review 2000*
  - 22 recommendations for improving out-of-hours primary care
- *Primary Care*
  - the debate about the introduction of revalidation, performance indicators, appraisal and accreditation of primary care
  - the new BMA contract (still being reviewed and debated by the General Practitioners Committee)

*With thanks to Sue Hawkett, DoH

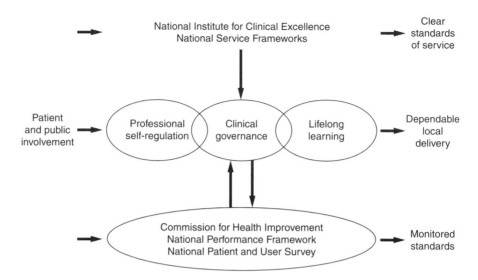

Figure 6.1: Inter-relationships of recent policy developments in England.

The Supportive Care Strategy for England and Wales

The Supportive Care Strategy for England and Wales is currently in development, but several initiatives are already having some effect (*see* Box 6.2). The National Council for Hospice and Specialist Palliative Care (NCHSPC) has suggested the following working definition of supportive care:

> *Supportive care is care designed to help the patient and their family cope with cancer and the treatment of it – from pre-diagnosis, through the process of diagnosis and treatment, to cure, continuing illness or death and into bereavement. It helps the patient to maximise the benefits of treatment and to live as well as possible with the effects of the disease. It is given equal priority alongside diagnosis and treatment.[3]*

Supportive care is provided throughout patients' and carers' care pathways. It is based on respect for the diversity of people with life-threatening disease and those close to them, creating a safe place in which they can explore and develop strategies for living and dying through utilising the external and inner resources available to them. It is a positive, sustaining and life-affirming concept that encompasses many areas of care, including communication, generalist and specialist palliative care, psychological support and other areas.

Supportive care is not a distinct speciality but is the responsibility of all health and social care professionals coming into contact with patients with cancer and their carers (*see* Figure 6.3). It is underpinned by specific communication skills and by organisations and teams who work in a coordinated and integrated way to ensure the smooth progression from one service to another.[4]

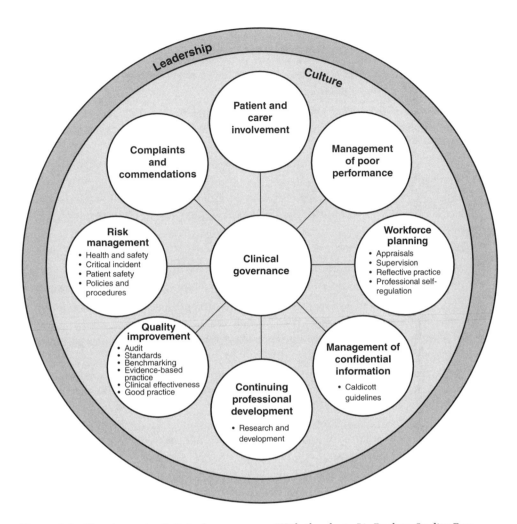

Figure 6.2: Key elements of clinical governance. With thanks to Liz Barker, *Quality Peer Review.*

Box 6.2 The Supportive Care Strategy

The Supportive Care Strategy in England and Wales is led by the National Cancer Director, Professor Mike Richards,[5] and aims to:

- improve the experience of care for all those affected by cancer
- have equitable provision of supportive and palliative care established in each cancer network
- provide service guidance and national standards supported by an evidence base
- establish a comprehensive strategy to improve the experience of care for those affected by cancer by coherence between strands, communication between project leads, support and advice, and coherent sequencing of projects within the overall strategy.

There are several initiatives:

- National Institute for Clinical Excellence (NICE) guidance and standards
- the development of a Supporting and Palliative Care Coordinating Group for England
- Cancer Information Advisory Group and the establishment of the Coalition for Cancer Information
- user involvement initiative, jointly run by Macmillan and the DoH to support user involvement in every network
- the Cancer Services Collaborative initiative, to include the Primary Care Strategy, with elements of supportive care throughout the cancer journey (the Gold Standards Framework is part of this)
- district nurse education and support programme, funded by the DoH, developing training for community nurses in every cancer network on the principles and practice of palliative care
- New Opportunity Fund (NOF) *Living with Cancer* programme, funding projects that can demonstrate improvements in, for example, home-based palliative care
- the development of national standards for specialist palliative care for cancer services
- advanced communication skills training.

NICE guidance topics
2002 – coordination and integration of care, communication and information, psychological support services, generalist palliative care, specialist palliative care, social support services
2003 – rehabilitation services, complementary therapy services, spiritual support services, carers and bereavement support services
It will be based largely within the supportive and palliative care networks under the auspices of the 34 cancer networks across England. Cancer networks are 'partnerships between commissioners of cancer care (health authorities and primary care trusts), service providers (at primary, secondary and tertiary levels), the voluntary sector, patient representatives and social services'.[5] They typically serve a population of 1–2 million people.

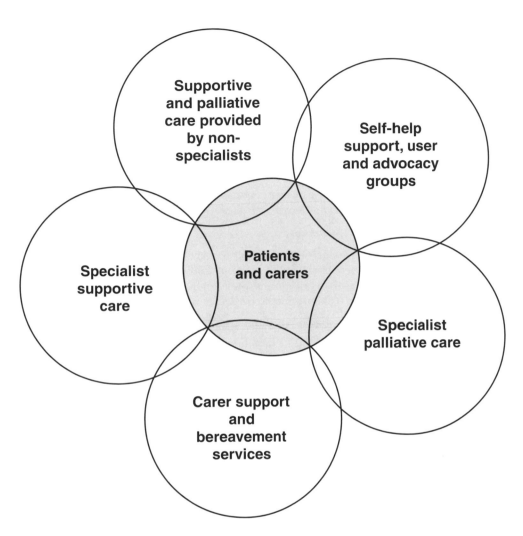

Figure 6.3: Supportive care.

Change management

Our dying patients deserve from us competence with compassion.

Dame Cicely Saunders

How do we cross the theory–practice gap for our patients and what skills are required to introduce changes that will have a positive impact on their care?

The head, hands and heart of improving community palliative care

It is suggested that excellence of care contains three main elements: the head (*clinical competence*), hands (*organisation*) and heart (*human dimension*) (*see* Figure 1.1, p. 8).

Clinical competence (head) entails:

- delivering our medical/nursing/other skills to the best of our ability
- ensuring the best clinical outcome for our patients that we can
- keeping updated, constantly learning and reinforcing our knowledge and skills, e.g. prescribing appropriately, diagnosing well, caring for wounds effectively, etc.

Organisational/medical 'systems' (hands) entails:

- the system around the delivery of this care and how it is organised
- how well each player keeps others informed, especially across primary/secondary/tertiary boundaries, i.e. information transfer
- the efficiency, spread and package of care delivered, e.g. the two-week rule for every patient with suspected cancer
- 'the key organising concept for an effective approach to improvement in the nature of a system'.[6]

'Every system is perfectly designed to produce the result it achieves.'[6] So if a system of care is not working well, what key changes can we make to improve things? For example, all may go well for a patient from Monday to Friday but then break down at a weekend, the patient is admitted to hospital in a crisis and dies there. However, with improved planning and communication, better access to advice, support and drugs, and an integrated out-of-hours protocol, perhaps this could have been avoided. By attempting to improve the system of care provision, the individual patient will benefit.

Human dimension (heart) entails:

- at all times maintaining our common humanity, the ability to view the situation from the patient/carers' perspective, as if we were the recipients of care
- compassion – being gentle with people at times of life-devastating events
- psychological support – ensuring the best psychological, social and 'non-clinical' support
- spiritual support – underpins all this – treating people with dignity and respect, encouraging their own autonomy and self-determination, and dealing with factors along the outer journey which allows the deeper, less tangible but crucially important issues of the 'inner journey' to be given a voice.

This ties in with the pillars of *clinical governance*

1 clinical effectiveness
2 risk management effectiveness } competence
3 patient experience
4 communication effectiveness } humanity
5 resource effectiveness
6 strategic effectiveness } organisational/systems
7 learning effectiveness

Modernising services

Whether you think you can or whether you think you can't – you're right.

Henry Ford

In this dizzy world of change, much skill is needed when attempting to introduce changes into any system. And when people do have 'the evidence', if it exists, how do they make the great theory-to-practice jump? For many people this is the challenge. The use of audit cycles, significant event analysis and many other developments have helped to cross this gap.

The principle is deciding and agreeing a clear 'high-level' aim, determining a specific change that you believe will move you in a direction consistent with that (based on a good understanding of the current situation and available evidence from the literature and, increasingly being informed by user groups), putting measures in place that will show if the change has brought about the hoped-for improvement and then moving to a means of implementing this change.

Don Berwick, founder of the Institute of Healthcare Improvement and a great inspiration to many, including myself, found that numerous reports from reputable mainstream organisations in the USA were being published in the late 1990s but that nothing was changing. Good individual people were struggling in a system that was set up to fail. He and others then developed the thinking behind system redesign, which has been extremely influential in the very successful Cancer Services Collaborative, and in other collaboratives and developments within the NHS Modernisation Agency in England.

> *The structure of a system significantly determines the performance of the system … Learning to move beyond events to see the structure in the system that underlies the problems is a start.*[6]

Redesigning systems

We are what we repeatedly do. Excellence, then, is not an act, but a habit.

Aristotle

'System redesign' involves a different approach that is not opposed to, but complements, that of the hard evidence-based 'double-blind random controlled trial'. It is felt by many to be more appropriate when trying to influence the provision of services rather than drug usage – both concepts have their place in medicine. It is my view, and that of a few other disillusioned renegades, that the world of evidence-based medicine leading to guidelines from on high (valuable as they are in defining good practice) has very obvious limitations which must be recognised (*see* Chapter 5). The art of medicine is in danger of being swallowed up and lost completely by the pseudo-science of evidence, and the rigid procedural timescales of publications are so inhibiting that there is little room for flexible adaptation of a developing idea. As we await a firm evidence base, patients may be dying with conditions we can treat.

With the more human and flexible Plan, Do, Study, Act (PDSA) model (*see* Figure 6.5), ideas are considered, tried out, tested, adapted and refined until they work in a much shorter timescale, with the acknowledgement that we learn more from our mistakes than our successes. This more 'bottom-up' transformational approach encourages other innovative approaches to service provision.

If you always do what you've always done, you'll always get what you've always got.[6]

Some particular key skills of the Collaboratives have been the introduction of:

- mapping of the patient's journey – '*process mapping*'
- the accurate estimating of *capacity and demand*
- the *PDSA* model of improving care with small well-evaluated steps
- the approach of '*measuring for improvement not for judgement*' – producing regular run-charts to demonstrate change
- examining the *human dimension of change.*

Why do change projects fail? The human dimension of change

People responsible for planning and implementing change often forget that while the first task of change management is to understand the destination and how to get there, the first task of transition management is to convince people to leave home.[7]

Many change projects fail and the most commonly cited reason is neglect of the human dimension of change. This neglect often centres around the lack of insight into why people resist organisational change and poor appreciation of the process of changing people as well as systems.

There are two approaches to improvement:

- the 'anatomical' approach – change is a stepwise process, typically initiated from top down, with objectives set (in stone!) and it goes wrong because of poor planning and project control
- the 'physiological' approach – outcomes cannot be predetermined, change is typically from the bottom up, there is no end-point and it goes wrong because of people issues.

In practice, both approaches are necessary:

- you need a plan to set direction but need to be flexible
- top-down support is needed for bottom-up change
- objectives need to be set and the team should be congratulated when each is achieved, but improvement never ends
- correct use of improvement tools and techniques should be planned and monitored, but gaining the commitment of people is vital.

If the people issues are not identified and managed effectively, the following problems may arise:

- strong emotions such as fear, anger, hopelessness and frustration can derail your project
- fall in morale and higher job dissatisfaction with increased sickness and absenteeism
- people become defensive and take exaggerated stances, e.g. blame others, overemphasise the benefits of the present working system
- there is constant complaining or scepticism
- people don't do what they say they will do
- conflicts can spiral out of control.

Change is not the same as transition. Change is situational: the new site, the new structure, the new team, the new role, the new procedure. Transition is the psychological process people go through to come to terms with the new situation. Remember that change is external and transition is internal.[8]

NB. There are many skills and tools available that help with these dimensions of change. For more details, please see the *Improvement Leaders' Guide to Managing the Human dimensions of change: working with individuals*, written by Jean Penny and the Redesign Team of the NHS Modernisation Agency, available on www.modern.nhs.uk/improvementguides/human.

Introducing a new project

Any change in behaviour may be resisted. However, as can be seen in the 'change equation',[9] if the dissatisfaction (D) with the present situation plus a vision (V) for a more desirable future is added to the knowledge of the first steps to take in moving towards that future (S) and the capacity (C) of sufficient resources to change, then the force for change (F) will overwhelm the resistance (R).

$$\text{i.e. for change to occur } F (D + V + S + C) > R$$

So if considering introducing for example the Gold Standard Framework into a practice, there are three elements to introducing this change of behaviour which will make resistance (R) less likely:

1   There is some dissatisfaction with the present situation and a vision of the ideal (sometimes GPs may not see the need to improve but cross-checking against certain criteria such as home death rate, user views, crises, out-of-hours problems can trigger this, e.g. with a SEA or baseline assessment) (D + V).
2   That the first steps towards implementation and a logical plan or framework is understood, owned, agreed and adapted (S).
3   That capacity is there, i.e. these changes reduce not increase the present burden and are efficient in time and workload (C). The 'what's in it for me' (WIFM) factors are satisfied by overall reduced workload from less crisis management.

To understand an organisation, the more people you can involve, and the faster you can help them understand how the system works and how to take responsibility for making it work better, the faster will be the change.

Marvin Weisbord

In the Collaborative approach (*see* Figure 6.4), the three fundamental questions for improvement are:

1   What are we trying to accomplish?
2   How will we know that a change is an improvement?
3   What changes can we make that will result in an improvement?

The PDSA model (*see* Figure 6.5) used by the collaboratives in the NHS Modernisation Agency has many advantages when attempting to change systems: it makes the processes and learning explicit, enables testing of ideas (customising changes to local conditions), minimises problems of getting started and promotes bite-sized chunks.

When introducing change, often the innovators will pick ideas up first, but it is recommended that the 'early adopters', the opinion leaders in the peer group, are particularly targeted.[10] It is estimated that once an innovation is adopted by about 20% of members in an organisation, it is then likely to tip over into routine accepted practice (*see* Figure 6.6).

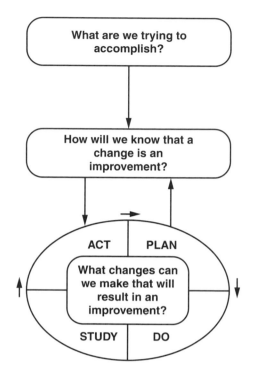

Figure 6.4: Model for improvement.

So if a primary care organisation or an individual practice were to adopt a project such as the GSF or any other, these factors need considering. The success of the GSF so far has depended on the fact that it has encouraged 'bottom-up change with top-down support'. By developing local ownership, adapting to suit the needs of the people and the area and demonstrating and celebrating the benefits this has allowed real rooted change, that in time will imperceptibly become part of the routine 'wallpaper' of the practice, long after the details can be remembered. It becomes standard practice: 'this is what we do for our palliative care patients'.

Effecting change in primary care

- Education in general practice.
- Personal/practice development plans.
- The use of significant event analysis.

A recent study of the needs of general practitioners in palliative care education confirmed that targeted teaching was important to GPs – learning as a team rather than the more detached learning from specific lectures.[11] With 'learn as you go' policies and building in teaching into the regular life of general practice using a variety of means, alongside the more traditional means of education, more effective learning can occur (*see* Chapter 16, C5). With this, and with the use of audit and reflective practice, will come the seeking of real practice-based changes.

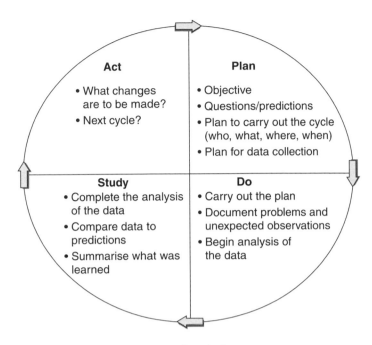

Figure 6.5: The Plan, Do, Study, Act (PDSA) cycle for improvement.

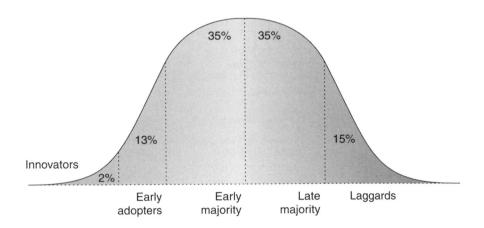

Figure 6.6: Diffusion of innovation.

The TARGET initiative, developed in Doncaster,[12] involves protected time for GPs' and whole practice teams' education during the day instead of the more usual evening or rushed lunchtime sessions. It has enabled the spread of protected learning times across the UK, and the development and implementation of very effective levels of change.

It wasn't long ago that a GP could continue in a solitary existence, without outside contact with colleagues, accountability or recourse to any educational sessions. Now, with the introduction of clinical governance, out-of-hours cooperatives and the rapid development of primary care organisations, we in primary care are benefiting from a much more shared collegiate way of working, familiar to many of our hospital colleagues. The structures in primary care are changing.

Similarly, the educational structures within primary care are changing with the phasing out of the Postgraduate Education Attendance (PGEA) 'brownie points'. Increasingly, practice multidisciplinary teams are being encouraged to work to produce 'personal development plans' and 'practice development plans'. Such PDPs will be a key feature of revalidation in the future.[13] They are a learning tool, drawn from what we do, and feed back directly into our work. Cancer and palliative care lends itself perfectly to this model as full multiprofessional and teamworking has to occur for best patient care. Maximising the team approach is an essential element in quality palliative care in the community – GPs and district nurses are far less effective in isolation or if working out of unison with each other. Real teamwork here bears much fruit.

Primary healthcare team meetings to reflect and decide on a practice's response and how and who should implement things, is a working example of such a PDP. Regular educational updates, case reviews, significant event analysis and audit, perhaps with a palliative care specialist (specialist nurse or doctor) present if possible, are good examples of means to develop improvements in primary care (*see* Figure 6.7[14]).

Use of significant event analysis

Reflective practice has long been a part of nurses' continuing education. Taking time to examine a particular case as it enfolds or after an event such as a death allows an objective

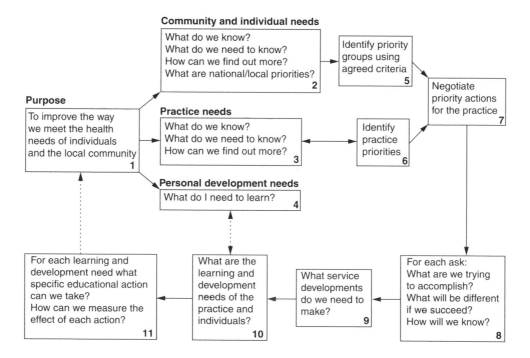

Figure 6.7: A guide to practice professional development planning.[14]

clarity to be shared around the facts of the case. It also stimulates discussion about the issues raised and how they can be best addressed. It is important always to consider what went well as well as what could be improved upon – to remember to celebrate the good aspects of care, of which there will always be many. Many practices use aids such as the traffic lights system of a page of green, orange and red sections representing what went well, average/near misses and what went not so well. The use of significant event analysis (SEA) has proved an invaluable tool for those wishing to improve the palliative care in their practice.

What is significant event analysis?

A significant event analysis is defined as occurring when 'individual episodes in which there has been a *significant* occurrence (either beneficial or deleterious) are analysed in a *system-atic* and detailed way to ascertain what can be learnt about the overall *quality of care* and to indicate changes that might lead to future *improvements*.'[15]

The underlying thinking relates to 'the blameless society' where, by examining the issues and systems of care rather than the person involved, there is less defensiveness, more honest admissions of problems or challenges, true assessments of risks or 'weakest links' and real measures to instigate improvements (*see* Figure 6.8).[16]

The SEA aims to look at the structure of the organisation and the processes of care. It is a qualitative form of audit which involves examining the way we do things rather than counting numbers. It is an enjoyable, constructive process that improves morale and builds teamwork, as well as leading to practical improvements in care.

Practical steps to a significant event analysis in palliative care[17]

- Ensure everyone understands the process is about looking at the way in which care is delivered rather than apportioning blame.

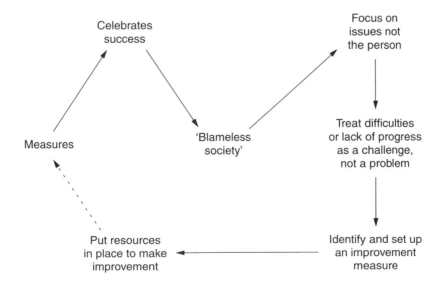

Figure 6.8: The blameless society.

- Set aside protected time – about an hour – distraction-free, drinks available, flip chart, etc.
- Choose a palliative care patient who has received a completed episode of care mainly in the community and involving several members of the team.
- Nominate a lead, keep focused on the task, ask for observations from those less involved and record important points and decisions (you could use an external facilitator).
- Use any guidelines, external resources, literature reviews or articles that are available to reflect on benchmarks of care.
- Draw up an action plan, decide who will do what and by when.
- Sum up, reminding first what went well, and recap the action points, deadlines and next steps.

Talking about a death three years ago, the SEA acted as a purge to my system emotionally. I had everything bottled up inside ... Talking about patient care in this way is good. In retrospect we could have got together and discussed this case as a significant event at the time. We really needed support with this patient.[17]

The benefits of significant event analysis

- Risk management
- Clinical negligence
- Positive approach to complaints
- Identifies learning needs
- Identifies audit and research topics
- Helps understanding of others' roles
- Builds and develops skills of teams
- Focuses on patient outcomes
- Promotes self-esteem and self-value
- Identifies communication opportunities
- Comprehensive nature
- Fulfils team potential
- Personal, professional and service development in an active way
- Key part of clinical governance.

Use of SEAs, practice development plans, targeted teaching and 'learn as you go' policies can move thinking on in a real way in practice teams, develop creative practical ideas and greatly enhance morale and a shared sense of each others' roles within the team. Our patients will undoubtedly benefit from this more concerted and thought through process, and we will too. *See also* Chapter 16, C5.

The tale of the hamster or significant event analysis made easy[18]

Trisha Greenhalgh, Professor of Primary Care at University College London, describes a familiar crisis over the death of the family hamster in terms of an exercise in significant event analysis. This amusing story has many parallels with the process a PHCT might go through when reflecting on their palliative care patients and is a model of reflective practice or SEA that we can all relate to ... especially when nobody changes the water!

She tracks the stages many might go through after a difficult death of a patient:

1 *Denial.* '... Their next reaction was to stage a cover-up. Don't tell the cleaner, they insisted. Their ill-informed plan was to leave the dead creature curled up in her cage, shifting her

position daily, and to walk past occasionally within the cleaner's earshot saying "Gosh, Smokey's asleep again". This plan was soon seen to be untenable, and our communal guilt surfaced.'

2   *Blaming.* 'We started to trade indictments. Who had abandoned the rota for cleaning her out?... Who had walked her along the piano keys? Whose friends had all had a go at Pokey Smokey? One of the kids decided that she had died of depression. He had been the only one who had ever understood her feelings. The rest of us, he claimed, had taken her for granted. "Rubbish," I said, "the culprit is Bart Simpson. It said in the guidelines (*Caring for your Hamster*) that you shouldn't keep them near the television, especially loud and violent programmes. If you kids hadn't kept playing that bloody video she would still be alive."'

3   *Reflection.* 'In the silence following the row, I regretted my outburst and reflected on the blame culture that we had allowed to develop. The hamster could not be brought back, but the event should be seen as a learning experience and processes put in place to prevent a similar disaster in the future. I found it hard to admit, even to myself, that I'd never read the guidelines properly nor had I arranged appropriate training for the principal carer. Lines of accountability were unclear, and, worst of all, the crucial task of changing the water was either everybody's or nobody's job.'

4   *Constructive improvements.* 'One week on, we are still slightly numb from the event, but we have all learnt a lot and we now have an evidence-based care pathway in place with essential roles assigned to named individuals who are appropriately trained and supervised; and six days on, young Ginger is still in the picture of health.'

Strategies for effective teamwork and productive meetings

In real life conflicts can arise between colleagues, causing a deterioration in both our own job satisfaction and in patient care. Difficult relationships between healthcare professionals are a reality and, for example, have been cited as one of the key sources of stress for clinical nurse specialists (particularly with GPs!).[19] Poor working relationships between interdisciplinary colleagues may negatively affect patient care[20] and this is one of the main triggers for staff changes. Conflict can arise from communication difficulties, differences in status, education, roles and a lack of agreed goals. The way we handle conflict is one measure of our maturity as adults, and an area in which we all can improve. The alternative to this resolution is that we become entrenched in static positions, with deepening grudges and deteriorating relationships which become harder to resolve. Generally, conflicts have two elements: the relationship between the people involved and the issue which is the basis of the disagreement. Preventing escalation, containing and positively handling conflict are important steps, but the main advice given is to acknowledge it, describe the issues and keep talking it through.[7]

If we are to work effectively as teams, we require skills of communication, collaboration and conflict resolution. Strategies to improve these skills can be learnt, but need practising. Some suggested strategies are listed in Box 6.3.[21] They can be applied to any scenario, including that of a typical lunchtime PHCT meeting, when a tension arises over a difference of opinion in patient care that may reflect a deeper agenda – a tricky but familiar picture. By breaking through this barrier of relationship conflicts, the spin-offs are a greater sense of respectful teamworking and better morale leading to much greater team productivity – the whole being far greater than the individual parts.

Box 6.3 Strategies for effective communication and collaboration in medical teams

1 *Be respectful and professional* in your interactions. Remember other people's histories and personal investments.

2 *Listen* intently to the other person. In active listening you learn about their underlying wants or needs and hidden agendas, and are more likely to reach a solution.

3 *Try to understand the other person's viewpoint.* Repeat back what you have heard and clarify until you have it right: 'It sounds like you are saying ... is that what you mean?' This is a real skill and greatly underused.[23]

4 *Acknowledge the other person's thoughts and feelings:* 'You seem upset'; 'That's another way to look at it'. Validating feelings builds trust and acknowledges that they have been heard.

5 *Be cooperative.* Assume good faith, think team. Use words like 'joint' and 'mutual' rather than 'either/or'.

6 *Look for shared concerns.* Start with smaller issues before moving on to the more difficult issues. Return to common interests if things begin to escalate.

7 *State your feelings.* Use words such as 'I feel' and 'I think' but rely on facts and information. Be consistent; surprises can erode trust.

8 *Don't take things personally.* Don't respond in kind to threats or personal attack. Take time out if needed. Defuse with a balanced neutral person if possible who will not fan the flames or escalate emotions.

9 *Learn to say 'I was wrong'.* Apologise when appropriate. This reduces personal agendas of winning and losing.

10 *Don't feel pressured to agree instantly* as this may be premature: 'Let's take time to consider the next step and find a time to meet again.' Breathing space allows perspective.

11 *Think about possible solutions before the meeting.* Consider your goals and what compromise you would be able to live with. Offer and ask for solutions. A third party might be helpful. Plan follow-up as a way to monitor resolutions.

12 *Think of conflict resolution as a helical process.* Conflicts are rarely resolved in one interaction. Returning later to the spiral, real progress is gradual, often step by step, with neutral stalling time in between.

Any improvement is a change, not every change is an improvement ... but we cannot improve anything unless we change it.[22]

This chapter has highlighted some of the current context of our healthcare system and provided some thoughts on the introduction of new ideas and change management, particularly in primary care. Much more is available from the sources quoted, including resources and courses run by the NHS Modernisation Agency in England or its equivalent elsewhere. The introduction of something new will always be a challenge and may at times feel a costly procedure not worth the hassle, but it is hoped that this will help and encourage those introducing such changes, keeping our focus firmly set on the goal of improving care for our seriously ill patients in the community.

References

1 Wilkinson J and Hatfield A (2002) The epidemiology of cancer. In M Baker (ed) *Modernising Cancer Services*. Radcliife Medical Press, Oxford.

2 National Council for Hospice and Specialist Palliative Care Services: minimum dataset. See also Eve A, Smith A M and Tebbit P (1997) Hospice and palliative care in the UK, 1994–5. *Pall Med.* **11**: 31–43.

3 P Tebbit, National Council of Hospice and Specialist Palliative Care Services Consultation, March 2002.

4 Draft Supportive Care Strategy Introduction, www.nice.org.uk

5 Richards M (2002) *Priorities in Developing the Supportive and Palliative Care Network Agenda*. National Council for Hospice and Specialist Palliative Care Conference, Bristol, May 2002.

6 Berwick D, Institute of Healthcare Improvement.

7 NHS Modernisation Redesign Team. Managing the Human Dimensions of Change. www.modern.nhs.uk/improvementguides/human

8 Bridges W (1995) *Managing Transitions: making the most of change*. Nicholas Brearley, London.

9 Upton T and Brooks B (1995) *Managing Change in the NHS*. Kogan Page Ltd, London.

10 Fraser S (2002) *Accelerating the Spread of Good Practice: a workbook for healthcare*. Kingsham Press, London.

11 Shipman E, Addington-Hall J *et al.* (2001) Educational opportunities in palliative care: what do general practitioners want? *Pall Med.* **15**: 191–6.

12 Coleman M and Dakin G, www.pltfoundation.com and target@doncastercentralpct.nhs.uk

13 Rughani A (2001) *The GP's Guide to Personal Development Plans*. Radcliffe Medical Press, Oxford.

14 Campion-Smith C and Wilcock P (2001) *Guide to Practice Professional Development Planning*. Department of Health and Community Studies, Bournemouth University.

15 Pringle M and Bradley C (1994) *Audit Trends*. Occasional Paper no. 70. Royal College of General Practitioners, London.

16 Stead J *et al.* (2002) *Significant Event Analysis*. Department of Primary Care, Exeter University.

17 Greenaway T (2001) *Making the Most of a Significant Event Analysis*. MAAG, Manchester.

18 Greenhalgh T (2001) Critical event audit: a hamster's tale. *BMJ.* **323**: 1195.

19 Newton J and Waters V (2001) Community palliative care clinical nurse specialists' descriptions of stress in their work. *J Pall Nurs.* **7**(4): 402–531.

20 Mackay L (1993) *Conflicts in Care: medicine and nursing*. Chapman and Hall, London.

21 Rider E (2002) Twelve strategies for effective communication and collaboration in medical teams [Career focus]. *BMJ.* **325**: S45.

22 Goldratt E (1990) *Theory of Constraints*. North River Press, MA.

CHAPTER 7

The key features of palliative care for patients with the common cancers

Susan Salt

Macmillan Consultant in Palliative Care
Calderdale & Huddersfield NHS Trust

This chapter includes:

1 Bladder cancer
2 Primary and secondary brain tumours
3 Breast cancer
4 Colorectal cancer
5 Gynaecological cancer
6 Head and neck cancer
7 Chronic leukaemia and myeloma
8 Lung cancer
9 Mesothelioma
10 Prostate cancer
11 Upper gastrointestinal cancer
12 Carcinomatosis of unknown origin.

The following pages contain some general comments about some of the palliative care issues that may be encountered by people suffering from the commoner cancers. The comments are not exhaustive but are a brief summary of some of the clinical situations that may be encountered by any healthcare professional working with these patients. Armed with the knowledge of possible problems relating to each cancer, greater anticipatory care can be instigated for patients in line with the GSF drive to improve assessment and advance planning.

Management plans have been included to help guide health professionals to the type of diagnostic procedures that they may need to initiate and subsequent treatment the patient may have to receive under specialist supervision. The summaries and management plans are a guide only and definitive management of the more complex symptoms should only be undertaken after discussion with your local specialist oncology and palliative care service.

With grateful thanks to Dr Mary Kiely, Consultant in Palliative Medicine, Huddersfield Royal Infirmary and Dr Liz Higgins, Consultant in Palliative Medicine, Kirkwood Hospice, Huddersfield who reviewed and amended the information.

Bladder cancer

General comments

Many patients will have had extensive investigations and treatment for polyps over a number of years before a malignant tumour occurs. *Surgical intervention* such as cystoscopy, cystectomy and urinary diversion may be appropriate. In addition *radical radiotherapy* and *intravesical chemotherapy* may help. The cancer journey is often long with many difficult symptoms which lead to exhaustion and an increased risk of *depression* in patient and carers alike.

Specific pain complexes

- **Bladder spasm** can be frequent and troublesome leading to frequency as well as pain. *Anti-cholinergic drugs* may help, but often specialist advice is needed.
- **Pelvic pain** is common in advanced disease due to tumour progression. This is often complex and only partially responds to opioids. Usually there is a neuropathic element which will require adjuvant analgesics in the form of *antidepressant and/or anticonvulsant medication.* Specialist advice is frequently needed to maintain symptom control.

Other complications

Recurrent haematuria is common and may be sufficient to cause *anaemia*. Discussion is needed about the appropriateness of repeated transfusion if the haematuria is persistent. Clot retention may result in acute retention which may be difficult to manage.

Urinary incontinence may occur. Many patients have long-term indwelling catheters, which increases the risk of *urinary tract infections*.

Lymphoedema of the lower limbs and genital area may occur and requires specialist management to prevent complications.

Fistulae may occur which are often amenable to surgery. These may be malodorous, cause skin breakdown and be very difficult to manage.

Renal failure may occur. Stenting the renal tract may be possible but may be inappropriate. Dialysis is rarely indicated. Specialist advice will be needed about maintaining symptom control in a patient with established renal failure.

Altered body image and **problems with sexual function** may arise. **Depression** is common because of the protracted time frame of the illness and chronic fatigue is often caused by nocturia in patients who are not catheterised.

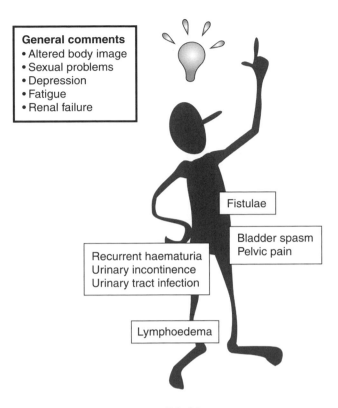

General comments
- Altered body image
- Sexual problems
- Depression
- Fatigue
- Renal failure

Fistulae

Bladder spasm
Pelvic pain

Recurrent haematuria
Urinary incontinence
Urinary tract infection

Lymphoedema

Figure 7.1: Key points in palliative care of bladder cancer patients.

Primary and secondary brain tumours

General comments

Benign tumours and some malignant ones are cured if they can be completely removed surgically.

Primary malignant brain tumours are treated with *surgery* where possible, but *radiotherapy* and *chemotherapy* may also be needed. The disease course may be protracted over many months and years with multiple problems. They do not metastasise outside the brain and spinal cord and hence the terminal stage may be prolonged.

Surgical resection of tumours may cause significant complications such as aphasia, paralysis, blindness, coma or death.

Secondary brain tumours are more common. *Surgical resection* of some isolated secondaries may be appropriate in breast, kidney and colon cancers. Otherwise *palliative radiotherapy* for those who are fit enough may help, depending on the sensitivity of the tumour.

Specific pain complexes

- **Headaches** due to raised intracranial pressure are usually controlled with *high-dose oral steroids* and *strong opioids* in the majority of patients. If there is evidence of hydrocephalus, neurosurgical referral for a shunt is needed.
- **Meningeal irritation** occurs in advanced disease and this may produce photophobia as well as neck stiffness. This may respond to *non-steroidal anti-inflammatory drugs (NSAIDs) and/or oral steroids*.

Other complications

Altered body shape, osteoporosis, skin fragility and mental effects of steroids commonly occur as patients are often on high-dose steroids for a long time.

Epileptic fits are common, but not universal. They may be difficult to control and advice from neurologists may be needed to ensure adequate control using *anticonvulsant medication*.

Disability with impaired mobility, incontinence and personality changes mean that patients often need intensive *multidisciplinary support* and *rehabilitation*.

Social and psychological issues are common. Many patients with primary brain tumours are young and may be the *main wage earner* in a family as well as having young children. *Children* often need specialist support before and after the patient's death, particularly if the patient has undergone personality and behaviour changes.

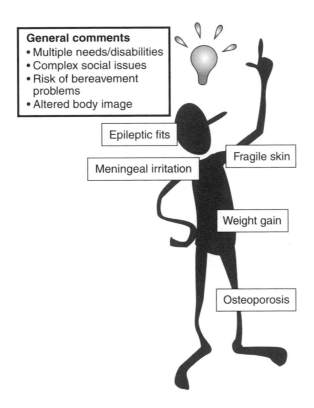

Figure 7.2: Key points in palliative care of patients with primary and secondary brain tumours.

Breast cancer

General comments

Late recurrence is common even after a number of years of disease-free survival. If a patient develops symptoms it is essential that investigations be carried out to make a firm diagnosis of their cause. This should include chest X-ray and liver ultrasound. If bone pain is a significant issue, plain X-rays of the affected area and/or a bone scan may be helpful. Disease-specific measures, including hormone manipulation, radiotherapy and chemotherapy, may achieve good palliation and should be considered in all patients, even those with advanced disease. Genetic counselling should be considered for those families with a strong family history of breast and/or ovarian cancer.

Specific pain complexes

Widespread **bone metastases** are common. Patients are at risk of:

- **Pathological fracture** that may occur without obvious trauma. This may need *orthopaedic intervention* (pinning or joint replacement) and/or *radiotherapy.*
- **Spinal cord compression** which requires prompt diagnosis, high-dose oral steroids in a single daily dose and *urgent discussion with a clinical oncologist.* The steroids should be continued at a high dose until a definitive plan has been made. They may then be titrated down in accordance with the patient's condition and symptoms.
- **Neuropathic pain.** Local recurrence of tumour or axillary lymph node spread may directly affect the brachial plexus. This may produce neuropathic pain affecting the arm and anterior chest wall. Such pain is partially opioid-sensitive but adjuvant analgesics in the form of *antidepressant and/or anticonvulsant medication* are usually required to supplement the effect of the opioid. Specialist advice is frequently needed to maintain good symptom control.
- **Liver metastases** often occur and may cause pain. These usually respond well to *NSAIDs* or *steroids*. Liver metastases may also lead to hepatomegaly that may cause squashed stomach syndrome with delayed gastric emptying and a feeling of fullness. This may respond to a prokinetic agent such as *metoclopramide.*

Other complications

Hypercalcaemia may occur. In many cases treatment should be considered with *intravenous (IV) hydration and IV bisphosphonates.*

Lymphoedema usually affects the arm involved in the original surgery. It can develop at any time in a patient's cancer journey. It needs to be actively managed if complications are to be avoided. Management includes good skin care, avoiding additional trauma to the affected arm (including taking of blood tests and blood pressure measurement) and appropriately fitting compression garments.

Lung and pleural disease are common and may cause breathlessness and cough. Consider draining a pleural effusion if present, although this may only afford temporary relief as the fluid may recur. *Surgical pleurodesis* may be appropriate.

Cerebral metastases are less common. Decisions about investigation and management may be complex and need to be made on an individual basis. There is a risk of epileptic fits and *prophylactic anticonvulsant medication* may be appropriate.

Superior vena cava obstruction (SVCO) can occur in patients with an indwelling venous catheter and less commonly in those patients who have extensive pulmonary disease. Management includes removal of the line (in consultation with the patient's oncologist), *vascular stenting, radiotherapy and high-dose steroids*. Long-term anticoagulation may be considered.

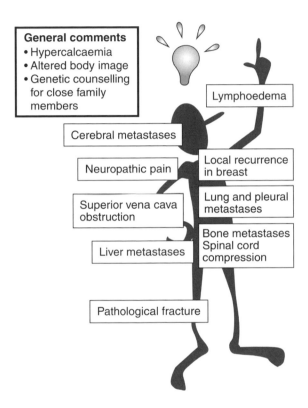

Figure 7.3: Key points in palliative care of breast cancer patients.

Colorectal cancer

General comments

Prognosis is closely linked to histological staging (Duke's classification). Adjuvant chemotherapy may be helpful in prolonging disease-free survival. Patients may present with bowel obstruction (see below). *Genetic counselling* should be considered for those with a family history of colonic cancer or who have polyposis coli.

Specific pain complexes

- **Liver metastases** often occur and may cause pain. These usually respond well to *NSAIDs* or *steroids*. Liver metastases may also lead to hepatomegaly that may cause squashed stomach syndrome with delayed gastric emptying and a feeling of fullness. This may respond to a prokinetic agent such as *metoclopramide*.
- **Perineal and pelvic pain** may be caused by advancing disease or be iatrogenic. There is nearly always a neuropathic element to the pain that will only be partially opioid-sensitive. Adjuvant analgesics such as *antidepressant and/or anticonvulsant medication* may be needed as well as more specialist interventions such as nerve blocks.
- **Tenesmus** is a unique type of neuropathic pain. It requires specialist assessment but may respond to drugs that have an effect on smooth muscle, including *nifedipine*.
- **Bone metastases** are rare but may occur. Management of subsequent pain may be difficult and specialist advice should be sought. These are becoming increasingly common, perhaps due to the role of adjuvant chemotherapy on the natural disease course.

Other complications

Bowel obstruction, unless it can be palliated surgically, should be managed medically using a syringe driver containing a mixture of *analgesics, anti-emetics and antispasmodics*. Naso-gastric tubes are rarely needed, and hydration can often be maintained orally if the nausea and vomiting are adequately controlled.

Fistulae between the bowel and the skin or bladder may occur. These can be very difficult to manage and require a multidisciplinary approach with specialist input.

Anorexia and altered taste are very common with advanced disease and difficult to manage, particularly for the family. *Small, frequent and appetising meals* may help as may supplement drinks. *Low-dose steroids* may temporarily boost the appetite.

Rectal discharge and bleeding are unpleasant and difficult symptoms to manage. They may respond to *palliative radiotherapy*. Seek specialist advice.

Hypoproteinaemia is common due to poor oral intake and poor absorption from the bowel and may lead to lower limb oedema. This may be complicated by pelvic disease causing lower limb **lymphoedema**. Early assessment by the specialist lymphoedema service is essential to maintain the patient's comfort and prevent complications.

Anaemia may occur due to chronic bleeding from the tumour. This may warrant regular blood transfusion to maintain quality of life and reasonable symptom control. Discussion is needed about the appropriateness of repeating transfusion if the anaemia is persistent.

Cerebral metastases are less common. Decisions about investigation and management may be complex and need to be made on an individual basis. There is a risk of epileptic fits and *prophylactic anticonvulsant medication* may be appropriate.

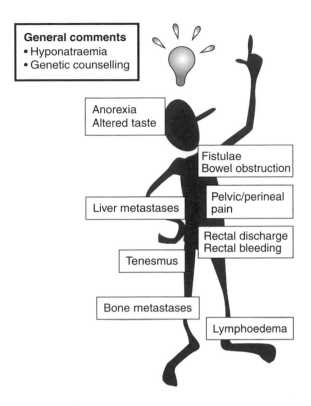

Figure 7.4: Key points in palliative care of colorectal cancer patients.

Gynaecological cancer

General comments

Primary treatment may have affected *sexual function, fertility and body image* and this will impact on coping strategies. Ovarian and vulval cancers often present late and so it may be appropriate for specialist palliative care input from the point of diagnosis. *Genetic counselling* should be considered for close female relatives of patients with ovarian cancer, particularly if there is also a strong family history of breast cancer.

Specific pain complexes

- **Perineal and pelvic pain** is common in all three of the common malignancies: cervical, ovarian and vulval carcinomas. There is nearly always a neuropathic element to the pain that will only be partially opioid-sensitive. Adjuvant analgesics such as *antidepressant and/or anticonvulsant medication* may be needed as well as more specialist interventions such as *nerve blocks*.

Other complications

Lymphoedema develops with uncontrolled pelvic disease. It can develop at any time in a patient's cancer journey and frequently affects both lower limbs. It needs to be actively managed if complications are to be avoided. Management includes good skin care, avoiding additional trauma to the affected leg(s) and appropriately-fitting compression garments.

Ascites is particularly common with ovarian cancer and can be difficult to manage. *Oral diuretics*, particularly spironolactone, in combination with a loop diuretic such as frusemide may help a little. Repeated paracentesis may be needed. Consideration of a *peritovenous (Leveen) shunt* may be appropriate in some cases where prognosis is thought to be longer than three months.

Complete or subacute bowel obstruction is often not amenable to surgical intervention and should be managed medically using a *syringe driver containing a mixture of analgesics, anti-emetics and antispasmodics*. Naso-gastric tubes are rarely needed, and hydration can often be maintained orally if the nausea and vomiting are adequately controlled.

Renal impairment can develop in any patient with advanced pelvic disease. It may be a pre-terminal event. Ureteric stenting may be appropriate depending on the patient's perceived prognosis, the patient's wishes and future treatment options. Renal impairment increases the risk of a patient developing opioid toxicity as renal excretion of opioid metabolites may be reduced.

Vaginal or vulval bleeding may respond to antifibrinolytic agents such as *tranexamic acid, radiotherapy and/or surgery*.

Offensive vaginal or vulval discharge can cause considerable distress to patient and carers. *Topical or systemic metronidazole* may help as can barrier creams. *Deodorising* machines may also help if the patient is confined to one room.

Vesico-colic and recto-vaginal fistulae need a surgical assessment. These can be very difficult to manage and require a multidisciplinary approach with specialist input.

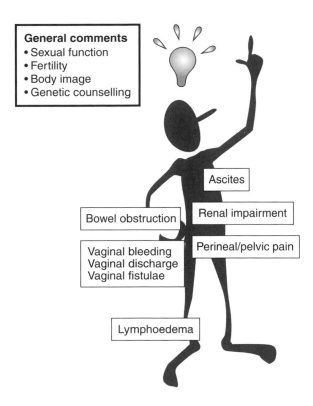

Figure 7.5: Key points in palliative care of gynaecology cancer patients.

Head and neck cancer

General comments

There are a wide variety of cancers affecting the head and neck, including the oral cavity, oropharynx, larynx, hypopharynx, nasopharynx, nasal cavity sinuses and salivary glands. They have two aetiological factors in common, namely cigarette smoking and heavy alcohol consumption. Many of the patients with these cancers have chaotic lifestyles that mean they find it hard to use the health service efficiently.

Frequently the patients present late when *curative surgery and radiotherapy*, which are the mainstays of treatment, cannot be undertaken.

Specific pain complexes

- **Neuropathic pain** affecting the head and neck and radiating to the upper arm is not uncommon. This can be the result of direct compression of nerves by the tumour or a result of treatment. There may be associated hypersensitivity of the skin and oral mucosa which may be so severe that the patient is unable to tolerate a light breeze or chewing food. The pain syndromes are often complex and only partially respond to opioids. Adjuvant analgesics in the form of *antidepressants and/or anticonvulsant medication* are usually needed. Specialist advice is frequently needed to maintain symptom control, especially as compliance with medication may be a problem.
- **Dysphagia** due to direct compression of a tumour mass or lymphadenopathy often means that feeding gastrotomies are needed to maintain nutrition and aid with the administration of medication via the oral route may not be available. There may be ethical dilemmas towards the end of life, particularly with regard to the administration of feeds in the last days of life.

Other complications

The tumour or the surgery performed often adversely affects a patient's **body image** in a site which is hard to hide from public view. Patients often become *socially isolated* as they feel disfigured and become reluctant to go out. **Depression** is a common feature. Relationship problems are not uncommon.

Difficulties with articulation and speech production are common. The quality of the voice may change significantly and make the patient self-conscious. All these problems need the regular input of specialist *speech and language therapists. Communication aids* may be needed after major surgery to enable a patient to express their needs and preferences.

Fungating and malodorous tumours can cause considerable distress. *Radiotherapy* may help in some cases, especially where there is bleeding. Topical antibiotics may help along with regular dressings sensitively applied to maintain dignity, but cover the most disfiguring parts of the tumour. The use of *deodorisers* in the patient's room may help.

Major haemorrhage. Patients with progressive tumours near the large blood vessels of the neck are at risk of a sudden massive bleed. This is rare but difficult to manage and the early involvement of specialists should be considered.

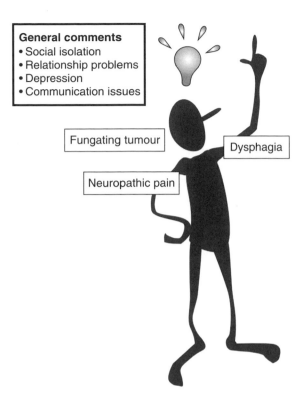

Figure 7.6: Key points in palliative care of head and neck cancer patients.

Chronic leukaemia and myeloma

General comments

The clinical course tends to be very variable but is characterised by a *protracted cycle of relapses and remissions.* This can cause considerable distress as the patients and their carers have to live with considerable uncertainty about the future. Both patient and the professionals involved with their care may find it hard to accept a patient is entering the terminal phase.

Infection is a frequent and unpredictable complication of both the disease process and its treatment. It can be fatal and this makes the prognosis even more uncertain.

Chemotherapy may continue in advanced illness because of the possibility of a further remission and/or useful palliation.

Specific pain complexes

- **Bone pain** due to infiltration of the bones and joints is very common. The pain is often worse on movement or weight-bearing which makes titration of analgesics very difficult. The pain often *responds well to radiotherapy and/or oral steroids. Non-steroidal anti-inflammatory drugs* may help but must be used with caution because they may interfere with platelet and renal function.
- **Pathological fractures** are particularly common in myeloma due to the lytic bone lesions. These often require *orthopaedic intervention* and subsequent *radiotherapy.* Prophylactic pinning of long bones and/or radiotherapy should be considered to prevent fracture and reduce the likelihood of complex pain syndromes developing.
- **Spinal cord compression** requires prompt diagnosis, high-dose oral steroids in a single daily dose and *urgent discussion with a clinical oncologist.* The steroids should be continued at a high dose until a definitive plan has been made. They may then be titrated down in accordance with the patient's condition and symptoms.
- **Wedge and crush fractures of the spinal column** can lead to severe back pain which is often associated with nerve compression and neuropathic pain. Such pain is partially opioid-sensitive but adjuvant analgesics in the form of *antidepressants and/or anticonvulsant medication* are usually required to supplement the effect of the opioid. Specialist advice is frequently needed to maintain symptom control.

Other complications

Bone marrow failure is usual. *Recurrent infections* and *bleeding episodes* can leave the patient and carers exhausted. Dependence on frequent blood and platelet transfusions may mean that difficult decisions about stopping transfusions must be faced at some stage.

Night sweats and fever are common, imposing a heavy demand on carers, particularly as it may mean several changes of night and bed clothes. Specialist advice may help in relieving the symptoms as there are a number of drugs that appear to be effective although not licensed.

Hypercalcaemia may occur, especially in myeloma. It should be considered in any patient with persistent nausea, altered mood or confusion, even if this is intermittent, worsening pain and/or constipation. Treatment with *IV hydration and IV bisphosphonates* should be considered for a first episode. Resistant hypercalcaemia may be a pre-terminal event when aggressive management would be inappropriate.

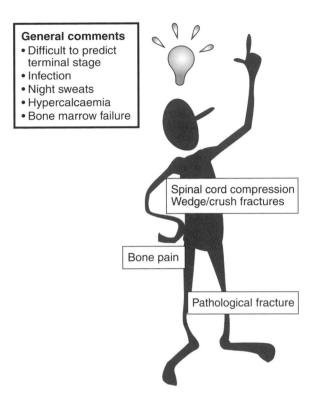

General comments
- Difficult to predict terminal stage
- Infection
- Night sweats
- Hypercalcaemia
- Bone marrow failure

Spinal cord compression
Wedge/crush fractures

Bone pain

Pathological fracture

Figure 7.7: Key points in palliative care of patients with chronic leukaemia and myeloma.

Lung cancer

General comments

This is one of the commonest cancers and because of its link with smoking (both active and passive) may be associated with emotional distress in the patient and their carers. Lung cancers often occur on a background of pre-existing lung disease which may alter the patient's perception of breathlessness and cough. On the whole the prognosis for lung cancers not amenable to surgery is poor with 90% of patients dying within a year of diagnosis.

Specific pain complexes

- **Pleuritic pain** may be associated with the tumour itself, metastases in the rib or local infection. This type of pain responds well to *NSAIDs*. It may also be helped by local nerve blockade.
- **Pancoast tumour** can produce severe neuropathic pain which will only be partially opioid-responsive and will need adjuvant analgesics such as *antidepressant and/or anticonvulsant medication*. Early referral for specialist help should be considered.
- **Bone metastases** may occur putting the patient at risk of *pathological fractures* and *spinal cord compression*. Management of subsequent pain may be difficult and specialist advice should be sought.

Other complications

Breathlessness is common and can be very distressing for carers. Treat reversible causes such as anaemia and pleural effusion where appropriate. Give clear explanations of what is happening. Ensure that practical measures such as sitting the patient up, opening windows and using fans have been discussed with the family. Regular doses of *short-acting oral morphine* every 2–4 hours may decrease the sensation of breathlessness. Other more specialist interventions such as *palliative radiotherapy, endobronchial laser therapy and stenting* may help some patients. Panic and anxiety are frequently associated with breathlessness and may be helped by *simple relaxation techniques*. A low dose of an *anxiolytic* such as diazepam may be helpful.

Haemoptysis is a frightening symptom. *Palliative radiotherapy* may be effective if the patient is fit enough. Oral antifibrinolytics such as *tranexamic acid* may help. Occasionally, frequent small episodes herald a catastrophic haemoptysis. This is a rare but difficult situation to manage and early involvement of specialists should be considered.

Cough can exacerbate breathlessness and pain, can affect sleep and a patient's ability to eat. Its management will depend on the cause but it is often appropriate to try and suppress the cough pharmacologically using *codeine or morphine linctus*. If not responding to simple measures refer for specialist assessment.

Hypercalcaemia may occur. It should be considered in any patient with persistent nausea, altered mood or confusion, even if this is intermittent, worsening pain and/or constipation. It may be a pre-terminal event when treatment with *IV hydration and IV bisphosphonates* would be inappropriate.

Cerebral metastases are common. Decisions about investigation and management may be complex and need to be made on an individual basis. Altered behaviour and personality as well as problems of comprehension and communication can be very distressing for relatives.

Persistent headache, worse in the mornings, and *unexplained vomiting* may be early signs of this diagnosis. There is a risk of epileptic fits and *prophylactic anticonvulsant medication* may be appropriate.

Hyponatraemia and other biochemical imbalances are particularly common in small cell lung cancer. Management can be complex and needs specialist input.

Altered taste and anorexia are common. *Good oral hygiene* and effective treatment of oral candidiasis may help. Carers may find it helpful to talk through different ways of encouraging the patient to eat, such as freezing supplement drinks to make lollipops, making small meals frequently, etc.

Superior vena cava obstruction (SVCO) can occur in patients who have extensive pulmonary disease, particularly small cell lung cancer. Management includes consideration of *vascular stenting, radiotherapy and high-dose oral steroids* in a single daily dose.

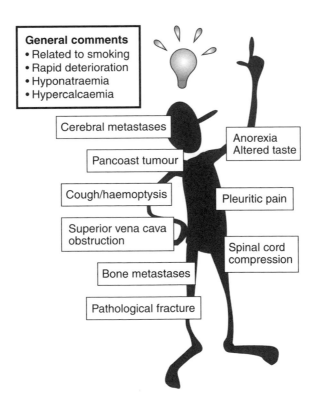

Figure 7.8: Key points in palliative care of lung cancer patients.

Mesothelioma

General comments

This usually affects the lung but can affect other parts of the body, particularly the peritoneum. It is associated with exposure to asbestos and there are clusters of cases around certain industrial sites. It is a relentlessly progressive tumour.

It is important that the patient is aware that they may be entitled to *compensation* and should consult a specialist lawyer about this.

All patients must have a *coroner's post-mortem* regardless of any compensation claims or litigation. The patient and family should be made aware of this to try and minimise distress at the time of death.

Specific pain complexes

- Mesotheliomas can produce **severe neuropathic pain** which will only be partially opioid-responsive and will need adjuvant analgesics such as *antidepressant and/or anti-convulsant medication*. Early referral for specialist help should be considered. *Local nerve blockades* can help in some cases.

Other complications

Pleural effusions are common, frequently bloodstained and become increasingly difficult to aspirate as the disease progresses. *Surgical intervention* to prevent reaccumulation of fluid may be helpful if carried out early enough.

The tumour may grow along the track of a biopsy or drainage needle to produce a cutaneous lesion. These areas can become painful and ulcerated and be difficult to manage. *Palliative radiotherapy* has a limited role to play in preventing the complication at the time of biopsy and also in managing established cutaneous spread.

Breathlessness can be severe due to pleural disease limiting the capacity of the lung as well as the occurrence of pleural effusions. Give clear explanations of what is happening. Ensure that practical measures such as sitting the patient up, opening windows and using fans have been discussed with the family. *Regular doses of short-acting oral morphine* every 2–4 hours may decrease the sensation of breathlessness. Panic and anxiety are frequently associated with breathlessness and may be helped by *simple relaxation techniques*. A low dose of an *anxiolytic* such as diazepam may be helpful. Other treatment options are limited.

Ascites occurs with peritoneal mesothelioma. The ascitic fluid is frequently bloodstained and becomes increasingly difficult to aspirate as the disease progresses.

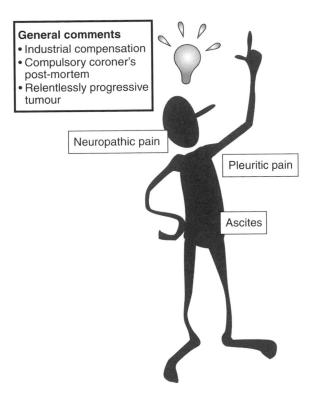

General comments
- Industrial compensation
- Compulsory coroner's post-mortem
- Relentlessly progressive tumour

Neuropathic pain

Pleuritic pain

Ascites

Figure 7.9: Key points in palliative care of patients with mesothelioma.

Prostate cancer

General comments

This is a common cancer that most often affects the elderly. The time course can be very variable, ranging from years with relatively few symptoms to an illness that lasts months with many symptoms. The mainstay of treatment is *hormonal manipulation* with *palliative radiotherapy*. A few patients present early enough for potentially curative treatment to be attempted using surgery and/or radiotherapy.

Specific pain complexes

Widespread **bone metastases** are common and are often present at diagnosis. Patients are at risk of:

- **pathological fracture** which may occur without obvious trauma. These may need *orthopaedic intervention* (pinning or joint replacement) and/or radiotherapy.
- **spinal cord compression** which requires prompt diagnosis, high-dose oral steroids in a single daily dose and *urgent discussion with a clinical oncologist*. The steroids should be continued at a high dose until a definitive plan has been made. They may then be titrated down in accordance with the patient's condition and symptoms.
- **neuropathic pain.** Local recurrence of tumour, pelvic spread or a collapsed vertebra may cause neuropathic pain. Such pain is partially opioid-sensitive but adjuvant analgesics in the form of *antidepressant and/or anticonvulsant medication* are usually required to supplement the effect of the opioid. Specialist advice is frequently needed to maintain symptom control.
- **bone pain.** If the tumour is hormone-sensitive then bone pain often responds to a change in hormone therapy. Skilled pain management is often needed and specialist advice should be sought about the appropriate use of *radiotherapy and radioactive strontium* as well as *nerve blockades.*

Other complications

Bone marrow failure may occur in patients with advanced disease. Typically the patient has symptomatic anaemia and thrombocytopenia. Support with *palliative blood transfusions* may be appropriate initially, but their appropriateness should be discussed with the patient and their family when there is no longer symptomatic benefit gained from them.

Retention of urine. Problems with micturition, including haematuria, may lead to retention of urine. This may be acute and painful or chronic and painless. If the patient is unfit for transurethral resection of the prostate (TURP) then consider a permanent *indwelling urinary catheter*. Chronic urinary retention can lead to renal failure.

Lymphoedema of the lower limbs and occasionally the genital area is usually due to advanced pelvic disease. It can develop at any time in a patient's cancer journey. It needs to be actively managed if complications are to be avoided. Management includes good skin care and using appropriately-fitting compression garments.

Altered body image and sexual dysfunction can result from any of the treatment modalities, hormone manipulation, radiotherapy or surgery. This may be exacerbated by apathy and **clinical depression** which are particularly common in patients with prostate cancer. Specialist mental and psychological health strategies may be required.

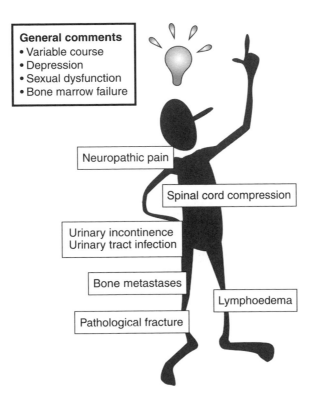

Figure 7.10: Key points in palliative care of prostate cancer patients.

Upper gastrointestinal cancer

General comments

Mild and non-specific symptoms often precede the onset of *dysphagia* for many months in oesophageal carcinoma. Stomach cancer often presents late and is frequently metastatic at presentation.

Specific pain complexes

- **Liver capsular pain** due to liver metastases is common. This is only partially opioid-responsive but responds well to *NSAIDs or oral steroids*.
- **Oesophageal spasm** may occur and can be difficult to manage. Specialist advice should be sought. It may be caused by *oesophageal candidiasis* which needs system treatment with *oral imidazole antifungals*.
- Involvement of the **coeliac plexus** causes a difficult pain syndrome with non-specific abdominal pain and mid-back pain. Blockade of the plexus using *anaesthetic techniques* can be very effective.

Other complications

Dysphagia can occur in both oesophageal and stomach cancer. It may be helped by stenting. *Oncological treatment* of the tumour may provide temporary relief. Advice about appropriate diet and consistency of the food taken may also help. *Feeding gastrostomies* can improve nutrition and quality of life but can cause ethical dilemmas towards the end of life with regard to when to stop treatment.

Anorexia is frequent and often profound. There may be a fear of eating because of pain. This may bring the patient and their carer into conflict about food and the 'need to eat'. Open and honest explanation can help to relieve anxiety and provide practical approaches to dealing with the situation.

Weight loss and altered body image can be profound with these cancers and can cause real problems for the patient and their family.

Nausea and vomiting can be persistent and difficult to control. Specialist advice is often needed and drugs may need to given by routes other than the oral one. *Small frequent meals* may improve the frequency of vomiting.

Haematemesis may be one of the presenting symptoms but can also occur as the tumour progresses. Where possible *local treatment* may help and, where available, *brachytherapy* and *laser therapy* to the tumour can reduce the incidence. There is risk of a major bleed. This is a difficult situation to manage and early involvement of specialists should be considered.

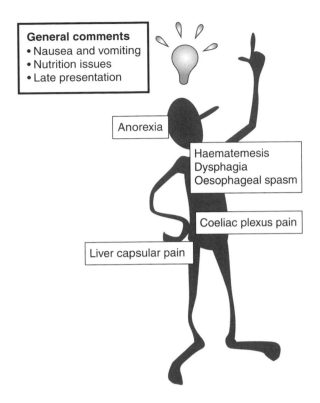

Figure 7.11: Key points in palliative care of upper gastrointestinal cancer patients.

Carcinomatosis of unknown origin

General comments

In 5% of patients presenting with metastatic cancer the site of origin is never established. Prognosis is generally poor. It is very difficult to anticipate the rate of disease progression and therefore to advise patients and their carers about symptoms and mode of deterioration which might occur.

It can be difficult to know how aggressively to pursue the primary cancer site. Cancers that respond to oncological intervention, such as breast, thyroid, lymphoma, ovary and testicular, should be considered.

Anxiety is common in this group of patients. Not knowing the site of the primary tumour causes considerable distress. Extensive investigations may raise false expectations and exhaust the patient. Equally, patients and carers may feel cheated of the chance to have effective treatment if the primary is not looked for.

Carers may find coming to terms with the patient's death difficult and are at greater risk of an adverse bereavement reaction.

Key points

- Anxiety
- Anger
- Risk of overinvestigation
- Adverse bereavement reaction.

CHAPTER 8

Tripwires in palliative care

Susan Salt

Macmillan Consultant in Palliative Care
Calderdale & Huddersfield NHS Trust

This chapter includes:

1   Pain
2   Nausea and vomiting
3   Intestinal obstruction
4   Breathlessness
5   Cough
6   Haemoptysis
7   Respiratory tract secretions
8   Spinal cord compression
9   Superior vena cava obstruction
10 Hypercalcaemia
11 Management of the last days of life
12 Terminal restlessness and agitation
13 Use of steroids
14 Miscellaneous problems
15 Indications for the use of a syringe driver in palliative care.

Sometimes it may feel to generalists that there are some palliative care 'tripwires' which may catch you out unexpectedly – some conditions and modes of drug usage that have become fairly commonplace in hospices but are rarely seen in general practice. There are a limited number of such tripwires and yet because we may see them rarely in primary care, we may feel unconfident and need to seek expert help in their management. The following was written by a consultant in palliative care, Dr Susan Salt, to provide information on such areas. Although many of the early stages of the following conditions can be managed appropriately by generalists, it is suggested that specialist advice is sought when needed. However, the following will forewarn generalists of particular difficulties, reassure you that the usual clinical skills of general practice medicine are of value here and educate and encourage you to seek further help from your palliative care colleagues and specialised texts, where appropriate.

Keri Thomas

Most palliative care is straightforward, relying on common sense and good general medical and nursing care. Good palliative care is as much about good communication skills, empathy and wisdom as it is about medical and nursing knowledge. For most patients who choose to remain at home it is carried out best by the people that know the patient and family well, in the place the patient feels most comfortable, i.e. at home with their family and friends being cared for by their primary care team.

The following pages contain some general guidance about some of the commoner symptoms experienced by people suffering from cancer. The guidance focuses on those areas where practice differs from other fields of medicine such as usual general practice, but it is not exhaustive. It is written as a guide to how to start managing those symptoms that may not be encountered very frequently in general practice. The chapter indicates when to seek specialist advice and support. It is not intended to replace the local specialist advice each primary care team has available to them.

It is good practice to ask the question 'why' when any patient with a life-threatening illness develops new symptoms or appears to deteriorate rapidly. As with all areas of medicine there are certain symptoms that should ring alarm bells and which demand a rapid response not only from the primary care team but also the specialists. If there is no straightforward explanation for a patient's deterioration or the patient has had radical radiotherapy or any form of chemotherapy, consider referral back to their oncology unit or centre. At the very least such patients should be discussed with the specialist services to ensure treatment-related conditions, such as neutropenic sepsis, have been excluded.

I have written these guidance notes for our local primary care teams as a specialist in Palliative Medicine. It is hoped they contribute to the ongoing education of staff and support them in the excellent work they do in managing complex and challenging patients at home. I offer my sincere thanks to Dr Mary Kiely, Consultant in Palliative Medicine, Huddersfield Royal Infirmary and Dr Liz Higgins, Consultant in Palliative Medicine, Kirkwood Hospice, Huddersfield who have reviewed and amended them.

Pain

Pain is what the patient says it is. Approximately 25% of all cancer patients will have pain at diagnosis. Up to 75% of all cancer patients will have pain in advanced disease. There are three main types of pain. These may co-exist and therefore it may be necessary to use more than one approach to achieve adequate pain control. The three different types are:

- visceral – tumour bulk, bowel obstruction
- bony – replacement of bone by tumour, pathological fracture
- neuropathic – nerve injury or nerve compression.

Always take a careful history and carry out an appropriate examination. Identify the likely pathological process(es) contributing to the pain, and where possible treat reversible causes such as infection or fracture. *Analgesia should not wait for investigations to be completed.* The pain associated with cancer and other life-limiting illnesses is usually chronic and needs regular medication to keep it under control. Adequate doses of analgesia on an 'as required basis' in addition to the regular medication must be made available. Where possible give analgesia by mouth, by the clock and by the WHO ladder. Unless there are problems with absorption from the small intestine, pain that does not respond to oral morphine is unlikely to respond any better to parenteral opioids. In this instance other approaches to pain management should be considered such as using adjuvant analgesics or anaesthetic approaches.

- Review the effectiveness of any intervention on a regular basis.
- Ensure all patients on a step 2 or step 3 analgesic are on regular laxatives and that the effectiveness of the laxative regimen is being adequately monitored.
- Remember the role of rest, relaxation, adequate sleep, explanation, heat pads, the TENs machine and massage in aiding pain control and encourage the patient to use self-help measures.

Visceral pain

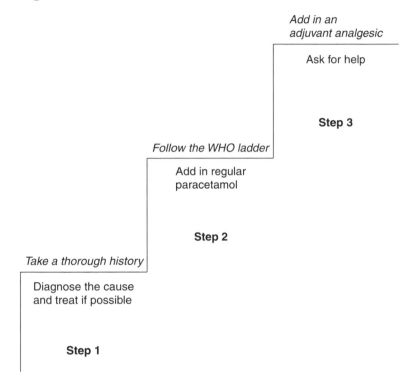

Figure 8.1: Visceral pain.

- **Paracetamol** may be particularly effective for some types of headaches and musculo-skeletal pain. In combination with codeine (30 mg) it is the step 2 analgesic of choice. Always prescribe a laxative if codeine is being used.
- **Short-acting opioids** are the drugs of choice for visceral pain. If a patient is already on the maximum dose of a step 2 analgesic then the starting dose of oral morphine sulphate is 10 mg every four hours, with the same dose for breakthrough pain. The dose should be titrated against the pain using increments set out in Table 8.1. Only consider starting doses of oral morphine sulphate of less than 10 mg if the patient is in renal failure, is very frail or has not been on a maximum step 2 analgesic. Once adequate pain relief has been obtained, convert the total dose of oral morphine sulphate taken in 24 hours

Table 8.1

4-hourly morphine sulphate dose increments	5 mg	10 mg	15 mg	20 mg	30 mg	40 mg	60 mg
	Renal failure	Normal starting dose					Seek specialist advice

(including breakthrough doses) to a long-acting formulation. Always ensure you have prescribed the equivalent four-hourly dose for breakthrough.

- Consider prescribing haloperidol 3 mg as an anti-emetic if the patient is at risk of opioid-induced nausea and vomiting. Warn patients about the possibility of short-term drowsiness as the morphine sulphate is started. For most patients this wears off after three to four days.
- There is no ceiling dose of oral morphine sulphate but specialist help should be sought if the 24-hour dose of morphine sulphate exceeds 360 mg (60 mg every four hours).
- Alternative opioids which may be used under the direction of a specialist are fentanyl, hydromorphone and oxycodone (with advice as needed from a specialist).

Bone pain

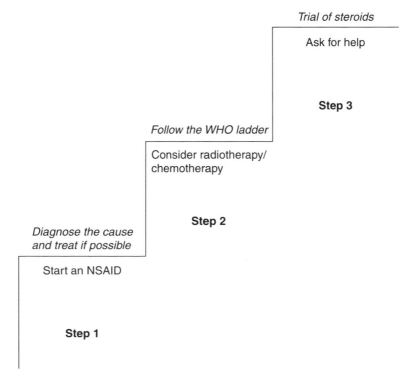

Trial of steroids

Ask for help

Step 3

Follow the WHO ladder

Consider radiotherapy/ chemotherapy

Step 2

Diagnose the cause and treat if possible

Start an NSAID

Step 1

Figure 8.2: Bone pain.

- Non-steroidal anti-inflammatory drugs (NSAIDs): start with the maximum dose of the NSAID. The dose may be titrated down if good pain relief is achieved. The choice of which NSAID to use will depend on the route of administration as well as a risk/benefits analysis. Use appropriate gastrointestinal (GI) protection with either a proton pump inhibitor or misoprostol in at-risk patients.
- Consider referral to a clinical oncologist for palliative radiotherapy.
- Orthopaedic intervention for large bone metastases may be appropriate and improve pain control.

Neuropathic pain

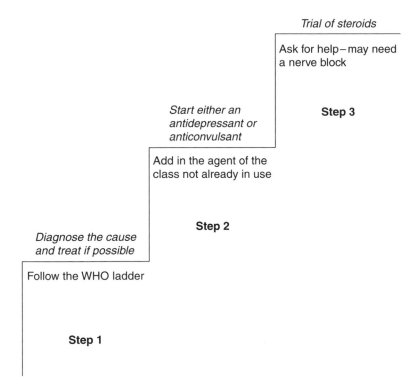

Figure 8.3: Neuropathic pain.

Neuropathic pain is partially opioid-responsive and so the patient should be titrated on short-acting oral morphine sulphate as for visceral pain. At the same time they should also be started on a neuropathic analgesic. The choice of what to use will depend on the side-effect profile and the risk/benefit assessment for each patient. Usually this type of pain is difficult to manage and the early involvement of the specialist palliative care team should be considered. The agents commonly used are:

- Amitriptyline, starting at 25 mg (10 mg in the elderly) in a single night-time dose and increasing by 25 mg every three days to a dose of 75–100 mg, depending on response.

- Sodium valproate, starting at 200 mg 12-hourly and increasing by 200 mg every three days to a maximum of 2.4 g, depending on response.
- Gabapentin, 100 mg 12-hourly, increasing by 100–200 mg every three days to a maximum dose of 1.8 g, depending on response. This is not the regimen recommended but in the author's clinical practice this has been tolerated better than the more rapid titration suggested by the manufacturers.
- Local nerve blockade may help. Pain anaesthetists may be able to give advice.

Nausea and vomiting

There are a number of basic causes of nausea and vomiting and if these can be identified then this will help with the choice of anti-emetic. It is not uncommon for the nausea and vomiting to be multifactorial, in which case a combination of anti-emetics may be helpful.

- Nausea and vomiting can sometimes be difficult symptoms to control. It is therefore important to seek out specialist advice early if initial measures fail.
- Remember that it may be necessary to use the subcutaneous route initially to ensure adequate absorption of the drug and thus control the symptom. Once the nausea and/or vomiting has settled, the drugs can be converted to the oral route.
- Assess the patient's bowel function and treat any constipation appropriately.

Chemical or drug induced

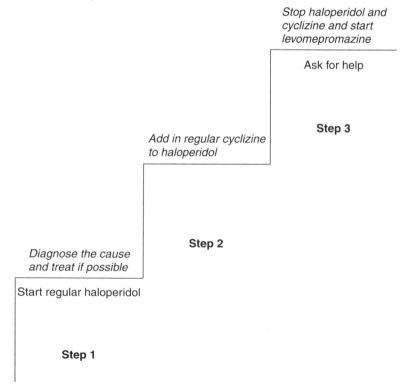

Stop haloperidol and cyclizine and start levomepromazine

Ask for help

Step 3

Add in regular cyclizine to haloperidol

Step 2

Diagnose the cause and treat if possible

Start regular haloperidol

Step 1

Figure 8.4: Chemical-induced nausea and vomiting.

This can be iatrogenic due to drugs such as morphine sulphate, NSAIDs or antidepressants, or due to biochemical abnormalities such as uraemia, jaundice or hypercalcaemia. All these affect the chemoreceptor trigger zone in the brain to produce nausea and/or vomiting.

Treat reversible causes where possible:

- drug of choice: **haloperidol** 2.5–5 mg subcutaneously initially then 3–5 mg orally as a single dose. This may be combined with cyclizine 75–150 mg over 24 hours in a syringe driver to maximise response
- second line: **levomepromazine** (otherwise known as nozinan or methotrimeprazine) 12.5–25 mg nocte or 12.5–25 mg over 24 hours subcutaneously in a syringe driver. Maximum daily dose needed to control nausea and vomiting is usually 75 mg.

Impaired intestinal motility

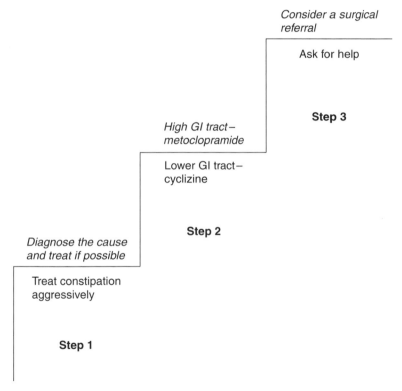

Figure 8.5: Nausea and vomiting due to altered bowel function.

This can be due to tumour compressing the lumen, altered intestinal flow or tumour bleeding and causing irritation (especially in the upper GI tract).

- If the patient is thought to have complete bowel obstruction then surgical intervention should be considered, although it may not be appropriate.
- If the problem is thought to be high in the GI tract consider **metoclopramide** 20 mg every eight hours, although it may make pre-existing colic worse.

- Consider **cyclizine** 25–50 mg every eight hours, although this will slow bowel transit time.
- If colic is a significant feature, **hyoscine butylbromide (Buscopan)** 60–100 mg in a syringe driver over 24 hours may help. Hyoscine butylbromide is not well absorbed orally and should only be administered parenterally.

Raised intracranial pressure

This may be due to a primary brain tumour, brain metastases and/or meningeal spread. High-dose oral steroid 12 mg **dexamethasone** given as single daily dose first thing in the morning (with appropriate GI protection) is the drug of choice. The dose should be titrated downwards over the subsequent days or weeks, depending on the patient's response. This may need to be combined with cyclizine or levomepromazine (as above).

Movement related

This may be due to a middle ear infection, vestibular problems or tumour at the cerebello-pontine angle. **Cyclizine** is the drug of choice (as above).

Regurgitation

This is common with oesophageal tumours or where there is mediastinal lymphadenopathy, causing extrinsic compression of the oesophagus. Interventions such as stent insertion, endoluminal radiotherapy and laser therapy, where available, may help. **Metoclopramide** is the anti-emetic of choice. **Antacids** combined with a **proton pump inhibitor** may help the gastritis and oesophagitis which occurs.

Anxiety

Fear and anxiety may contribute to nausea and vomiting. Stress-relieving measures such as relaxation techniques as well as anxiolytics such as **diazepam** may help. Acupuncture may help some people. Occasionally some patients undergoing chemotherapy or radiotherapy develop anticipatory vomiting. This often needs specialist input to ensure that compliance with therapy as well as good symptom control is achieved.

Intestinal obstruction

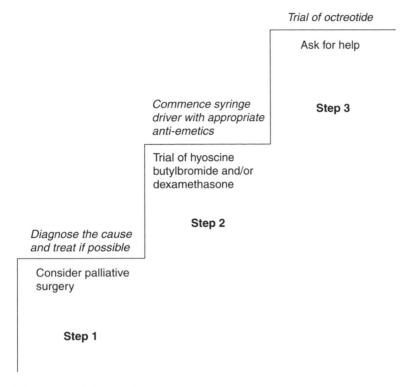

Figure 8.6: Intestinal obstruction.

Any patient with cancer that affects the abdomen or pelvis may develop bowel obstruction, but it is most common in patients with ovarian and colorectal cancers.

Common signs and symptoms

- Large-volume vomits often with little or no preceding nausea. May vary in frequency.
- Abdominal colic, which often varies in frequency and intensity.
- Abdominal distension, which may be absent.
- Constipation or reduced number of bowel movements.

In many cases there are multiple levels of obstruction, which means patients may not present with all the classic symptoms. It should be considered in any patient with advanced malignancy who is vomiting.

Investigations

The diagnosis is based on the clinical picture. Investigations may help but are not needed for appropriate management to be initiated.

- Plain abdominal films may show the classic fluid levels of obstruction.
- Computed tomography (CT) of abdomen and pelvis may be helpful in detecting tumour recurrence.

Management

- If a single level of obstruction is possible, as in colorectal cancer, then a surgical opinion should be sought if the patient's general performance status is good.
- Vomiting will rarely be abolished whatever the level of obstruction, but can be reduced to a tolerable frequency in most cases.
- It is rare for a patient with malignant bowel obstruction to need nasogastric tube insertion and parenteral fluids. The nausea and vomiting can usually be controlled (although not completely eliminated) using appropriate medication in a syringe driver. This often needs specialist input to establish the correct drug combination:
  - in high-level obstruction consider metoclopramide 60 mg subcutaneously over 24 hours in a syringe driver
  - if colic is a significant feature use hyoscine butylbromide 60 mg subcutaneously over 24 hours in a syringe driver
  - if nausea is a significant symptom use haloperidol 5 mg subcutaneously over 24 hours
  - with frequent large-volume vomits, consider using octreotide 600–900 micrograms subcutaneously over 24 hours in syringe driver, titrating the dose up or down depending on response.

Patients may eat and drink what they wish: sufficient absorption across the GI tract can take place to prevent absolute dehydration. Patients will tolerate some degree of dehydration provided careful attention is paid to mouth care.

Breathlessness (dyspnoea)

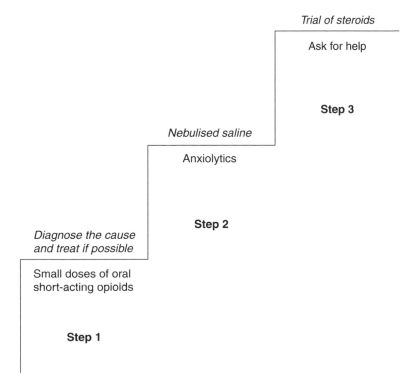

Trial of steroids

Ask for help

Step 3

Nebulised saline

Anxiolytics

Step 2

*Diagnose the cause
and treat if possible*

Small doses of oral
short-acting opioids

Step 1

Figure 8.7: Breathlessness.

- The impact of dyspnoea on patients will vary. Patients with a history of chronic obstructive pulmonary disease whose respiratory capacity is already limited may be less affected than someone with no such history.
- Identify and, where possible, treat reversible factors such as anaemia, bronchospasm and pleural effusion.
- Identify and address the patient's and family's concerns and expectations about breathlessness. Patients and families are frequently fearful that the patient will choke to death (unlikely) or literally run out of breath (unlikely).
- Teach self-help measures such as use of fans, open windows and relaxation/breathing techniques. Modify lifestyle to minimise physical exertion, e.g. moving the bed downstairs, sitting down to wash and shave, etc.

Drugs which may be used in breathlessness

- **Short-acting opioids** decrease the sensation of breathlessness. Start with 5 mg of oral morphine sulphate solution on an 'as required' basis (2.5 mg if the patient is particularly frail or there is concern about renal function). Remember to co-prescribe a laxative and anti-emetic. Long-acting opioids probably have a similar effect but there is less evidence for their effectiveness.

- **Anxiolytics** may help when there is considerable anxiety exacerbating the breathlessness. Possible drugs which can be used include diazepam 2–5 mg three times a day, lorazepam 0.5–1 mg twice a day and buspirone 5 mg twice a day (although its effect may take up to two weeks).
- **Nebulised saline** may improve the sensation of breathlessness although it will have no effect on lung function. Use 2.5–5 ml of normal saline for injection in a standard nebuliser.
- **Nebulised bronchodilators** may help if there is associated bronchospasm, identified by an inspiratory wheeze on auscultation. Salbutamol 2.5–5 mg as often as two-hourly may be needed, but the patient may find the subsequent tremor unacceptable.
- **Oral high-dose steroids** may help where there is evidence of lymphangitis or bronchospasm. Consider dexamethasone 8 mg in a single daily dose in the morning. If effective, titrate the dose down to the minimum dose that controls symptoms in the subsequent two weeks (usually 2–6 mg). Use appropriate GI protection with either a proton pump inhibitor or misoprostol in at-risk patients.
- **Oxygen** has a limited role to play in the dyspnoea of advanced lung cancer, but if a patient has been shown to be hypoxaemic by pulse oximetry, the judicious use of oxygen at flow rates between 2–4 l/min may be of benefit. In some cases of lymphangitis, higher flow rates may be needed to maintain oxygenation.

Cough

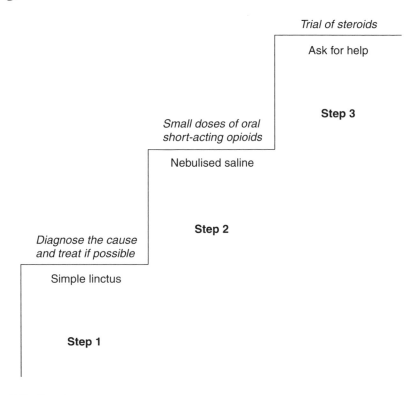

Figure 8.8: Cough.

- Cough affects up to 90% of lung cancer patients at some point in their cancer journey. It can affect patients with other primary diagnoses such as oesophageal carcinoma and those with metastatic lung involvement, particularly breast cancer.
- It can be very debilitating, particularly if spasmodic.
- Identify treatable causes such as acute infection and bronchospasm or iatrogenic causes such as ACE inhibitors. Remember the possibility of cough induced by aspiration or gastro-oesophageal reflux.
- Consider the use of postural drainage and physiotherapy.

Drugs which may be used in cough

- **Simple linctus**, which acts as a peripheral anti-tussive, may help.
- **Nebulised saline**: use 2.5–5 ml of normal saline for injection in a standard nebuliser.
- **Short-acting oral opioids**, which act as a central anti-tussive, may help some patients.
- **Oral steroids** may help if there is associated lymphangitis: starting dose 8 mg dexamethasone as a single dose in the morning. Titrate downwards after one week to the minimum dose that controls the cough. If there is no effect after one week, stop. Use appropriate GI protection using either a proton pump inhibitor or misoprostol in at risk-patients.
- **Nebulised local anaesthetic** may occasionally be used, but should only be commenced after assessment by a specialist in palliative care or respiratory medicine.

Haemoptysis

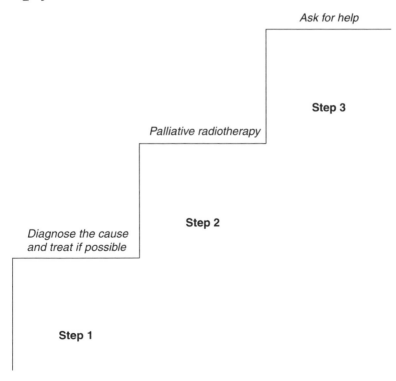

Figure 8.9: Haemoptysis.

Haemoptysis can be due to acute or chronic infection as well as tumour progression. It is essential to consider the possibility of a pulmonary embolus. If an embolus is suspected and the patient is felt to have a reasonable or uncertain prognosis then acute management should be started immediately, usually via admission to hospital. Remember that expectorated blood may not have come from the lungs but can come from the nasopharynx or upper GI tract.

Management

- In all cases acknowledge and explore the patient's and family's ideas and expectations. Deal with fears honestly.
- **Radiotherapy**: both external beam and endobronchial are effective in reducing the frequency and severity of haemoptysis. External beam radiotherapy has a response rate of 80% for haemoptysis associated with lung cancer, but can only be given to the tolerance of the lung tissue.
- **Laser** treatment is available in a limited number of centres and is highly effective and can be repeated indefinitely.
- **Antifibrinolytics**, such as tranexamic acid 1 g tds, may help some patients and should be considered when the patient is unfit for other interventions.
- **Oral steroids** can help when the haemoptysis is due to tumour progression. Start dexamethasone 8 mg as a single morning dose and titrate downwards after one week to the minimum dose that controls symptoms. If there is no effect after one week, stop. Use appropriate GI protection using either a proton pump inhibitor or misoprostol in at-risk patients.

Management of catastrophic haemoptysis

In approximately 1% of all haemoptyses, the bleed will be the terminal event. In such cases there has usually been a number of smaller 'herald' bleeds.

Managing such cases is difficult and traumatic for all involved. If there is concern about a large haemoptysis, decisions about place of care need to be made with the patient and family. The family need to know what they can do and who to contact.

- Consider having a portable suction machine in the house and show the family how to use it.
- Ensure the patient is comfortable, which is usually in the sitting position leaning forward with the head and neck well supported. Use green towels to mask the amount of blood lost.
- Ensure all those involved with such a traumatic death have chance to talk about the events and their feelings.

Respiratory tract secretions

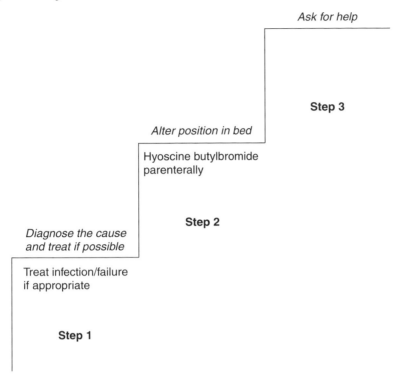

Ask for help

Step 3

Alter position in bed

Hyoscine butylbromide
parenterally

Step 2

*Diagnose the cause
and treat if possible*

Treat infection/failure
if appropriate

Step 1

Figure 8.10: Respiratory tract secretions.

- A clear explanation to the family (and the patient) about the cause of the secretions may help to minimise the impact of the noise on the family.
- The secretions can often be managed by adjusting the patient's position in bed.
- Occasionally the use of gentle suction may help, but this will stimulate more secretions to form and so has to be an ongoing process.
- Hyoscine butylbromide (Buscopan) will dry up the production of secretions although it will not get rid of secretions already formed. Give a stat. subcutaneous dose of 20 mg, which can be repeated after 15 minutes if there is no effect. A subcutaneous infusion via a syringe driver will need to be set up within the next four hours to ensure control is maintained. Use 60–120 mg of hyoscine butylbromide over 24 hours.
- Hyoscine hydrobromide (hyoscine) may be used in a similar way to hyoscine butylbromide, but it is more sedating and can occasionally cause paradoxical agitation so should be used as a second-line agent.

Care needs to be taken that both the doctor and the nursing staff are aware of which formulation of hyoscine they are using and why. It is easy to draw up the wrong formulations of hyoscine as the vials are similar.

Spinal cord compression

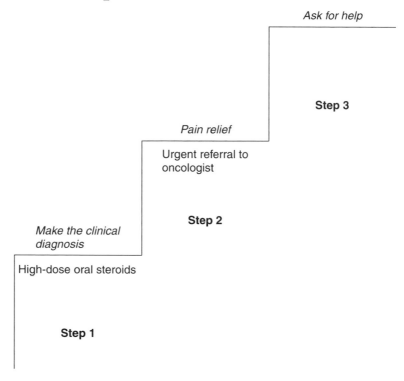

Figure 8.11: Spinal cord compression.

Spinal cord compression occurs in approximately 3% of all patients with advanced cancer, most commonly those with breast, lung and prostate cancer. Less common cancers such as renal cell, lymphoma, myeloma, melanoma and sarcoma account for the majority of others. It is usually caused by metastatic spread to a vertebral body or pedicle, although rarely can be due to direct invasion through the intervertebral foramina.

Common presenting signs and symptoms of spinal cord compression

- Pain that is made worse by movement, straight leg raising and coughing. May be described as being 'like a band'. May precede other symptoms by weeks or months.
- Weakness in limbs that initially may be subtle. The patient may describe struggling to get up out of a chair, altered balance or legs giving way.
- Altered sensation, often with a definable level on clinical examination. The patient may describe having heavy legs, feet that feel like cotton wool, tingling or altered bladder and/or bowel habit. The patient, until formally examined, may miss this. Disturbance of sphincter function occurs late. There may be painless bladder distension.

- Reflexes will be absent at the level of the lesion and increased below the level of the lesion. The patient may have up-going plantar reflexes. In some cases there is clonus.

The diagnosis is a clinical one based on history and examination. *It needs to be considered in anyone who has 'gone off their legs'.* In the majority of cases, plain X-rays of the spine will show evidence of metastatic disease. *However, normal plain X-rays of the spine do not exclude the diagnosis.* MRI is the investigation of choice but management should start as soon as the diagnosis is suspected.

Management

- High-dose oral steroids, 12 mg dexamethasone given as a single dose as soon as the diagnosis is suspected and continued until the diagnosis is confirmed and subsequent treatment is in place. If the patient is at risk of GI side-effects, start appropriate GI protection at the same time in the form of a proton pump inhibitor. Once a management plan has been established the steroids should be reduced as dictated by the patient's condition.
- Contact the local clinical oncologist the same day to discuss the need for hospital admission, investigation and palliative radiotherapy. Occasionally, neuro-surgical intervention is required. The aim is to maintain function.
- Institute adequate pain relief measures.
- Catheterise if there appears to be sphincter involvement.

Prognosis

There is no guarantee of restoration of function after treatment, so if the diagnosis is delayed this has an adverse impact on outcome. In general, those with a rapid onset and paraplegia do badly and those with a paraparesis do better. Treatment should be considered in all cases for pain control purposes, even if function has already been lost. Remember pressure area care.

This is an oncological emergency and requires urgent investigation and treatment.

Superior vena cava obstruction

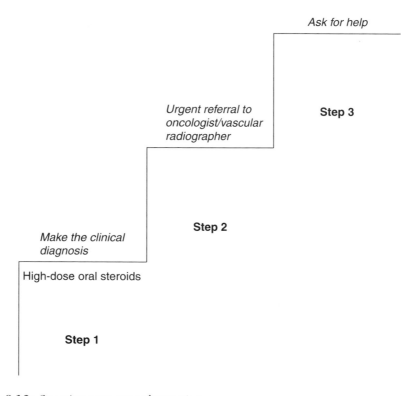

Figure 8.12: Superior vena cava obstruction.

Superior vena cava obstruction is caused by tumour in the mediastinum preventing venous drainage from the head, arms and upper trunk. It usually occurs over weeks or months, allowing for collateral circulation to develop. Occasionally it occurs acutely, when urgent treatment is needed to control symptoms and prevent death. It is most commonly seen in patients with lung cancer, particularly small cell lung cancer, lymphoma and those with large lung metastases, such as those seen in breast cancer and renal cell cancer. Patients with central intravenous lines are also at risk due to clot formation.

Common signs and symptoms

- Persistent headache and feeling of fullness in the head. This may initially be mistaken for sinus problems.
- Oedema of the face and arms that is usually bilateral, is usually worse in the morning and may fluctuate over the day. Early morning oedema of the eyelids, making it hard for the patient to open their eyes, is an early sign.
- Dusky colour to the skin of the chest wall, arms or face with distended superficial veins.
- Breathlessness that is worse on lying flat.

Investigations

- Chest X-ray may be helpful in identifying the mass.
- CT scan of the chest may identify the mass.
- Venography may help define the site of the obstruction and will be necessary if a stent is to be inserted.

Treatment

- Always consider admission to hospital to allow adequate investigation and treatment to improve symptom control and prevent the development of stridor.
- Whilst waiting for a definitive management plan the patient should be started on 12 mg oral dexamethasone as a single dose. If the patient is at risk of GI side-effects, start appropriate GI protection using a proton pump inhibitor. This should be continued until other interventions have been carried out, and then the steroids should be tailed off as dictated by the patient's condition.
- Discuss with the local oncologist and/or specialist in palliative medicine about the use of an SVC stent inserted under radiological control and/or the role of oncological treatment to reduce the size of the tumour.
- Manage symptoms, particularly headache and breathlessness. Both may warrant oral opioids.

Prognosis

Superior vena cava obstruction may recur as the disease progresses. There may be a role for long-term anticoagulation to prevent recurrence in patients with a reasonable life expectancy.

Hypercalcaemia

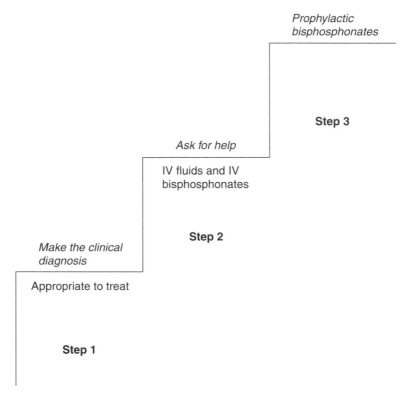

Figure 8.13: Hypercalcaemia.

- Any patient with cancer can develop hypercalcaemia but those with breast, lung, genito-urinary, myeloma and lymphoma are the most at risk. The patient may *not* have any demonstrable bone metastases as this condition is a paraneoplastic phenomenon.
- It is not always appropriate to treat hypercalcaemia as it may be a pre-terminal event. The decision to treat must be made on clinical grounds.
- Diagnosis can only be made if a raised adjusted calcium backs the clinical suspicion.

Symptoms

Symptoms are variable and give no indication of the calcium level. In general, the more rapid the rise in calcium level the more poorly and symptomatic the patient is. *It may be very difficult to differentiate hypercalcaemia from a general deterioration in a patient's condition.* If untreated, hypercalcaemia is fatal.

Common symptoms that *may* indicate a raised adjusted calcium level include:

- fatigue and lethargy
- nausea and/or vomiting
- anorexia

- increasing pain, particularly bone pain, but the pain can be non-specific
- intractable constipation
- drowsiness, confusion that may be intermittent, leading ultimately to coma.

Indications for treatment

- All patients considered for treatment must have venous access and be willing to have IV therapy. It may be difficult to obtain informed consent as the patient may be confused.
- For treatment to be considered the patient must have a measured adjusted calcium of 2.8 mmol/l (normal range 1.8–2.6 mmol/l), have been symptomatic with a reasonable quality of life prior to the current deterioration and not have been treated for hypercalcaemia in the preceding six weeks.
- If a patient does not want to be admitted to an institution, either hospice or acute medical ward, it may be inappropriate to investigate further as the management of hypercalcaemia involves IV rehydration followed by a bisphosphonate infusion, which may be difficult to supervise in the community. However, it can sometimes be arranged as a day patient.

Management

If the decision is made that the patient is too poorly to treat then it is inappropriate to check the calcium level. Appropriate symptom control measures should be instituted. This will include managing nausea and vomiting, ensuring adequate pain control and considering sedation if the patient is agitated. The situation may well warrant the use of a syringe driver.

If the decision is made that it is appropriate to treat if the patient is hypercalcaemic then admit to an appropriate institution for the following treatment.

- IV rehydration with at least two litres of normal saline (more if the patient is clinically dehydrated). Slow the rate of hydration if there are signs of fluid overload developing.
- Give an appropriate dose of a bisphosphonate such as pamidronate or zoledronic acid as directed by local guidelines.
- If successful in improving symptoms and the patient's physical state allows, check the calcium level after five days. The calcium level should then be checked every six weeks and, if increasing, a bisphosphonate infusion repeated with prehydration with a litre of normal saline.
- If there is no improvement in the patient's condition, review the decision to treat. If it is still felt to be appropriate, repeat a bisphosphonate infusion. If resistant to this second dose, discontinue treatment.

Prognosis

If the patient has two or more episodes of hypercalcaemia, or has metastatic breast cancer, consider either:

- regular monthly or bimonthly bisphosphonate using the maximum dose as directed by local guidelines
- regular oral bisphosphonates, although compliance due to side-effects may be an issue.

Management of the last days of life

This is a difficult time for all concerned. Professional carers may need a way of being able to acknowledge and share their feelings. The mutual support of working in a multiprofessional team can be very important.

It may be hard to recognise when death is imminent but it is usually heralded by a more rapid deterioration in the patient's general condition and the following:

- profound weakness with the patient bed-bound and drowsy for long periods
- disorientated in time
- limited attention span of a few minutes
- disinterested in food and drink and the world around them
- too weak to swallow medication.

If the approach of death is recognised, this allows the withdrawal of unnecessary treatments such as antihypertensives, appetite stimulants, etc. It also allows the family and in some instances the patient to prepare for death. It can be difficult to ask directly about the patient and family's perceptions of how close death is, but if it is possible to do so it allows for the most appropriate management plan to be negotiated. This will include looking at the preferred place of death and whether this is achievable with the resources (both professional and informal) available. The wishes of the patient may already be known to the primary care team and the family, but they should be checked again as death approaches. Many patients and carers have unfinished business. This may be legal (drawing up a will), financial, inter-personal or spiritual. Be prepared to ask broad questions and help the family and patient to access the appropriate help from the appropriate 'expert'.

Physical care

- Good regular mouth care to eliminate dry mouth and reduce the sensation of thirst. This may be something that some families like to be actively involved with.
- Ensuring that appropriate pressure-relieving mattresses are in place and their effectiveness regularly monitored.
- Consider catheterisation, using convenes or pads to maintain dignity and avoid incontinence.
- Only continue medication needed for symptom control, but ensure that the family is aware of why other medications have been stopped. Review the route of administration and plan ahead so that an alternative route is available if the oral route becomes impossible.
- Anticipate possible symptoms and ensure there is a means of addressing them quickly both in hours and out of hours. For instance, is the patient at risk of a fit? If so, can the family be taught to use rectal diazepam and is it in the house?
- Patients are dying from their disease and not from lack of fluid or food. Artificial hydration of any sort does not usually contribute to a dying patient's comfort. This needs to be sensitively explained to the carers and patient.

Terminal restlessness and agitation

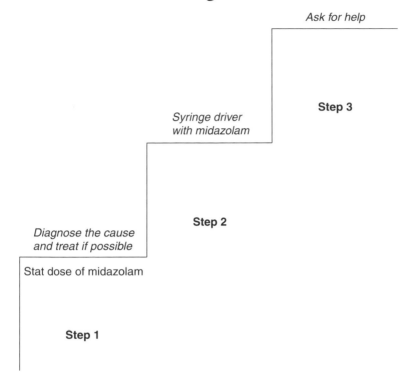

Figure 8.14: Terminal restlessness.

How people die lives on in the memory of those left behind.

Dame Cecily Saunders

No matter how well pain and other symptoms are controlled, agitation and restlessness occur as a pre-terminal event in the final hours or days of life in about 10% of patients. Respiratory tract secretions can also accumulate in the final hours or days of life. This is more likely to happen with lung pathology, whether primary or secondary, and those who have cardiac problems. Such secretions cause distress to the relatives and occasionally to the patient and may need to be actively managed.

Exclude treatable causes for agitation:

- urinary retention – palpable bladder?
- faecal impaction – loaded rectum?
- increased or undertreated pain – has the patient had their usual analgesics? Is the syringe driver working?
- opioid toxicity – is there evidence of myoclonus, twitching, cognitive impairment including hallucinations?

Correct any treatable causes where possible and where the intervention is acceptable to the patient and family.

If opioid toxic, reduce the opioid dose by 50% and review the effect. Consider the use of haloperidol as outlined below.

Generalised agitation

Give a stat. dose of midazolam 5 mg subcutaneously. Repeat a 5 mg dose after 15 minutes if necessary. After another 15 minutes give 10 mg if there was no or only a partial response to the initial two injections. A subcutaneous infusion via a syringe driver will need to be set up within the next two hours to ensure control is maintained as midazolam has a very short half-life. Dose range will be between 20–60 mg over a 24-hour period. Ensure an adequate p.r.n. dose of midazolam 5–10 mg is prescribed and available for use.

Agitation associated with visual hallucinations and/or paranoia

Give a stat. dose of haloperidol 5 mg subcutaneously. This may have to be combined with midazolam 5 mg to get the patient settled initially. A subcutaneous infusion via a syringe driver will need to be set up within the next four hours to ensure control is maintained. Use 10 mg of haloperidol over 24 hours.

Remember that open and honest communication may help avoid long-term complications. Children, parents and grandparents may feel excluded in the last few days of life and may need to be actively involved by the professionals. Specialist advice might be needed when young children are involved. Look for those members of the family at risk of an abnormal and prolonged grief reaction and organise appropriate support. It may be appropriate for such support to start before the death.

Use of steroids in palliative care

Steroids are frequently used in palliative care to help with symptom control. The risks and benefits to the patient should always be considered before they are started, but in patients with a limited prognosis they can help considerably in improving quality of life.

In all cases the dose should be titrated down as quickly as possible, depending on the patient's condition, to the lowest dose that controls symptoms. All patients at risk of GI side-effects should have either a proton pump inhibitor or misoprostol prescribed along with the steroid.

Steroids can be used:

- in oncological emergencies – spinal cord compression, SVCO. Give 12 mg dexamethasone in a single dose before admitting to hospital.
- to reduce inflammation associated with the disease process or treatment (NSAIDs may have a similar role). Starting dose of dexamethasone is 12 mg in a single daily dose. For:
  - liver capsular pain
  - lymphangitis
  - post-radiotherapy
  - brain tumours causing neurological symptoms or headache associated with raised intracranial pressure.

- as an anti-emetic. Dose of dexamethasone is usually between 4 and 8 mg daily for a finite number of days. For:
  - pre- and post-chemotherapy anti-emetic regimens
  - radiotherapy
  - anti-emetic regimens where part of the bowel is irradiated
  - in bowel obstruction.
- as an appetite stimulant. Starting dose of dexamethasone is usually between 4 and 6 mg daily. They should be stopped after two weeks if there is no improvement. Benefits:
  - temporarily increases appetite in some individuals
  - patients may experience an increased sense of well-being. This may be due to better nutrition or a direct central effect of the steroids.

Side-effects are common. The key ones to look out for are:

- oral and oesophageal thrush
- Gastro-intestinal irritation or bleeding
- Agitation and poor sleep – give steroid dose in the morning
- muscle wasting, especially the thighs and upper arms
- skin fragility leading to increased risk of bedsores, wound breakdown
- vaginal or penile thrush.

Miscellaneous problems

Liver capsular pain

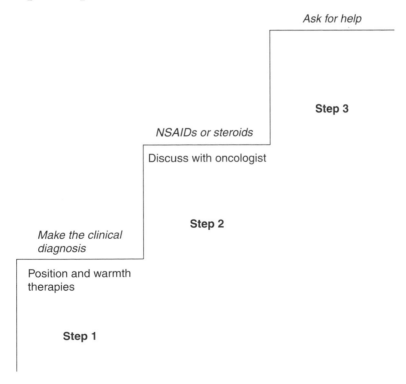

Figure 8.15: Liver capsular pain.

Liver capsular pain usually presents as a persistent dull ache in the right hypochondrium, sometimes radiating to either shoulder or through to the back. It is frequently pleuritic in nature, made worse on sitting forward. It is often associated with anorexia and a feeling of fullness. Sometimes there is associated dyspnoea as the enlarged liver splints the diaphragm.

- Explain the likely diagnosis to the patient and organise investigations if appropriate.
- If a new diagnosis of liver metastases has been made, discussion with the oncologist or specialist in palliative care may be appropriate. In some instances palliative chemotherapy to reduce the size of metastases should be considered, e.g. breast cancer.
- Warmth therapies using wheat bags or heat packs help some patients.
- Start an appropriate NSAID with appropriate GI protection in the form of a proton pump inhibitor or misoprostol.
- The pain also responds to oral steroids, and if there are other symptoms requiring steroids, such as concurrent brain metastases causing headache, this should be first line. Suggested drug is dexamethasone 12 mg as a single daily dose, titrating down to the minimum dose that keeps the pain and other symptoms under control. Appropriate GI protection should be concurrently prescribed.

Squashed stomach syndrome

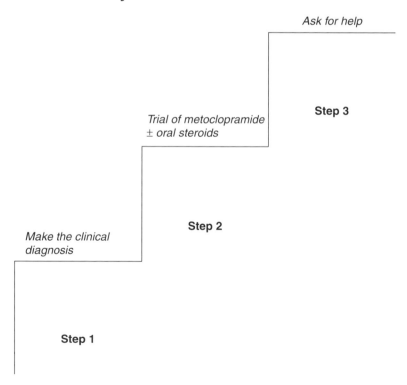

Figure 8.16: Squashed stomach syndrome.

Squashed stomach syndrome is characterised by a combination of anorexia, a feeling of fullness in the hypochondrium, pain and rapid satiation during a meal. Some patients may also vomit or regurgitate rapidly after meals. It is often associated with liver metastases and/or upper gastrointestinal surgery. There is a combination of partial obstruction of the gastric outlet and reduced capacity of the stomach.

- Advise small, regular, high-calorie snacks and supplement drinks rather than big meals.
- Try a combination of metoclopramide 20 mg every four to six hours with oral dexamethasone 8 mg as single daily dose. Remember to prescribe appropriate GI protection. If the patient is vomiting, the drugs may have to be administered parenterally using a syringe driver.

Hiccups

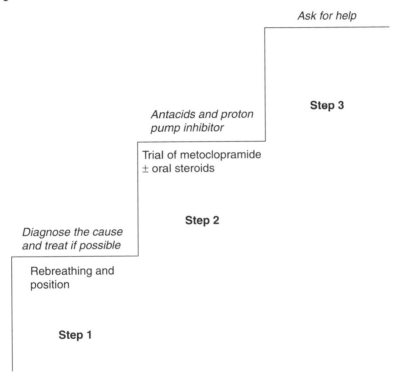

Figure 8.17: Hiccups.

Intractable hiccup is uncommon but usually occurs in patients with cancer affecting the thorax or upper abdomen, including mediastinal lymphadenopathy and liver metastases. Hiccups can be very difficult to manage and early involvement of specialists in palliative care should be considered.

- Simple techniques such as re-breathing using a brown paper bag may help as may altering a patient's position.

- Antacids prescribed with proton pump inhibitors may reduce inflammation in the upper GI tract and thus the frequency and pain associated with the hiccups.
- Oral metoclopramide 20 mg every four to six hours acts as a prokinetic and may help, particularly if there are associated liver metastases causing a squashed stomach.
- Oral steroids (dexamethasone 4–8 mg as a once-daily dose) with appropriate GI protection may help to improve both the hiccups and anorexia if present.
- Baclofen 5 mg every eight hours may help, but this is beyond its product licence and needs to be discussed with the specialist palliative care service.
- Major tranquillisers, such as chlorpromazine, in small doses have found to be helpful in some patients but must be used with caution and under the direction of a specialist.

Sweating

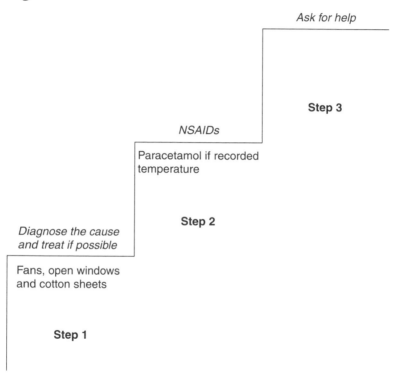

Figure 8.18: Sweating.

Sweating can be viewed as severe when a patient needs to change clothing and/or bed linen on a regular basis. In some cancer patients it is a paraneoplastic syndrome, although it is also associated with pyrexia, exercise, a high ambient temperature and/or emotion.

- Practical measures such as using fans, opening windows and using cotton bed linen and clothes may help.
- If there is a fever, paracetamol 1 g orally or rectally every six hours may help. Consider using an antibiotic if there is infection.

- NSAIDs can help with sweating which is persistent and due to a paraneoplastic syndrome. Their impact on the sweating will take at least two weeks and up to one month.
- If the sweating is secondary to hormone manipulation as in breast or prostate cancer, consider trying megesterol acetate 40–80 mg daily or clonidine 50 micrograms twice daily, increasing to 75 micrograms twice daily after two weeks. Both these interventions will take at least two weeks and up to a month to reduce the sweating.

Itch

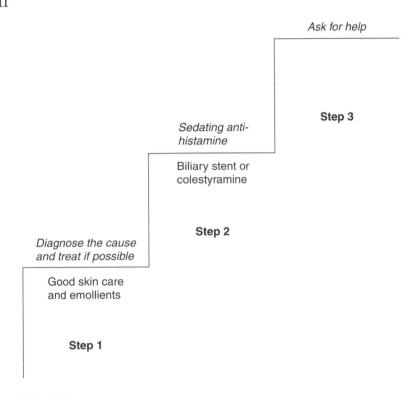

Figure 8.19: Itch.

Try and identify the cause of the itch. If secondary to obstructive jaundice, biliary stenting may be appropriate. Exclude common causes such as changes in washing powder, additives to the bath, etc. Review medication and, where possible, stop drugs that may be contributing to the problem. If morphine sulphate is a suspected cause, consult the local specialist palliative care team about alternative opioids.

- Encourage good skin care and regular use of emollients.
- Consider using a sedating antihistamine such as chlorpheniramine 4 mg every four to six hours as needed, or as a single dose of 4 mg at night.
- If jaundiced secondary to biliary obstruction and where biliary stenting is not an option, cholestyramine 4–8 g as a daily dose may help, although many patients cannot tolerate it.

- If the itch persists, consider starting stanazolol 5–10 mg as a once-daily dose. Other options include oral ondansetron 4–8 mg daily. Both drugs are being used beyond their product licence and should only be initiated after discussion with the specialist palliative care service.

Anorexia

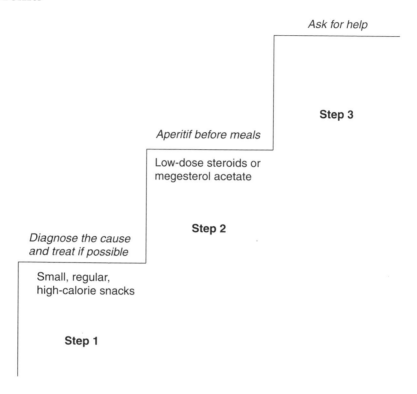

Figure 8.20: Anorexia.

A loss of appetite is often a sign of advancing disease. This is a very common symptom and difficult to manage. Honest discussion with the carers about their desire to meet a basic human need and the patient's inability to accept the offer of food needs to be sensitively handled. The carer may feel rejected and hurt that their loved one is not trying and the patient may feel overwhelmed by the pressure exerted on them to eat. It is important to exclude treatable causes of anorexia such as a sore mouth, oral thrush and ill-fitting or lost dentures. It may be appropriate to treat biochemical abnormalities such as hypercalcaemia in order to restore appetite.

- Practical advice should be given to carers about providing regular, small, high-calorie snacks rather than a single big meal.
- Ensuring a meal is well presented on a small plate so it is not overwhelming may encourage a patient to eat.
- Carers may be unaware that taste changes are common in advanced disease and need to be accommodated.

- In addition, if supplement drinks appear too filling when taken from the carton they may be frozen and used like lollipops.
- Simple strategies like giving an aperitif such as sherry before a meal may help some patients.
- Low-dose steroids (dexamethasone 4–6 mg in a single daily dose) with appropriate GI protection may temporarily stimulate a patient's appetite for a few weeks. If there is no improvement in appetite they should be stopped after a two-week trial.
- Megesterol acetate 80 mg in the morning and at lunch-time may also temporarily stimulate the appetite for a few weeks or months and may have some anti-cancer effect. This use of megesterol acetate is beyond its product licence and should only be initiated after discussion with the specialist palliative care service.

Dry mouth

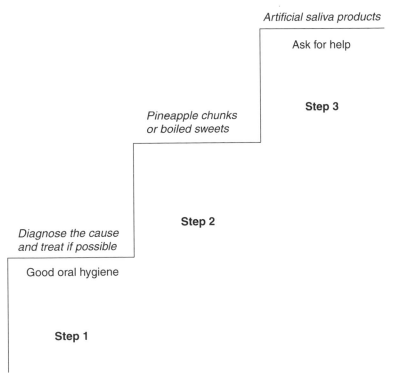

Figure 8.21: Dry mouth.

This is a very common complaint and can adversely affect both appetite and mood. It is important to exclude infection as this can often be treated. Ensure good and regular oral hygiene is being carried out. Dentures that do not fit may aggravate the problem. Dry mouth can also occur as a consequence of mouth breathing and as a long-term consequence of anti-cancer treatments.

- Dry mouth is a common side-effect of many of the drugs used in palliative care, particularly the strong opioids and tricyclic antidepressants. If it is possible to stop or alter medication to diminish side-effects without compromising other symptoms, this should be done.

- Ensuring that the patient has regular small drinks may be sufficient to restore comfort. Simple measures such as chewing fresh pineapple, which stimulates the natural production of saliva and concurrently cleanses the mouth, may be effective. Sucking boiled sweets or chewing sugar-free gum can achieve adequate moistness in many cases.
- Artificial saliva sprays, pastilles and tablets replace natural saliva and offer temporary relief. They may restore a patient's ability to enjoy the taste of food. However, their effect is often short-lived and the patient may need to use the spray as frequently as every hour or so to get sustained relief.

Fatigue

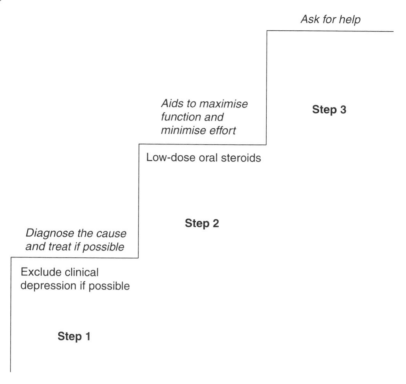

Figure 8.22: Fatigue.

A lack of energy and concentration leading to a sense of disinterest in the world and events around them is very common in patients with advanced disease.

- Identifying and treating where appropriate reversible causes such as anaemia must be the first stage of management.
- It is essential to identify and treat clinical depression, although this may be very difficult.
- Ensuring patients have adequate amounts of good quality sleep may also help.
- Providing aids to maximise function and minimise effort are a cornerstone of management. There may need to be regular review to ensure the aids provided remain appropriate.

Advice about conserving energy, carrying out tasks in stages and pacing activity may help.
- Oral steroids (dexamethasone 4–6 mg in a single daily dose) may temporarily increase a person's sense of well-being, but may cause loss of muscle bulk in the long term. They are best restricted to a two-week course.
- Specialists may consider using low-dose amphetamines if there are short-term goals to be achieved, but there are few helpful pharmaceutical interventions currently available.

Indications for the use of a syringe driver in palliative care

Indications for the use of a syringe driver in palliative care include:

- uncontrolled nausea and/or vomiting
- bowel obstruction
- severe weakness
- dysphagia
- maintenance of symptom control in the dying phase.

Except in the case of poor absorption, pain that is non-responsive to oral morphine sulphate will be non-responsive to parenteral diamorphine sulphate.

If a patient is well symptom controlled using other routes of administration and these can be maintained in the dying phase, a syringe driver does not have to be set up as a matter of routine in the terminal phase.

CHAPTER 9

Bereavement

This chapter includes:

1 Consequences of grief
2 What helps?
3 Listen
4 The process of grief
5 What is abnormal grief?
6 Staff need support too.

Death is part of life. We all realise this, but death and loss can cut through our defences and be the most devastating event of our lives – and yet somehow also one of the most refining. As GPs and district nurses we are often exposed to grief but may be unprepared to deal with it. I was a young GP trainee, fascinated by the subject of bereavement, when I became a widow at the age of 25. Suddenly, the neat theories and clinical labels exploded in my face, leaving a crater of confused emotions. The loss of a close loved one can be the greatest psychological trauma that many of us will experience in our lifetime – and yet grief is a normal process.

As doctors, we meet death more often than most – an estimated 20 patient deaths per GP per year – and we should never underestimate its impact. Unresolved grief can have significant consequences in terms of psychological and physical symptoms. Loss takes many forms but there are common themes in our reactions to it, as Bowlby reminds us:

> The loss of a loved person is one of the most intensely painful experiences any human being can suffer, and not only is it painful to experience but it is also painful to witness.[1]

If we are unsure how to help when exposed to the raw grief of the recently bereaved, then our natural tendency is to avoid the situation. Then we may feel guilty and miss the chance to help the bereaved person, who may appear perfectly normal outwardly but have the desperate wound of grief burning in their chest as they present small clues as cries for help – 'not waving but drowning'.

Consequences of grief

Evidence of a bereavement–mortality relationship is extensive and consistent. Comparative mortality rates, matching the bereaved with control groups, reveal that men fare worse than women, young worse than old and the first few months are the most critical.

The most common causes of death after bereavement are liver cirrhosis, heart disease, suicide, road accident or other violent deaths.[2] It is therefore important to enquire about suicidal thoughts: 'Have things ever got so bad that you've thought of ending it all?' Increased morbidity is caused by increased levels of clinical and subclinical depression, with up to a third of bereaved people developing a depressive illness.

Emotional pain can also commonly be expressed as physical pain – the 'pit' in the stomach, palpitations, anorexia or even physical symptoms similar to those of the person who died. However, by easing the associated strains of grief, the bereaved can be buffered against the most dire consequences of loss. Many studies have shown that the right help given to people at the right time can be effective in reducing physical and mental symptoms and can improve the quality of life before and after bereavement.[3]

The aim when helping people grieve is that they will achieve some restitution and adjustment to a new way of being, 'emotionally relocating the deceased'.[4] They will be permanently changed, but many will be stronger and wiser after grief and may wish to use their experience to help others.

Timescales are difficult to estimate. Two years is considered average, although many, especially parents, may need much longer – either way we should be alert to long-term consequences.

What helps?

When a death is anticipated, helping those closest prepare for bereavement can greatly improve outcomes. It is possible to implement a useful bereavement protocol in primary care as a form of active outreach.[5] Useful suggestions that take little organisation but can be so greatly appreciated are:

- **initiated visits**, both early on and after three to six months, when many will be at their lowest
- at the initial bereavement visit, a relationship of trust and open access is confirmed and a **follow-up plan** formulated. It is often very difficult for some to respond to the request to 'pop back any time' – usually they won't as there is a natural sense of inertia and transitional existence – and so an initiated proactive date for further contact can be greatly appreciated
- good **note-keeping** to alert the GP during a consultation so they are prompted to ask the right question at the appropriate time (many will present with physical symptoms when the pain and distress become overwhelming)
- flagging up the patient's notes, especially around the **anniversary** of the death or at critical times, so that contact can be made at that vulnerable time
- keeping a **practice directory** of local contact details for bereavement counselling, e.g. through the hospice, hospital chaplain, etc. This could include local clergy, chaplains and other religious leaders, social services, voluntary self-help groups, etc.
- keeping these patients' details as former carers from the Supportive Care Register, and maintaining some contact; setting up a carers' database enables this.

On one occasion, I was worried about the recently bereaved husband of a patient of mine, who had not been coping very well, but I ran out of time on my visits and didn't pop in. The following week I was called to find he had hanged himself in the barn. You never forget that kind of thing. I always watch out now and try to initiate visits if I can. You develop a sense for when things are alright and when they are not.

GP, Shropshire, GSF Phase 2

We should train ourselves to hear the clues of past losses in day-to-day consultations as well as at the bedside of the dying, and make an effort to listen – we can make a real difference. This is a special role of those of us in primary care – if we don't do it, invariably no one else will.

Listen

The key to bereavement counselling is listening. If you only have five minutes, giving 100% attention with eye contact and body language for that time is valued. People often need longer, so suggest an end-of-surgery appointment and plan follow-up. While the bereaved are explaining their feelings to us they are also explaining their feelings to themselves.

Despite grief being a normal process, things can go wrong and there are some indicators of 'pathological grief' (*see* Box 9.1).

Box 9.1 Risks for poor outcome or pathological grief

- Ambivalent or dependent relationship
- Multiple losses
- Previous mental illness such as depression
- Sudden traumatic death
- Long terminal illness (more than six months)
- Suicide
- Level of perceived social support
- Ability to perform valued rituals is curtailed

What is abnormal grief?

One important role for the GP is in the detection of abnormal grief, although this is rarer than expected. As the expression of grief is so affected by cultural and personal factors, assessing whether grief is abnormal or normal is complex.

Abnormal grief is 'the intensification of grief to the level when the person is overwhelmed, resorts to maladaptive behaviour or remains in a state of grief without progression of the mourning process towards completion'.[2]

There are four types of abnormal grief reactions:

- chronic – the most common
- delayed – no grieving, followed by a later reaction
- exaggerated – perhaps leading to the development of phobias
- masked – such as by alcoholism.

Antidepressants and short-terms hypnotics may play a useful role and referral is recommended if pathological trends seem to be developing (*see* Box 9.2). Refer to local support groups if appropriate, or with an interested staff member – such as a district nurse – a practice support group can be initiated.

Children should not feel excluded at this critical time, and should be encouraged to attend the funeral if they wish to. Grief work may need to occur at several stages in their development. Parents are often the best people to talk to their children about this, but may need support, recommended books or referral to special advisory groups (*see* Box 9.3).

Box 9.2 Sources of help

- Local hospice, hospital, clergy, counsellor, community psychiatric nurse, psychologist
- CRUSE Bereavement Care, tel: 0870 167 1677; fax: 0208 940 7638; www.crusebereavementcare.org.uk
- CRUSE Scotland, tel: 0131 551 1511
- CRUSE Northern Ireland, tel: 028 9079 2419
- Compassionate Friends (parents) 0117 953 9639; www.tcf.org.uk; e-mail: info@tcf.org.uk
- SANDS (stillbirth), tel: 0207 436 5881
- National Association of Bereavement Services, tel: 0207 247 0617
- Jewish Bereavement Counselling Service, tel: 0208 349 0839

Box 9.3 Children's grief: ways to help[6]

- Be calm – crying is fine, distress is frightening.
- Explain the situation clearly in language they'll understand.
- Reassure them about their own future and the continuing care for them.
- Sit down and really listen to their questions and their fears.
- Don't assume you know what they mean or want to know or want to ask.
- Don't overprotect or try to make it better – allow them to express their sad feelings.
- Set the stage for continuing discussions about the person who died, the death itself, feelings, changes, etc.
- Explain simply what will happen now, e.g. the funeral – allow them to decide how much they'd like to be involved.
- Give some information about grief and what they might expect.
- Keep to your routine and avoid too many changes.
- Encourage remembering, rituals and traditions – don't avoid family events but do plan ahead ways to deal with them.

The process of grief

It can be difficult to categorise the emotional processes of grief, but it is helpful to have a frame of reference. Parkes suggests bereavement is a process through different stages.[3] Other authors describe the daily swing from loss to restoration, with a gradual tendency to the latter over time (*see* Box 9.4).[4,7,8] It is not a neat clinical process, so beware of pigeon-holing. The emotional pain of loss has to be faced in the bereaved person's own particular manner and time, if they are to move on. Some people find it helpful to be reminded that this is a pain but it is not meaningless, it is the other side of love – 'everything has its price and the price of love is pain' – and there are ways in which we learn deep lessons through the pain.

Box 9.4 Stages of grief

Stage	Common emotions and experiences	Task
Initial shock	Numbness, disbelief, heart and head in conflict	Accept the reality of the loss
Pangs of grief	Sadness, anxiety, vulnerability, anger, guilt, regret, hypersensitivity, preoccupation, social withdrawal, inertia, restlessness, transient hallucinations, nightmares	Experience the pain of grief
Despair	Loss of meaning and direction in life – lack of will to live	Adjust to a new environment in which the deceased is missing
Adjustment	Develop new interests, relationships and outlook – moving on	Emotionally relocate the deceased to an important but not central position

Your pain is the breaking of the shell that encloses your understanding.

Kahlil Gibran

In my experience, many have found the 'amoebic' pictures (*see* Figure 9.1) helpful in representing the progression towards healing, with the internal wounds enlarging the inner person. Some emotions may be heightened, such as raging anger, and some dulled. Perhaps most significant of all is the loss of the relationship.

Staff need support too (*see also* Chapter 17)

If it is alright for our patients to grieve, it should be acceptable for us to grieve also. Any caring team must build in staff support, such as debriefing sessions, to 'de-stress the distress'. What resources do we have to draw upon ourselves as GPs and do we know our limits?

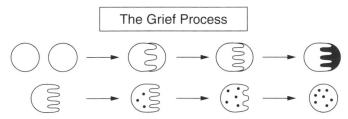

The Grief Process

An 'amoebic' picture such as this might help patients understand the grief process; the inter-relationship. The crater of loss when one half dies, but the gradual healing of the wound in the movement back towards wholeness.

Figure 9.1: The grief process.

In the PHCT meetings it can be helpful to undertake a significant event analysis after a death, to reflect on the care provided but also to ensure that the staff involved have unloaded any baggage of residual feelings, especially if the death has been traumatic.

The vital role of primary care

In grief, the GP and the PHCT are often in the most suitable position to help, either directly or by referral to others. Bereavement is a significant life event but there is much that can be done to reduce morbidity and enable the healing of the wounds of grief. Intervention at this time can have a significant positive impact for patients.

The principles of grief counselling can also be applied to other kinds of loss, such as altered body image, divorce, loss of ability or role – anything that has caused a restructuring of the internal model of the world. Improving our communication skills in this area will have far-reaching benefits elsewhere.

Bereavement care is rewarding as well as challenging. Parkes *et al.*[9] point out that 'with proper training and support we shall find that repeated griefs, far from undermining our humanity and our care, enable us to cope more confidently and more sensitively with each succeeding loss'. Many have found that working with bereaved people can teach us to value our close relationships and to give them our time and energy.[10] We are reminded that love is a precious gift that we should appreciate while we can.

References

1 Bowlby J (1980) *Attachment and Loss*, Vol. 1. Penguin, Harmondsworth.

2 Stroebe M S, Stroebe W and Hansson R O (1999) *Handbook of Bereavement: theory, research and intervention*. Cambridge University Press, Cambridge.

3 Parkes C M (1996) *Bereavement: studies of grief in adult life* (3e). Tavistock, London.

4 Worden J W (1983) *Grief Counselling and Grief Therapy*. Routledge, London.

5 Charlton R and Dolman E (1995) Bereavement: a protocol in primary care. *Br J Gen Pract*. **45**: 427–30.

6 Downing M *et al.* (1998) *Handbook of the Victoria Hospice Society*. British Columbia, Canada.

7 Stroebe W and Stroebe M S (1987) *Bereavement and Health?* Cambridge University Press, New York.

8 Sheldon F (1998) Bereavement. *BMJ*. **316**: 456–8.

9 Parkes C M, Relf M and Couldrick A (1996) *Counselling in Terminal Care and Bereavement*. BPS Books, London.

10 Penson J (2000) Bereavement. In: J Cooper (ed) *Stepping into Palliative Care*. Radclife Medical Press, Oxford.

CHAPTER 10

Sources of help and words of wisdom

This chapter includes:

1 Networks
2 Specialist palliative care eligibility criteria
3 Other sources of help for healthcare professionals
4 A few words of wisdom.

Networks (in England)

Your Cancer Network Primary Care Group or Palliative and Supportive Care Network Group (in England) will probably have already produced some of the following, which may be of help to you:

- a *directory* of all involved in cancer and palliative care in the Network with contact details
- a *formulary* of agreed drug uses and dosages
- *some guidelines* on common symptom management
- *out-of-hours palliative care policy* across the Network
- your Network Primary Care Group who may be collating the *baseline review of services* which will indicate further needs and your starting point for any improvements
- there may be a *primary care project manager* within the Network, working on areas of primary palliative care, linked up with the Cancer Services Collaborative. The *Cancer Services Collaborative Primary Care Group* have developed a strategy for improving cancer care in two main areas:
  - service provision
  - supportive care.
  This covers the four areas of:
  - rapid referral, diagnosis and treatment
  - communication between primary, secondary and tertiary care
  - primary palliative care. The Gold Standards Framework programme was jointly funded by the Cancer Services Collaborative and Macmillan in Phase 2, and is being promoted as a key way of improving supportive care, initially in the palliative care phase but later moving up towards diagnosis
  - user group involvement.

Specialist palliative care eligibility criteria

Some palliative care groups have developed eligibility criteria which help the inter-working of specialist and generalist palliative care.[1] Box 10.1 gives an example of criteria for referral to specialist palliative care services which are based on patient need, not diagnosis.

Box 10.1 Calderdale and Kirklees Palliative Care Group: Eligibility criteria for referral to specialist palliative care services

Eligible patients have:

1 any active progressive and potentially *life-threatening* disease

2 *anticipated or actual unresolved*, complex needs that cannot be met by the caring team, i.e. physical, psychological, social, spiritual needs such as complicated symptoms, specialist nursing needs, difficult family situations, ethical issues regarding treatment decisions, etc.

3 been recently *assessed* by a member of one of the specialist palliative care teams.

Other sources of help for healthcare professionals and patients

- *Macmillan Cancer Relief*. UK-wide charity working to improve the treatment and care of people with cancer and their families from the point of diagnosis. Produces useful leaflets containing information for patients, carers and professionals. Also highly recommended are the charity's following publications: *Directory of Patients' Information Materials* with illustrated leaflets available, *Out-of-Hours Palliative Care Report* (2001), *Directory of Complementary Therapy Services in UK Cancer Care* (2002) and *The Cancer Guide* which contains a list of helpful organisations and contact details for patients, etc. Macmillan Cancer Relief is based at 89 Albert Embankment, London SE1 7UQ. Information line: 0845 601 6161; tel: 0207 840 7840; www.macmillan.org.uk

- *Cancer Services Collaborative* (joint funders of the GSF programme, Phase 2). Part of the NHS Modernisation Agency. A publication list is available from 4th Floor, St John's House, East Street, Leicester LE1 6NB. Tel: 0116 222 1415/5110; www.modern.nhs.uk/cancer; e-mail cancerservicescollaborative@npat.nhs.uk
  NB. Improvement Leaders' Guides on subjects such as *Measuring for Improvement*, *Managing the Human Dimensions of Change*, etc. are highly recommended and available from improvementguides@npat.nhs.uk or www.modern.nhs.uk/improvementguides

- *National Council for Hospice and Specialist and Specialist Palliative Care Services*. Produces informative booklets and guidance. These are available from 1st Floor, 34–44 Britannia Street, London WC1X 9JG. Tel: 020 7520 8299; www.hospice-spc-council.org.uk; e-mail enquiries@hospice-spc-council.org.uk

- *St Christopher's Hospice Information Service*, London. Produced a *Directory of Hospice and Palliative Care Services* and offers central support for a large range of enquiries about palliative care from across the world. Tel: 020 8778 9252; www.hospiceinformation.co.uk; e-mail info@his2.freeserve.co.uk

- Other useful websites include:
  www.doh.gov.uk/cancer
  www.cancerbacup.org.uk

www.cancersupportuk.nhs.uk
www.cancercare.uk
www.carersuk.demon.co.uk
www.cancerblackcare.org
www.mariecurie.org.uk
www.nationalcanceralliance.co.uk
www.patients-association.com
www.bristolcancerhelp.org
www.changingfaces.com
www.crossroads.org.uk
www.crusebereavementcare.org.uk
www.nhsdirect.com
www.roadsscot.fsnet.co.uk
www.nagpc.com
www.palliativedrugs.com
www.palliative-medicine.org
www.eapcnet.org
www.sign.ac.uk
www.nelh.nhs.uk
www.bmj.com
www.nice.org.uk

A few words of wisdom

In an age when a surfeit of data and information is hitting us from all sides, when knowledge, or the lack of it, cries out to us from all sources and multiple divergent choices confuse us when they purport to help, what we seek in essence is some pure wisdom, some guidance on the right direction, some greater knowing – a map. How often do we find ourselves lost, both practically or in a more metaphysical way, and carry on in the wrong direction because we haven't craned our necks to see from a higher standpoint the better course. We need maps. We need the penny-dropping feelings of that innate knowledge, when something chimes with our natural instinct and we know it to be right. We hear the resonance of wisdom in our deepest core.

Sometimes this comes in moments of quiet whilst visiting a somnolent patient or perhaps on the journey home, or sometimes it comes sideways at us through poetry, a sea skyline or a smile. We as healthcare professionals are patients and carers too – the boundary is gossamer thin. We need time and space and guidance at times to see the possible road ahead, to spot the waving not drowning figure, to reflect on the bigger picture. We need to recognise wisdom in each other, particularly in our experienced colleagues and in our dying patients and their grieving families. As we are honoured to travel with them as they approach the end, may we be worthy of the task and ever open-hearted enough to be good 'companions on the journey'.

The following personal choices each express different aspects of the hidden depths to me and through their words some deeper illumination of wisdom filters through.

You can shed tears that she has gone
or you can smile because she has lived

You can close your eyes and pray that she'll come back
or you can open your eyes and see all she's left

Your heart can be empty because you can't see her
or you can be full of the love you shared

You can turn your back on tomorrow and live yesterday
or you can be happy for tomorrow because of yesterday

You can remember her and only that she's gone
or you can cherish her memory and let it live on

You can cry and close your mind, be empty and turn your back
or you can do what she'd want: smile, open your eyes, love and go on

Anon.
(Read at the funeral of the Queen Mother, April 2002)

The Bright Field

I have seen the sun break through
To illuminate a small field
For a while, and gone my way
And forgotten it. But that was the pearl
Of great price, the one field that had
The treasure in it. I realise now
That I must give all that I have
To possess it. Life is not hurrying
On to a receding future, nor hankering after
An imagined past. It is the turning
Aside like Moses to the miracle
Of the lit bush, to a brightness
That seems as transitory as your youth
Once, but is the eternity that awaits you.

RS Thomas

Our deepest fear is not
that we are inadequate.
Our deepest fear is that we are
powerful beyond all measure.
It is our light, not our darkness,
that frightens us most.
We ask ourselves, who am I to be
brilliant, gorgeous, talented and fabulous?
Actually, who are you not to be?
You are a child of God.
Your playing small doesn't serve the world
There's nothing enlightened about
shrinking, so that other people
won't feel insecure around you.
We were born to make manifest
the glory of God that is within us.
It's in everyone!
And as we let our light shine,
we unconsciously give other people
permission to do the same.
As we are liberated from our own
fear, our presence automatically liberates others.

Marianne Williamson, quoted by Nelson Mandela

Death: the horizon is in the well

We are wrong to think that death comes only at the end of life. Your physical death is but the completion of a process on which your secret companion has been working since your birth ... How does death manifest itself to us in our day-to-day experience? Death meets us in and through different guises in the areas of our life where we are vulnerable, frail, hurting or negative. One of the faces of death is negativity. In every person there is some wound of negativity; this is like a blister on your life. You can be quite destructive towards yourself, even when times are good. Some people are having wonderful lives right now, but they do not actually realize it ...

Negativity is an addiction to the bleak shadow that lingers around every human form. Within a poetics of growth or spiritual life, the transfiguration of this negativity is one of our continuing tasks. This negativity is the force and face of your own death gnawing at your belonging in the world. It wants to make you a stranger in your own life. This negativity holds you outside in exile from your own love and warmth. You can transfigure negativity by turning it towards the light of your soul. This soul light gradually takes the gravity, weight and hurt out of negativity.

Another face of death, another way it expresses itself in your daily experience, is through fear. There is no soul without the shadow of fear.

Many people are terrified of letting go and use control as a mechanism to order and structure their lives ... But too much control is destructive ... When you begin to let go, it is amazing how enriched your life becomes. False things, which you have desperately held on to, move away very quickly from you. Then what is real, what you love deeply, and what really belongs to you, comes deeper into you. Now no-one can ever take them away from you.

Other people are afraid of being themselves. They play a continual game, fashioning a careful persona which they think the world will accept or admire ... One of the most sacred duties of one's destiny is the duty to be yourself. When you come to accept yourself and like yourself, you learn not to be afraid of your own nature ... Life is very short and we have a special destiny waiting to unfold for us. Sometimes through our fear of being ourselves, we sidestep that destiny and end up hungry and impoverished in a famine of our own making.

Death is the great wound in the universe and the great wound in each life. Yet, ironically, this is the very wound that can lead to new spiritual growth. Thinking of your death can help you to radically alter your fixed and habitual perception. Instead of living merely according to the visible or possessible within the material realm of life, you begin to refine your sensibility and become aware of the treasures that are hidden in the invisible side of your life.

Imagine if you could talk to a baby in the womb and explain its unity with the mother. How this cord of belonging gives it life. If you could then tell the baby that this was about to end. It was going to be expelled from the womb, pushed through a very narrow passage finally to be dropped out into vacant, open light. The cord which held it to this mother-womb was going to be cut and that it was going to be on its own for ever more. If the baby could talk back, it would fear that it was going to die. For the baby being born would seem like death ... and yet in fact it was being given life.

John O'Donohue, *Anam Cara: spiritual wisdom from the Celtic world* (1997)
Bantam Press, London.

A Blessing for Death

I pray that you will have the blessing
   of being consoled and sure about your
   own death.
May you know in your soul that there is no need
   to be afraid.
When your time comes, may you be given every
   blessing and shelter that you need.
May there be a beautiful welcome for you in the
   home that you are going to.
You are not going somewhere strange. You are
   going back to the home that you never left.
May you have a wonderful urgency to live your
   life to the full.
May you live compassionately and creatively
   and transfigure everything that is negative
   within you and about you.
When you come to die may it be after a long life.
May you be peaceful and happy and in the
   presence of those who really care for you.
May your going be sheltered and your welcome
   assured.
May your soul smile in the embrace of your
   anam cara.

John O'Donohue, *Anam Cara: spiritual wisdom from the Celtic world* (1997)
Bantam Press, London.

There is a place deep in the soul, that neither time nor space, nor any created thing can ever touch.

Meister Eckhart

There is a hard law … that when an injury is done to us, we never recover until we forgive.

Alan Paton

Companions on the Journey

We are not meant to walk this path alone
There is a fundamental need within our souls
To have companions on the journey as we move
Along this shared chronology of time.
If we can be that good companion, that trusted friend,
We will receive far more than ever we will give.
The stark horizon throws our lives in sharp relief
And we will see our empty fears as nothing more than ghosts
The Emperor's clothes will vanish from our sight
We are most human and yet still most divine
And we will hear, within the inner whisper of the soul,
That this is the reason we have come.

Keri Thomas

Loving medicine

'Loving medicine' is a term we may be shy to use with our white-coated scientific mindset, but it is a driving force for many in this area of work. As you mull over the words in this book, and begin to use it as a practical manual, my hope is that something resonates with you, deepens your wisdom, and that you are encouraged, enabled and inspired to continue in this noble and privileged work as a companion on the journey. In seeking to improve the 'head' knowledge and the organisation of the 'hands', we are better able to affirm loving medicine and to put back some of the 'heart' in the care for our patients in the last stages of their lives.

... And prayer is more
Than an order of words, the conscious occupation
of the praying mind, or the sound of the voice praying.
And what the dead had no speech for, when living,
They can tell you, being dead: the communication
of the dead is tongued with fire beyond the language of the living.
Here, the intersection of the timeless moment
Is England, and nowhere. Never and always.

From *Little Gidding* by TS Eliot

Reference

1 Bennett M, Adams J, Alison D, Hicks F, Stockton M (2000) Leeds Eligibility Criteria for specialist palliative care services. *Pall Med.* **14**(2): 157–8.

PART 3

The Gold Standards Framework – A Handbook for Practices and the Macmillan GSF Programme

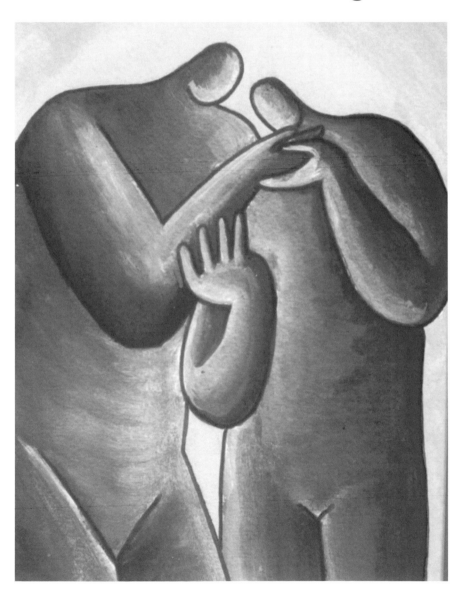

The Handbook for Practices:
the Gold Standards Framework

This section forms The Handbook for Practices, a practice tool kit for those undertaking the Macmillan Gold Standards Framework (GSF) Programme, currently on-going across the UK. Included in this section is the background and structure of the GSF and Standards C1–7 in more detail, with practical recommendations on 'next steps' and 'getting going'.

CHAPTER 11

Background to the Gold Standards Framework

The GSF has brought about a real culture shift in our work: it is now more patient-focused, more proactive, with better teamworking, more caring. These real deep-seated changes can never be tangibly measured but are more real than anything we can measure.

GP, Scotland, GSF2

Another way of looking at this framework: it's rather like a game of snakes and ladders in which you try to remove all the snakes and maximise the ladders.

Participant from Cornwall, GSF Phase 3, summer seminar

The Gold Standards Framework project is the only thing in palliative care over the last few years that has really made a difference.

District nurse, Glasgow, GSF Phase 2

The care of all dying patients should be raised to the level of the best.

NHS Cancer Plan

This chapter includes:

1   Background thinking and underlying messages
2   History and structure of GSF projects
3   Needs-based care and key themes
4   Benefits in taking part
5   Stepwise changes.

The clear aim of the Gold Standards Framework is to support, encourage and enable primary healthcare teams to develop improvements in the supportive care of patients in the last stages of life.

Background thinking and underlying messages

The Gold Standards Framework for community palliative care has developed from the struggles of real-life grass-roots primary care, in the current context in the UK. It aims to support and facilitate the whole practice team as they work together to 'raise their game' towards highest quality care for patients with any diagnosis in the last stages of life. It has begun with cancer patients, but the principles of supportive care should then extend to those with non-malignant end-stage illnesses and, if suitable, to all cancer patients from diagnosis or urgent referral.

The name 'Gold Standards' developed in the initial 'think tank' as an attempt to crystallise our aspirations of best practice in community palliative care, in the knowledge that in the real world this is not always possible. We felt that this group of patients, above all, deserved our best standard of care. We tried to picture the model of best practice and the way it might actually look in primary care, knowing that often, in reality, silver or bronze standards might actually be good enough and be the best we could achieve with the resources available.

However, aspiring to the best will enable some change, and sometimes small changes in attitude, emphasis and detail can make a huge difference in patient care.

The word 'Framework' represents the fact that this has grown not as a didactic 'top-down, must-do' but as a 'bottom-up, try this' approach to a sometimes difficult aspect of primary care that many feel is vitally important. It is a practical guiding framework for each practice or area to use and then fill in the gaps, customise and personalise, using previously researched, thought through and piloted suggestions. Using the experiences of those with an interest in this area, it enables practices to start from a higher base – and just as in the climbing frame, it's fun! There is less re-invention of wheels and more sharing of good practice, as no matter where we live or what our health structures are, it affirms that caring for seriously ill people in the last stages of life is important to us all.

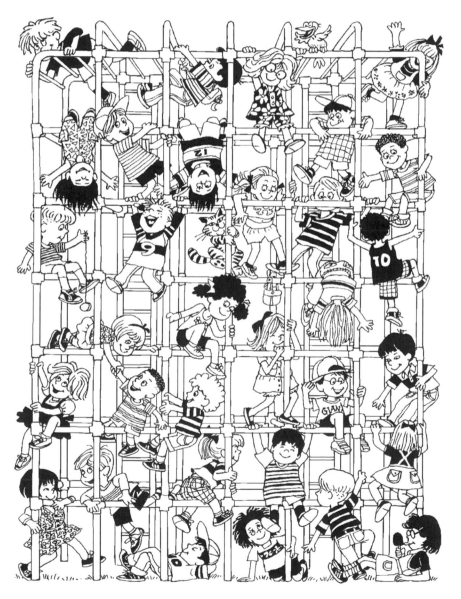

Figure 11.1

This work aims to be part of the solution not part of the problem. If the weight of the current workload or staff changes becomes too great, it's important to prune back to the basics of this improved care rather than abandon it altogether. Of the benefits gained from using this framework, many have found that it is the almost imperceptible re-emphasis on patients' needs, better communication and teamworking and a built-in change of mind-set towards planning care that have made a difference, even though these are hard aspects of care to measure.

Underlying messages

There are several important 'subtexts' in this work which emerge repeatedly in the evaluation from pilot practices:

- A key guiding light is the increased *patient-centredness*, involving *empowerment* of patients and carers to become active members of the team, and to retain control and autonomy as much as possible, in a world gone mad with the devastation of the news of a life-threatening illness.
- Another key feature is the *encouragement* of the primary healthcare team, the building up of confidence (especially of the district nurses in the team) to lead to real *sustainability* and continuous developments in their primary palliative care. This is an area in which we do well, but we could do even better. Trying this out with a small group of patients then leads to an extended approach to improving the system of supportive care offered to all patients from diagnosis and with any end-stage illness. This can feel like a neglected area of primary care, and yet it absorbs a large amount of time and energy from those within the team.
- Key outcome features are the development of a *sense of security, comfort and support* for patients and carers at home.
- In the light of increasingly disabling bureaucracy and political directives, this work affirms the role of primary care in supporting patients as a worthwhile and valued activity – as Gomas said 'sometimes caring, always relieving, supporting right to the end'.[1]
- The three main processes of development are in:
  - *identifying* these patients
  - *assessing* and responding to their needs
  - and *planning* care,
  with better *communication* running through all areas.
- *Increased awareness of these patients.* Raising palliative care patients higher on the practice agenda by identifying them specifically, e.g. in the register. They are special patients.
- *Focusing on the patient by better assessment*, using suggested tools to clarify and record patients' priorities, problems and needs as well as those of the carers.
- A move from reactive to *proactive care.* Advanced planning is a crucial element in this – scanning the horizon for any predictable issues and pre-empting them.
- Better *teamworking and communication* underpins the work and better valuing of each other's roles.
- Better *dovetailing* with specialists in palliative care and understanding of roles and contributions. There's plenty of work out there for all of us, but we must maximise our skills and effectiveness and work together well.
- A sense of improved team *morale, enjoyment and job satisfaction* from a job well done. We may forget staff support and morale at our peril – our staff are our greatest resource and as any 'one-minute manager' will tell you, those who feel good about themselves do the best work.[2]

- Most of all it's *people-centred, relationship-based care*, using tools and structures to develop this.

See the Appendix for a description of 'reactive' and 'proactive' patient journeys.

The history and structure of the GSF projects so far

The first two phases were structured as follows.

Phase 1

- This was based on practice visits to over 70 practice teams and several workshops run by the author as Macmillan GP Facilitator in Cancer and Palliative Care, Calderdale and Kirklees Health Authority, Huddersfield, West Yorkshire.
- There was a multidisciplinary reference group of primary care and palliative care specialist doctors and nurses, debating and researching the key issues in community palliative care and mapping the patient journey.
- A Gold Standards Framework handbook was then developed with wide consultation amongst colleagues. (There were only six standards initially.)
- It was piloted in 12 practices in West Yorkshire over one year from February 2001 and was facilitated by the author.
- Each practice had a coordinator (usually the DN but alternatively the practice manager or practice nurse) and lead GP.
- There were two initial teaching sessions plus repeat practice visits, with monthly feedback sessions for facilitators (over lunch).
- It was evaluated as part of a research project (for more details, *see* Chapter 19, p. 271) examining in particular its acceptability and compatibility with real life primary care. This entailed:
  - baseline questionnaires, before and after, on intervention and matched practices
  - focus groups initially setting the goals, and then repeated after three months of assessing progress
  - a semi-structured interview with GPs one year later.

Phase 2

- A central team was required to coordinate and oversee the project. This was derived from the joined support of the project by Macmillan Cancer Relief and the Cancer Services Collaborative of the NHS Modernisation Agency, and was composed of a national clinical lead and representatives of the above groups, with project management, analysis, research and administrative support.
- It involved 76 practices in 18 project areas across the UK, and each had a facilitator.
- There was a facilitator in each project area (mainly Macmillan GP Facilitators already in post or primary care trust Cancer Leads in England). The facilitator explains, develops and supports this work with teaching sessions and regular feedback meetings involving the practice coordinators and interested GPs. *This is an essential part of the back-up support offered and a large reason for the success of the framework*, in bringing together motivated and interested enthusiasts who encourage each other and share examples of good practice. It also helps develop local ownership of each project and gives local flavour to the framework, which varies in each area, whilst retaining the same basic model.
- The facilitators are supported by the central team with resources, teaching, regular contact by phone and e-mail, national feedback conferences, list-serve, conference calls and some visits. They are the links between the central team and the practices (*see* Figure 11.2),

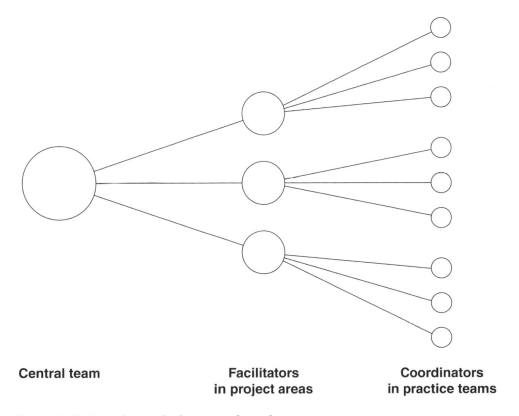

| **Central team** | **Facilitators in project areas** | **Coordinators in practice teams** |

Figure 11.2: Central team, facilitators and coordinators.

for example for the dissemination of resources and information to practices and evaluations from practices. They are most successful when backed up by administrative support (an essential ingredient).

- Each practice had a coordinator, running the project in their practice team (*see* Chapter 13, C2).
- Each practice received a number of resources: a flyer to introduce the project, a Supportive Care register, the handbook, home packs and a resource pack consisting of useful textbooks, articles, CD-roms, videos, etc.
- There was usually a practice review/audit meeting after six months, using evaluation and significant event analysis tools to develop an action plan for improvement and a practice protocol.
- The evaluation in Phase 2 (*see* Chapter 19) consisted of:
  - a baseline questionnaire, repeated after six months, with feedback to individual practices
  - brief monthly key outcomes sheets, producing run charts for each project area showing incremental improvements
  - qualitative assessment using independent university researchers, examining the views and ideas of GPs, district nurses and carers in intervention and matched practices in four project areas across the UK.

- Meetings were held – all facilitators were invited to workshops before and after the six-month pilot to share ideas, evaluations and examples of good practice.

The successful implementation of the framework across so many areas of the UK was largely related to the enthusiasm and hard work of the facilitators and dedication of the primary care teams.

My everlasting admiration and thanks go especially to the stalwart group of district nurses I have worked with over the years. Their commitment and personal self-effacing dedication has been such an inspiration and encouragement to me. If the district nurses feel there have been improvements, then I'm satisfied – they are the real touchstones of care for the dying in the community.

It's enabled me to do the job of district nurse I'd always wanted to do.

DN, Halifax, GSF Phase 1

Also contributing enormously were the original Phase 1 Yorkshire GPs and the wonderful band of Phase 2 GP facilitators across the UK, who were so helpful in their constructive feedback and comments to me. I am indebted to them, and hope this evolving resource for others is testimony to their hard work and enthusiasm.

Needs-based care and key themes

It is important from the outset to clarify clear goals – to 'begin with the end in mind'.[3] These must be based on patient need. From the previous discussion relating to the head, hands and heart of care (*see* Chapter 4), it is seen there must be a balance between the clinical competence required, the organisation of services and the expression of humane patient centred care, based on the needs of the patient and their families.

Relating to this previous discussion, it is helpful to clarify the needs of our patients (meeting these needs is the desired outcome) and the structure and process required to achieve this, i.e.:

- patient/carer/staff needs
- outcome desired
- process required
- structure to help delivery of outcome.

The main needs we are focusing on are those of improving the comfort, security and support of patients and their carers in the community (*see* Table 4.1).

The overall goal of the GSF is better care for palliative care patients provided by primary healthcare teams.

Based on appropriate *need*, the desired *outcome* is for patients and carers to feel comfortable, secure and supported, i.e. symptom-free, and to be given appropriate information to allow autonomy and control so that they may continue their journey towards emotional and spiritual peace at the end of their lives.

The *process* of doing this involves undertaking the tasks of the GSF by:

1 *identifying* clearly this group of patients and their carers
2 *assessing* their needs
3 *planning* their care

with better *communication* throughout the process; and then the *structures* provided – the people and the papers and the suggested examples of means to do this, such as register, home packs, assessment tools, templates, etc.

> *We felt safer because the GSF project provides a system of care to make it less likely that people will slip through the net. It has formalised what we were trying to do in a very haphazard way before, a more watertight organised service which gives more patients better care and gives us more job satisfaction.*
>
> GP, Halifax, GSF Phase 1

During the pilot phase of the GSF project, the key themes to better palliative care to emerge from the focus groups and discussions were:

1 advanced planning/proactive care
2 a sense of teamwork, continuity and better communication
3 symptom control for patients in the community
4 support for carers and patients (and also for staff).

These formed the basis of the development of tasks or gold standards – the 'seven Cs' and their later evaluation (*see* Chapters 12–18). Within each of the seven sections are suggested means of achieving these outcomes, but others are being developed by individual practices as they consider how best to respond to the needs of their patients. These are by no means exhaustive lists of ways to improve primary palliative care.

A further milestone would be the development of your own **practice protocol for palliative care patients**, building on your practice's experience of the GSF project so that the best of care becomes standard practice. The collective writing of the protocol is a large reason for its success.

What is presented here is a tried and tested framework that has helped to kick-start changes in practices in different ways, involving about 3000 patients in a great variety of settings across the UK. In settings as varied as Halifax, Glasgow, Dorset, Shropshire, Aberdeen, outer London and inner Londonderry, it has been taken up with enthusiasm and used and adapted in different measures to improve the experience of care for patients and their families. A few had difficulties continuing with it, although most of them would say it has still been of some help in focusing on this issue. None of us would say that we have always achieved the 'gold standard' of care for all our patients during these pilot projects, but all have made some changes that have begun in a small way to improve care for our patients in the last months of life.

There are many 'maps' and many routes to the same destination: the GSF saves on some of the 'wheel reinvention' but encourages more localised ideas too. Although common-sensical and apparently simple, it is the beginning of a process which can, if encouraged, lead to radical changes. The differences between the practices who received greatest benefit and those who faltered were many and varied, but the collective impression is that it had to do with extraneous workload, staff changes, time pressures, difficulties holding practice meetings and the overall atmosphere of resourcing and encouraging good practice (*see* Chapter 19).

In this current climate of increasing primary care workload pressures with inadequate community resources, for anything to be successful it must be quite obviously beneficial and easily implemented and supported. However, some areas may particularly struggle due to staff changes and factors or pressures beyond their control.

It sounds simple but it's like the hub of the wheel – everything else grows from it. And we can continue to improve all the time.
    Chris Martland, Huddersfield, GP – one of the original inspirations and Phase 1 participants

Benefits of being part of the Macmillan Gold Standards Framework programme

NB. Details of future phases are still to be confirmed at the time of going to press but the proposals are as follows – see the website for current details.

These are the benefits we aim towards, most of which are achievable most of the time, once a better system of care has been established. Although in the real world there will always be exceptions, the level of care for all can be improved with a wider planning of supportive care in practice teams and attention to detail (*see also* Chapter 19).

Benefits to you in the primary healthcare team

- Make life easier for yourself in general practice palliative care.
- Join the national programme, using the tried and tested framework which has been piloted in a variety of situations, with adaptations in response to pilot Phases 1 and 2.
- Receive templates for you to adapt to local needs.
- Receive training, support and encouragement from the central team and others in the GSF programme.
- Link with the central team who have built up expertise in this area, are involved in other project areas across the UK and who can cross-reference your problems or ideas to other areas, e.g. common issues in other rural areas, etc.
- Receive the Supportive Care register.
- Receive Home Packs, including examples of booklets.
- Receive support from your facilitator, who will be connected to others across the UK undertaking this work.
- Improved teamwork, both in the practice and across teams.
- It enables and encourages you to make localised improvements in care.
- Networking with other interested coordinators in your area at lunch-time meetings.
- Enjoyment from better job satisfaction and watching improved service development – FUN!
- Possible financial reward, e.g. from BMA new contract, Network, etc. Cost neutral in most areas.
- Feedback of your audit/findings, supplying you with evidence to develop local commissioning of improved community service, e.g. through your PCO budgets/health board budgets.

Benefits to your patients

- Overall, a better sense of comfort, security and support to enable a better quality of life in the last months and a good 'quality of death'.
- Dying is more likely in the preferred place of choice, with less likelihood of crises.
- Supported by a strong well-coordinated, multi-professional team to give support – 'companions on the journey'.
- Greater sense of control and joint working with professionals – a feeling of being listened to and having their opinion valued.

- Greater acknowledgement of the patient and carers' own needs, agendas and preferences, e.g. preferred place of care, and better planning towards its fulfilment.
- The team, including those involved in out-of-hours care, is well informed of the patient's condition, needs, medication and preferences.
- Better symptom control.
- Better practice organisation of care and clarification of roles and contacts.
- Better inter-working with specialists and hospital/hospice care.
- Better information to patients and carers to enable shared decision making and reduce anxiety about the future.
- Better needs assessment and support for carers themselves.
- Better advanced planning of management and fewer crises, especially out of hours, leading to more time spent at home and less in hospital.
- More attention to non-medical and spiritual needs.
- Better advice on finances and benefits, access to equipment and other practical matters.
- Better bereavement care.
- Improved services in the community in response to the practice's evaluation and local needs assessment, e.g. more night sitters.

Benefits to the central team

- National improvements in community supportive and palliative care across the UK, in line with national policies, e.g. NHS Cancer Plan and Supportive Care Strategy.
- Developments are in line with strategic planning and policies of supporting agencies, i.e. the Macmillan Policy on community developments and the Cancer Services Collaborative Primary Care Section strategy on supportive care across the cancer journey.
- The sharing of a variety of ideas and improvements and the collective experience of community palliative care across the UK.
- Helping the development of creative new ideas and creative people.
- The seeking of further funding to resource supportive care.
- The central collection of some levels of information, leading to refining the key indicators for change and the criteria for good community palliative care, which in turn leads to better standard setting and benchmarking.
- Indicators of need and areas for future development – real information from grass roots primary care to feed back to the DOH, with possible resourcing implications.
- Guidance on further areas for research for academic departments.
- The development of a strong primary care group to interlink with secondary and specialist palliative care services.

Stepwise changes

The longest journey begins with a single step; the hardest part of beginning anything new is getting started. It's important to build up one step at a time, at a pace that feels comfortable, with an overview of the direction of the whole framework from the start. There is no rush to do it all at once, and developments will be better sustained if slowly rooted and owned by the whole team. Some suggest progressing in three or four steps (*see* Figure 11.3), at intervals of a few months, as seems appropriate and to take these steps in the combination and order that suits you best. Six-monthly reviews/audit meetings allow time and space for reflection, the building of team spirit and a perspective of vision, enabling gradually the aspiration of the gold standard of care to become more of a reality for our patients. Others prefer to take all standards on in one go, in a concentrated effort of radical redesign.

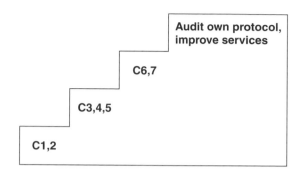

Figure 11.3: Step-by-step development of the seven Cs.

Remember to do a baseline assessment before instigating any changes and to be honest about your current position, and to measure again after a fixed interval, e.g. six months, to demonstrate changes. This forms a useful part of your assessment, triggers discussion and will be a satisfying demonstration of changes made. It will be of use in clinical governance measures and when applying for further funding – for example in awards, bids to PCTs and others, etc. – to provide local evidence that your efforts have made a difference, and to clarify further areas of development. Additionally, key outcome scores will track progressive improvements. As with any integrated care pathway evaluation, these should be as global, relevant and useful as possible and should not forget the more intangible aspects of care.

Pre-project work for facilitators

This involves stimulating interest, raising awareness, developing a group of motivated practices and setting up some administrative support. The suggested stepwise development could be taken in any order (after step 1) and at any suitable pace – there is always room to continuously improve.[3]

Step 1 (C1 and C2)

Set up the **register**, organise the **PHCT meetings** and clarify the role of the nominated coordinator – this is the bulk of the work.

Step 2 (C3, C4 and C5)

Add in better **assessment of symptoms** and clinical management, improving **out-of-hours** continuity with handover forms, etc., and build in targeted **learning**, e.g. invite the Macmillan nurses to discuss cases with you. Measure continuously and reflect on developments. Use significant event analysis when appropriate.

Step 3 (C6 and C7)

Add the use of improved information for **carers** (e.g. using Home Packs) and better support for carers. When reaching the terminal stages, examine your agreed protocol for the **last days of life** and use suggestions made.

Step 4

- **Review/audit** meetings six-monthly.
- Reflect back analysis of data to local commissioners to improve services.
- Develop your own **practice protocol** with local details, allocated personnel, etc.

Use your findings and reflections to examine the care you provide and how it could be improved. Collaborate with your facilitator, primary care organisation/Network to commission better services for your patients. Continue to measure (for improvement, not for judgement) and discuss as a team any new ideas and suggestions on how you will routinely provide supportive care for your seriously ill or dying patients. Then embody this in a practice protocol to set your own idealised patient pathway – your own gold standard of care for your patients.

Possible further steps

If appropriate, add in care for patients with **non-malignant conditions** (maybe using a different register if there are too many) and consider extending similar supportive care to all patients from diagnosis or fast-track referral. Some have developed the nursing role to make contact with patients at diagnosis and offer support from the PHCT at this devastating time of a patients journey, but this obviously takes more time than the implementation only of the GSF in practices.

Most practices have found the first step (C1 and C2) takes the most time and once established the later steps fall automatically into place. Introducing too much at once though can be a great disincentive and cause the destructive feeling of being overwhelmed, so adding to each step at the pace that feels right to you is preferable. However, the steps are meant to be seen as a whole in an attempt to cover all aspects of primary palliative care.

> Once the first step is done (C1 and C2), it becomes easier as some of the later steps fall automatically into place. For example, at the PHCT meetings, discussion of the patients in the register (C1) will automatically involve aspects of C3 (symptom control), C4 (out of hours if needed), C5 (learning, e.g. a Macmillan nurse may suggest a treatment the GP had not thought of, so he might think of it next time), C6 (the family may be involved and already have expressed concerns) and C7 (if in the dying phase, issues will be raised at the meeting). This should help practices a lot when they formalise the later steps. The beauty of the 7 Cs is that they are all interlinked and interact with each other, and all should be considered if we are to provide complete palliative care.
>
> Dr Hong Tseung, Facilitator, Halton PCT, GSF Phase 2

Preventing patients slipping through the cracks

The GSF offers a way of structuring and formalising many of the things you are already doing, encouraging you to fill it with your own ideas, relevant details and local colour to enable it to best fit your local situation.

- *Practice protocol.* The short-term goal is that, using the GSF as a template, you modify and adapt it and gradually grow it into an accepted practice protocol or system of care for the dying in your practice. In introducing ways of measuring or auditing care we must remember the function of these figures – 'measuring for improvement not measuring for judgement'. These are not for some nebulous higher source but are only of use if they will eventually benefit the patient in front of you.

- **Audit and local service improvement.** The longer-term goal is that, having reviewed and audited your care, using your own experience backed up by local measurements, you also help to mould the kind of service provision in your area that you and your patients need. For example, if you have had 32 deaths in the last six months and 17 died in their preferred place of choice, but with 11 there were problems with accessing night sitters, with 15 difficulties accessing drugs out of hours, with three problems getting commodes, etc., you now have some ammunition, pooled with other practices' findings, to make real changes. With better real life information about your area, your PCT, Network or other commissioning body will be more likely to respond to your request for improved services and you and your patients will benefit from targeted improvements.

- **Begin with palliative care for cancer patients** – the DS1500 and the 'surprise question'. There is as yet no easy all-embracing trigger for palliative care, but one suggested trigger in the community is from consideration of the completion of the DS1500 attendance allowance form. This should not act as a barrier at all, so if someone is not eligible for the DS1500 this does not mean they will be excluded from register. If you consider applying for fast-track attendance allowance for a patient and their estimated prognosis is six months or less, complete the DS1500 (Read-coded appropriately) and then enter them on the register.

  Some physicians developing an 'Improved care' programme in the US found that there were not enough appropriate early referrals for palliative care until they asked what came to be known as 'the surprise question'. They suggested that the trigger was: 'Which patients are sick enough that you would not be surprised if they died in the next year?' This question then opened the gates and appropriate early referrals for palliative care began coming in.[4] Perhaps this should be part of our regular thinking as we follow patients along the cancer journey, to ensure they receive maximum support at the appropriate time.

- **Later, consider extending to supportive care from diagnosis and include non-cancer and chronic cancer patients,** as previously discussed. It is obviously a little false to suddenly introduce the concepts of palliative care in primary care at a certain point, and it makes more sense in some ways to consider the more far-reaching concept of supportive care from diagnosis for all patients with a life-threatening illness. Referral to specialist palliative care could be after consideration of certain eligibility criteria.

- **Comprehensive care – starting small but not cherry picking.** The Framework has undergone continuous modification in its detail, offering a medley of options and ideas to use, own and adapt, but the overall structure has remained constant and should be seen as a whole, as the seven key areas – the seven Cs. Picking only one or two areas or topics is unlikely to fulfil the potential of the challenge, but a gradually developing and continuously improving system of care for the dying in a practice will ensure that practices are empowered and enabled to provide the best service more often – the excellent becoming the routine standard of care.

- **The problems of meetings.** You may find that holding PHCT meetings is difficult in certain practices, such as those with many partners working different shifts or on different sites. This is very understandable, but good effective compromises have been reached in these practices with real developments still made in patient care. It is not 'sink or swim' whether your practice can hold a PHCT meeting, even if it *is* preferable – a 'silver standard' will often do very well! It's very important to take the bigger view of why we are trying to make improvements and not to get overwhelmed in paperwork or structures for the sake of them. Improving patient care is the goal. However, holding a meeting is preferable if at all possible, as many will endorse, especially those who have moved from never having held clinical meetings to beginning them, and experience of multi-disciplinary team meetings (MDT) in hospital confirms this. District nurses in particular value these meetings. They have to be well run, efficient, focused and productive, however, and the use of the summary sheet in the register helps this process.

- *Use of information technology* – getting the best of both worlds. For those adept at information technology (IT) and electronic information sharing, using paper may seem a retrograde step. However, it still has its uses and on occasions, I would argue, it still exceeds the value of clever whiz-bang electronics. If the ethos of better communication is developed using paper versions, e.g. the Supportive Care register and the faxed handover form, then electronic versions can follow on smoothly. Electronic forms have fewer restrictions in the amount written, can be automatically updated and of course speedily transferred. Nurses have less regular access to computers, so practices may want to begin with paper versions such as those supplied and then, once established, adapt to electronic versions. It is helpful to share these developments with others across a Network or a PCT, e.g. common agreed Read codings, etc. An example is the combined use of the front-sheet of the register as a handover form and carer's register/database also in one form, which could be electronically transferred and adapted as needed. The skill is in managing to balance the best of electronic systems, e.g. rapid transmission, data collection, etc., with the steady old-fashioned paper versions, e.g. tangible accessible handover forms, a register in one place, patients' contributions to body charts or review sheets, etc.

- *Confidentiality* is a topical and complex issue in the light of the current Caldicott and other NHS Information Authority requirements. Both the Data Protection Act of 1998 and the European Bill of Human Rights, incorporated into English and Welsh law in October 2000, confirm that individuals are entitled to privacy and confidentiality in respect of their lives. Therefore obtaining informed consent is important, particularly regarding evaluations/audit. There has to be a balance between improving communication about patients across boundaries of care for their clinical benefit, whilst still maintaining their dignified and rightful need for confidentiality of information. Looking after palliative care patients involves many people. Opinions can sadly can grow into fact, whether true or not. We need to ensure that information is handled sensitively and confined only to those that need to know. The inappropriate sharing of private conversations of peoples' inner thoughts occasionally happens, and can merge imperceptibly into something resembling gossip, especially in small communities; this is a danger we must all guard against. Ideally, information, for example on the handover form, should be discussed with the patient and family and permission sought to pass it on to other professionals involved; most handover forms do include a consent box.

So, with your eyes fixed on the gold standard of best quality care for your patients in the last year of life, the kind you might wish for yourself or your family, the milestones are that:

1 you gradually build up improvements in a stepwise form, reflecting on your practice and constantly adding to the range of ideas and improvements (*see* Chapter 19)
2 you develop your own practice protocol for palliative care

3   you measure and audit your care after a period of time, e.g. six-monthly, and use your findings to help develop services in your area by submitting them, with others maybe, to your local commissioning bodies.

The GSF, still with ongoing evaluation but validated and borne out by real-life primary care experience, offers a possible way forward when you feel your practice, primary care organisation, network or hospice community wants to move from the struggles of real-life disorganised entropy to the more systematised order of the integrated care pathway.

When devastation hits a family in the form of a diagnosis of cancer or another end-stage illness, what can we offer our patients as they begin to face the end of their lives? What we can offer is ourselves; but also we can offer a structured, well-planned system that puts the patient and carer at its heart, listening to them and revolving around their needs, building up the strengths of the team and their sense of worth together, and ensuring that the best of care becomes normal practice. As Joanne Lynn put it:[5] we try to reduce the chance of this happening by sheer good luck, and make excellent care routine. In primary palliative care, we do well but we can always do better. Death is one certainty we all face: if we can do it for airlines, we can surely begin to do this for care of the dying at home.

The following pages are effectively the handbook that was used by practices when introducing the Gold Standards Framework, with certain modifications. It can be dipped into as needed, as a guide and reference, or read comprehensively for an overview. It has been adapted in the light of much experience but the basic framework has remained much the same. Some developments, reflections, ideas for improvement and examples of good practice are also included, but more can be added and updated on the website or in future versions as we continuously learn how to improve our care of the dying at home.

References

1   Gomas J M (1993) Palliative care at home: a reality or 'mission impossible'. *Pall Med.* **7**(11): 45–59.

2   Blanchard K and Johnson S (1983) *The One Minute Manager.* Harper Collins, London.

3   Covey S (1992) *The Seven Habits of Highly Effective People.* Simon and Schuster, London.

4   Trandrum G (2000) Asking the surprise question – the Franciscan Health System finds a way to reach dying patients sooner. Accelerating Change Today, The National Coalition of Health-care, Tacoma, Washington. *The Institute for Healthcare Improvement Magazine,* October 2000. www.nchc.org; www.ihi.org

5   Lynn J (2000) Sick to death and not taking it any more! Accelerating Change Today, The National Coalition of Healthcare, Tacoma, Washington. *The Institute for Healthcare Improvement Magazine,* October 2000. www.nchc.org; www.ihi.org

The light-hearted 'Reduced Shakespeare' summary of the Gold Standards Framework

There are three elements (with communication in each):

1   *Pick out and identify* the palliative care patients – lift them above the rest, using a register to centralise information. Discuss them as a team regularly – build in better communication tools and give someone in the practice the task of coordinating the care (C1 and C2).

2   Use tools to better *assess* patient and carer choices, needs, symptoms and problems; listen more closely *and respond* to these; refer appropriately (C3). At intervals, reflect on your practice, linking in learning with palliative care specialists, e.g. local Macmillan nurse, and audit your care to determine where to target changes in your practice and requests for resources. Link with clinical governance, measure for improvement and celebrate success and teamwork (C5).

3   Build in advanced/proactive *planning* and better *communication* in everything. Plan in response to patient and carer need, and 'horizon-scanning' of what might happen next. Send a handover form to the cooperative/out-of-hours team and leave drugs and equipment they might need in the home (C4). Consider carers' needs and give them useful information and contact details, especially for a crisis (C6). Ensure good care in the last days of life (check-list); consider bereavement care (C7). Agree a practice protocol for all dying patients so that the best of care becomes normal practice – 'this is what we do for our palliative care patients'. Use tools to improve communication. Maybe, extend this support from diagnosis and for patients with conditions other than cancer. Enjoy your work!

The seven Cs

The Gold Standards Framework for palliative care in primary healthcare teams

C1 Communication

Practices maintain a supportive care register (paper or electronic) to record, plan and monitor patient care, and as a tool to discuss regularly at their monthly PHCT meetings. The aims of the meetings are to improve:

- the flow of information
- advanced planning/proactive care
- measurement and audit, to clarify areas for improvement in future at patient, practice, PCT and network level.

C2 Coordination

Each PHCT has a nominated coordinator for palliative care (e.g. district nurse) to ensure good organisation and coordination of care in a practice by overseeing the process, i.e.:

- maintaining the register problems/concerns, summary care plans, symptom sheets, handover forms, audit data, etc.
- organising PHCT meetings for discussion, planning, case analysis, education etc.
- using tools such as a check-list, e.g. PEPSI COLA, to cover all areas of care.

C3 Control of symptoms

Each patient has their symptoms, problems and concerns (physical, psychological, social, spiritual and practical) assessed, recorded, discussed and acted upon, according to an agreed process. The focus is more on the patient's agenda.

C4 Continuity

Practices will transfer information to the out-of-hours services for palliative care patients, e.g. using a handover form and out-of-hours protocol. This builds in anticipatory care to reduce crises and inappropriate admissions. Information should also be passed on to other relevant services, e.g. hospice/oncology dept (e.g. using patient-held records/medication cards). Record and minimise the number of professionals involved, i.e. note lead GP, lead DN, etc.

C5 Continued learning

The PHCT will be committed to continued learning of skills and information relevant to patients seen – 'learn as you go'. Using practice-based or external teaching, lectures/videos, significant event analysis or other tools, the practice and personal development plans and audits/appraisals are implemented. A practice reference resource is assembled. Learning is clinical, organisational/strategic and also attitude/approach, e.g. communication skills.

C6 **Carer support**

- *Emotional support*. Carers are supported, listened to, kept fully informed and encouraged and educated to play as full a role in the patient's care as they wish. They are regarded as an integral part of the team.

- *Practical support*. Practical hands-on support is supplied where possible, e.g. night sitter, respite, commode, etc.

- *Bereavement*. Practices plan support, e.g. practice protocol, visits, notes tagged, others informed, etc.

- *Staff support* is inbuilt and nurtured, leading to better teamwork and job satisfaction.

C7 **Care of the dying** (terminal phase)

Patients in the last days of life are cared for appropriately, e.g. by following the Liverpool Integrated Care Pathway. This includes stopping non-essential interventions and drugs, comfort measures, psychological and religious/spiritual support, bereavement planning, communication and care after death being assessed, recorded and acted upon.

CHAPTER 12

Communication: Gold Standard 1

C1

Practices maintain a Supportive Care register (paper or electronic) to record, plan and monitor patient care, and as a tool to discuss regularly at their monthly PHCT meetings. The aims of the meetings are to improve:

1 the flow of information
2 advanced planning/proactive care
3 measurement and audit, to clarify areas for improvement in future at patient, practice, PCT and network level.

Why?

- The Supportive Care register improves communication, information flow and updating within the PHCT.
- The register acts as a central place to keep all facts to hand for team discussion.
- It is a vehicle for PHCT meetings (in ward-round style) to discuss patients regularly and keep them in mind – the summary sheet can act as a focus to keep discussion directed and efficient.
- It acts as a prompt in proactive planning of palliative care needs and highlights trouble areas – this then leads to actions such as leaving drugs in the home. This is particularly important as the terminal phase is approached.
- It measures certain factors leading to audit – this can provide evidence for the need for changes either in the practice, or be recommended to the PCT/hospice/pharmacists/ Network, e.g. lack of night sitters, accessing drugs, etc.
- Without such measurements, real change is difficult – cumulative numbers from practices/PCTs can provide strong ammunition to drive improvements in care.
- Six-monthly special review meetings are recommended for practices, to take an overview examination of their care, reflect on needs and feed back to PCTs via their PCT cancer lead, and thereby to the Cancer Network, who could help implement change. Use of significant event analysis/'traffic lights' approach at such meetings can be valuable.
- Communication involves many areas (*see* Figure 12.1). There may be many gaps in communication, e.g. between primary care and hospitals, etc. Constant observation of the flow of information and areas of need is required to help plug potential gaps.
- With better communication, patients and carers can be more active in decision making and feel that they are retaining some degree of control, whilst teams can better anticipate needs and initiate the appropriate care.

One particular concern that was mentioned often was that patients wanted somebody to take the initiative rather than leave it all up to them.

Report from patients' and carers' views from the
North West Region Project in Primary Cancer Care[1]

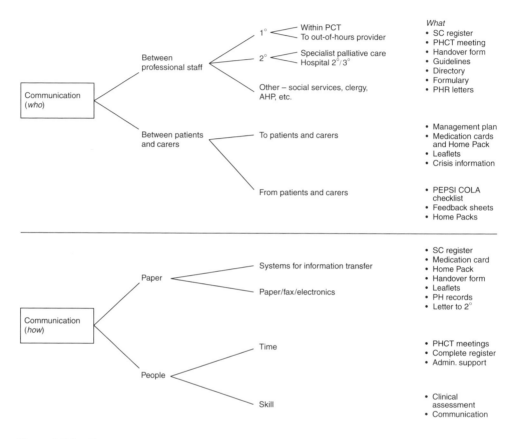

Figure 12.1: Communication.

What?

- The Supportive Care register is for those patients in the last 6–12 months of life, i.e. the suggested point of entry is the need for DS1500, but this should be interpreted loosely and all approaching the end of curative treatment or the last year considered.
- Initially we suggest starting with cancer patients, but once developed, extending it to all seriously ill with non-cancer illnesses, e.g. motor neurone disease, end-stage heart failure, etc.
- A different section or folder could be used for those with more chronic cancer or other serious illnesses, if more practical. Most people find the distinction 'active and inactive' or 'poorlies and pending' a useful division, but this may not correspond exclusively with those in the terminal stages – some may be in the active section when recently discharged from hospital or undergoing aggressive treatment.

- The Supportive Care register is a loose-leafed, paper-based folder that can be assembled for you to use and adapt as you see fit. It is a central collection of information for the practice, but it can act as several forms in one to reduce paperwork (*see* Appendix for enclosures; further copies of sheets are available at www.radcliffe-oxford.com/caring).

We can identify clearly who the patients are ... when we are discussing with the GPs at the meetings ... We have got them all in one place, so we can reflect on the deaths that we have had in the last month ... We can then add people to the register that the GPs want to tell us about in the meeting, so having it all together keeps them special if you like, and the GPs are doing that now – they are treating their patients as a bit more special.

DN, coordinator, GSF Phase 2

- Alternative electronic versions are being used in practice computer systems, which will obviously be the way forward in future, with electronic health records, etc. However, the paper version promotes the concept of a means to identify and single out these palliative care patients, and the systematic recording of relevant information.
- There is a front-sheet for every patient which acts as (1) a summary of treatment, problems and concerns with contact details, but could also be used as (2) a handover form if faxed to the out-of-hours provider, and (3) for a carers' database, collecting together all carers' details, as recommended in the National Carers' Strategy.[2]
- Behind the front-sheet can be kept the problems/concerns overview, the *aide-mémoire* PEPSI COLA check-list (*see* Boxes 13.1 and 13.2), the other handover form if used, the body charts, the significant event analysis, 'traffic lights', etc., as practice teams prefer (*see* Chapter 14).
- The lead GP and lead DN are noted for each patient, with second on-calls to cover absence, to reduce the number of different people that the patient sees. It has been estimated that some patients can see about 75 different healthcare professionals in the course of their illness; we want to minimise this in primary care.

Patients are getting better care because they are seeing, or they are more likely to see, the same GP or the same nurse at each visit, so it's easier to follow things through and continue care.

DN, Coordinator, GSF Phase 2

- National cancer datasets are developing and are likely to become statutory requirements in primary care (according to the NHS Cancer Plan). Information from the Supportive Care register will feed into and cross-reference these. The figures will work for us in our routine practice, helping us to actively manage patients and triggering measures of quality care. The Cancer Information subgroup of the NHSIA[3] has been consulted in the Supportive Care register's production, and there is much overlap. (The register templates may alter in line with national recommendations – details are on the website). Information can be held electronically, and so could feed into the PCT and Cancer Network's requirements for data collection, which would then provide information for the commissioning and management of services. These could be Read-coded with commonly agreed codes. But initially, for the purposes of this project, a register will help develop this ethos of improved teamworking, planning and audit. There are many current developments, and much potential for advance using electronic methods, so this is an area to watch in future. One such development is a Macmillan project in Ellesmere Port which has developed an electronic practice register that triggers good care at all stages of the cancer journey.[4]
- It is recommended that practice teams go through this register briefly as part of the monthly PHCT meetings, although as things move fast in care of the dying, weekly PHCT meetings would be even better. It need only form part of the meeting, occupying

perhaps a regular 10 to 20-minute slot to discuss the practice's most seriously ill patients. Then at three- to six-monthly intervals, special review meetings can be held to reflect on cumulative measures and audit against standards (*see* www.radcliffe-oxford.com/caring for suggested formats for such meetings).

- Use of the register at regular PHCT meetings has become one of the most fruitful and important parts of the whole project, and forms the hub of the wheel around which everything else develops. However, some practices find regular meetings hard to achieve for various reasons. Improvements in care can still be made in these practices and occasional review meetings may still be possible.

Having a regular meeting to discuss these patients was a great improvement for us and we, as nurses, very much value the opportunity to discuss them and share the burden of care with the whole team. We can think ahead of possible problems and put things in place to prevent crises and allay the fears of the relatives. We didn't have meetings like this before and we wouldn't be without them now.

DN, Coordinator, Huddersfield, GSF Pilot Phase 1

- If you meet resistance, wait, and later it may be worth exploring with the team how they prioritise the many demands on their time and which patients are most needy and could benefit most from good quality primary care. It is easy to feel overwhelmed and 'lose the wood for the trees'; palliative care is a good example of an area in which we operate at maximum effectiveness when we share care as a team – no one individual can do it all themselves. When we 'think team' we are maximising the potential of the support we are able to offer to patients and ourselves. There are many hidden benefits in team-building and a greater appreciation of each others' roles. District nurses appreciate the chance to learn of patients earlier in their journey, share ideas and plan anticipatory care. Other team members can pick up ideas of problem management and will become better informed of their partners' patients, which helps if they have to deal with them later.

A positive outcome was the fact that when I went to see my partner's patient out of hours, I was able to say: 'Dr A. has told me about you and I understand that X and Y are your main difficulties.' Patients really appreciate the continuity of care and the fact that we have cared enough to discuss them as a team.

Northern Ireland GP, GSF Phase 2

- We have to prioritise these patients in the last year of life, reorganise to put some time aside to develop roles and good functioning of the team. The development of multidisciplinary team meetings has been one of the most productive aspects of the Quality Standards for hospital cancer care since it became a requirement for all secondary services in January 2001,[5] and there are many examples of it being one of the most important developments. We in primary care have perhaps been a little slack in developing the proactive rather than reactive aspect of care, and some in secondary care find this lack of planning meetings surprising; good communication and teamwork are now recognised as crucial in all settings.

We are a big practice with 10 doctors in two sites. Even though we weren't able to have regular meetings in our practice, one of us did discuss each patient with the relevant GP, at regular intervals and after a death, using the register and the 'traffic lights' page. Everyone wants to keep out of the red areas! We all feel that care has really improved, despite not having meetings, since starting the GSF work.

DN, Coordinator, Calderdale, GSF Phase 1

- Other members of the team know about patients on the register, perhaps by listing them on a white board in the surgery, so that receptionists might speed up prescriptions for them, are sensitive to the needs of carers and the rest of the team are aware that a serious event is happening to that family, when other family members attend the surgery.

How/who/when?

- The nominated coordinator should ensure the register is completed and kept up to date and that patients are discussed at PHCT meetings.
- The coordinator should organise monthly (or weekly) PHCT meetings, e.g. with invited Macmillan nurses, plus at least six-monthly review meetings.
- Communication skills training is highly recommended when available – this involves skills in breaking bad news, etc.

Talking to members of the practice team, there is consensus that there is improved communication across the practice about ill patients. The clinical team is more aware of the problems patients are experiencing. There is a more systematic approach to recording data and making sure tasks on the check-list are completed. Recording data provides an opportunity to audit outcomes such as place of death, whether wishes of patients were recorded and if wishes were achieved.

GP Facilitator, Liverpool, GSF Phase 2

What if ...: potential benefits

What if:

- every seriously ill patient approaching their last months of life received the benefit of all the coordinated skills and care available in the primary care team, dovetailed with those in hospital or specialist care. This is the ideal of seamless care.
- the care of all seriously ill patients was discussed in team meetings (with specialist advice available), thereby improving communication within the team, building in anticipation of needs plus a chance for audit, reflection and debriefing. This could lead to implementing further improvements, e.g. requesting more night sitters to improve care on a wider scale. This team preplanning and initiating care should lead to fewer crises, more anticipation, better carer support and more dying well in their place of choice.
- patients and carers are seen as integral members of the team, with their views and needs listened to, noted, communicated and responded to appropriately.
- patients and carers feel that someone is taking the initiative rather than leaving it all up to them, that there are some 'companions on the journey'.

Discussion

Benefits of a supportive care register

The benefits of a register include:

- communication within the PHCT and keeping in mind patients' needs
- valuing different skills of the multidisciplinary team
- proactive planning, especially carer support, leading to fewer crises
- improved education/significant event analysis
- audit and review, leading to changes and constant development.

Patient-held records

- Many examples of patient-held records are developing across the country. They can become an invaluable vehicle for promoting good communication, especially across the boundaries of care between primary, secondary, tertiary and specialist palliative care services. However, where they sometimes have foundered has been in the necessary duplication of doctors and other staff writing in notes – too much paperwork is a killer to good ideas! To avoid this, some used a single set of notes or patient-held records.[6,7]
- The overall aim of patient-held records is to improve communication:
  - *to* the patients and carers
  - *from* the patients and carers
  - *between* professionals.

The Home Pack

The *Home Pack*, available in the tool kit or on the website, is for patients to keep at home as a means of facilitating better communication with patients and carers. Enclosed in the pack, which can be customised according to each patient's requirements, are contact details and individualised notes and booklets, with a Weekly Review sheet for patients and carers to feed back their views. The folder can also contain means to improve communication between professionals, i.e. the *handover form* (*see* Chapter 15), the *medication record card* (*see* below), etc. There are many excellent booklets available from Cancerbacup, Cancerlink, Macmillan, etc. – for more details see the excellent resource directory produced by Macmillan, which contains details about all available information materials relating to cancer.[8] Patients with other conditions can be supported with material from the appropriate support agency.

> *Access to appropriate information can empower patients to express their treatment preferences and help to improve the information base of clinical decisions.*[9]

The medication record card

The medication record card is a simple card (*see* the tool kit or www.radcliffe-oxford. com/caring) which can be kept by patients in a plastic folder and taken on all hospital or hospice trips. It is important to keep it updated with current treatments to be able to judge better changes in medication as needed. It can be used to help empower patients and explain the reasons and functions of medications, and colour-coding bottles with the card clarifies which ones are the 'little white tablets' and which should be taken at what time. It also functions as a useful trigger for doctors as potentially dangerous drug combinations will be highlighted, preventing, for example, the frail patient already on steroids and morphine having a NSAID such as naproxen added without being covered by a gastric protector such as omeprazole, which would make a gastric bleed a real possibility. Also, as morphine is increased, laxatives are not always increased proportionately, and ensuing constipation can be more troublesome than the original pain. Again, this can be clearly charted on the medication card.

> *This was a very simple idea that made a really big difference. Patients liked knowing more about their treatment and having some control, and we felt safer with better documentation of their drugs. When the patient said they were on the little white tablets, we knew which ones they meant and could give advice accordingly.*
>
> GP, GSF Phase 1

Communication to other teams

It is important to ensure good two-way communication across teams in other areas, e.g. hospices and hospitals, occupational therapists, social services, etc. Keeping records in the home pack or patient-held record can help improve this. Practices should have policies and protocols to inform relevant agencies after a death, e.g. the out-of-hours provider (who may be accumulating handover forms!) and hospitals to cancel appointments etc., but these may need updating and maybe formalising at times. Hospital services are also trying to improve two-way communication with specified primary care information requirements at the point of diagnosis, standardised discharge letters, etc.

It has been suggested by the Cancer Services Collaborative Primary Care Group that all information, particularly at diagnosis, should contain the following:

D   Diagnosis and prognosis as general guidance
O   Options regarding treatment
C   Care plan, timescales and follow-up
T   Told what the patient and carer have been told
O   Other agencies involved
R   Review who, where and when.[10]

Many hospital staff would like to improve communication with primary care teams, e.g. at the point of discharging a patient or at diagnosis, but are not sure who to contact. Many say that it is difficult to get past receptionists to those in primary care who need to know. Therefore, if the hospital knows who the coordinator (*see* Chapter 13) is in the practice, and their contact details, direct information can be passed more efficiently, and a better dialogue set up, to improve patient care.

References

1 North West Region Primary Care Cancer Standards, www.nwrocancer.org.uk

2 Department of Health (1999) *A National Strategy for Carers*. The Stationery Office, London.

3 More details are available on www.cancer.nhsia.nhs.uk/dataset

4 Further details are available from a.dawson@macmillan.org.uk

5 NHS Executive (2000) *Manual of Cancer Services*. Department of Health, London.

6 Measham Practice's Beacon award-winning patient-held records. Available from Orest Mulka on mmu@tesco.net or 01530 270667.

7 For more details of the Hadley Practice patient-held records in Dorset, contact Chris McCall cmcall@btinternet.com or adawson@macmillan.org.uk

8 Macmillan Cancer Relief (2000) *A Directory of Information Materials for People with Cancer 2001/2*. Macmillan Cancer Relief, London.

9 King's Fund (1998) *Informing Patients: an assessment of patient information*. King's Fund, London.

10 Jones P (2002) *Communication Pathway. Primary Care Group of Cancer Services Collaborative.* www.modern.nhs.uk/cancer

CHAPTER 13

Coordination: Gold Standard 2

C2

Each PHCT has a *nominated coordinator* for palliative care (e.g. district nurse/manager/practice nurse) to ensure good organisation and coordination of care in the practice by overseeing the process, i.e.:

- maintaining the register, care plans, symptom sheets, handover forms, audit data, etc.
- organising PHCT meetings for discussion, planning, case analysis, education, etc.
- using check-lists, tools and protocols to cover all areas of care, e.g. PACA scale, PEPSI COLA, end-of-life care, etc.

Why

Coordination is a real skill and vitally important in the complexities of the modern healthcare system. Patients and their carers appreciate the sense that someone is acting as a guide and understands their way round the system. Most problems arise from a lack of coordination and communication – people can slip through the net too easily.

In developing a more comprehensive system of care for dying patients, one person in the team should overview the process – ask everyone to do it and it won't get done, give one person (usually a nurse or manager) a task and it will happen! Deficits and duplication of tasks occur easily in practice across the boundaries of care. It is easy to think someone else has done something, e.g. completing DS1500 forms, and thus to inadvertently omit them (*see* the example of changing the hamster's water on p. 94). The coordinator ensures these key tasks are carried out by overseeing improvements in organisation of the system of care and being responsible for its coordination. They do not have to do everything themselves, for example if the coordinator is a DN they may need admin back-up to fulfil their tasks, e.g. sending handover forms.

NB. This is not the same as the 'linkworker', or primary care oncology nurse, who may coordinate care for individual patients. This person does not replace the 'key professional' named on the register frontsheet, who is the clinician (GP or DN) involved in that patient's care. The role of the coordinator relates to the practice team's organisation of care, rather than the individual patient's, although this may well overlap. Some teams develop the idea of the nurse's role being extended from diagnosis and following the patient's journey, so being the main point of contact for patients and acting as advocate and reference point during contact with secondary and tertiary care. This latter role of 'cancer coordinator' or primary care cancer nurse is being piloted in some areas, but does entail more work and dedicated time than is required of the practice coordinators for the GSF.[1]

What

The coordinator acts as the 'conductor of the orchestra'! They also act as a link with other groups, e.g. hospital staff, social services, specialist palliative care, clinical nurse specialists, clergy or religious leaders, etc. The lead GP backs them up, but by improving the system of care, there should be little extra work for the GPs, i.e. more effective and efficient use of time and effort. The coordinator's time input is greatest in the set-up period, but then levels off as the work becomes a standard part of practice routine. The six-monthly audit meetings will require more time for preparation, ideally helped by administrative staff.

There are three specific tasks involved in the coordination:

1 to assemble the supportive care register (paper and/or computer)
2 to organise the regular PHCT meetings and six-monthly review meetings
3 to check that paperwork is completed and updated to allow better assessment and planning, e.g. handover form, summary sheets, etc.

In doing this there is a raising of awareness of the needs of these seriously ill patients – prioritising and moving palliative care patients up the agenda.

We also have to watch for the overwhelming nature of paperwork – it is there to serve us, not to take mastery over us! Only use what is useful and if your present system works well for all the team, gradually add anything else you find most helpful. Be constantly vigilant and reduce duplication. However, such paperwork can lead to better assessment and planning and better communication – so seek to maintain the balance.

Who/how

Asking one person in a team to be a coordinator reduces the chance of things slipping through the net or duplication of care. They should be encouraged and supported in their role.

The coordinator checks the Supportive Care register regularly (weekly at least), checking assessments have been made, handover forms sent, drugs available, etc. The PHCT meetings are organised, prepared for and kept efficient and effective by them – good chairing may be needed to avoid too many tangents (see Figure 13.1).

An area often omitted is the provision of *customised information* to patients and carers. The Home Pack (see the GSF tool kit and the website) is one suggestion. Enclosed is a suggested template – add your own information and contact details here to make this localised and relevant for you. Add in any booklets/factsheets found useful or write your own. Introduce this at a time and at a pace that's appropriate – they are back up to the information you're giving verbally, plus more resources if wanted. Information provided promotes a sense of security at home, a feeling of control and a helpful resource in a crisis. Encourage real listening – use the feedback sheets from patients and carers if helpful. The Home Pack folders also could keep the medication cards, handover forms, management plans or other information of use to professionals involved in the care – this then becomes a dynamic patient-held record. Sometimes carers need this even more than patients – the folder could be used to hold any relevant papers or information for the patient, as distinct from the DN notes which are geared more for health professionals.

What if ...

What if a practice functions as a team, orchestrated by a key coordinator who ensures that communication and teamwork are improved. With a well-organised coordinated system, time

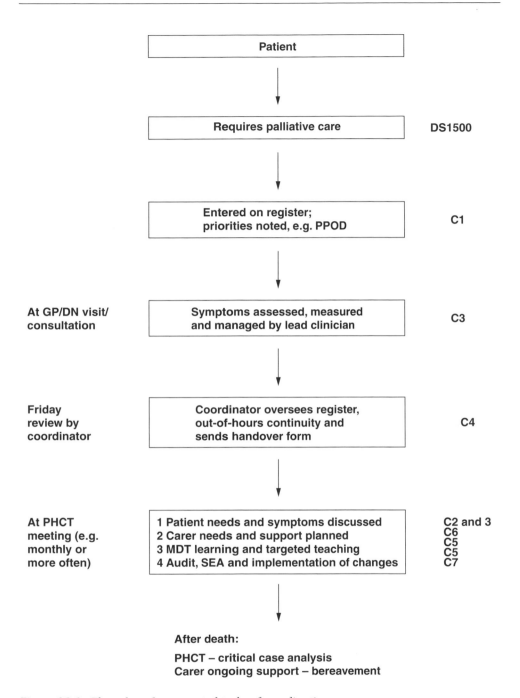

Figure 13.1: Flow chart for suggested tasks of coordination.

is saved by keeping records in one place, routine care is at the best standard, the practice interlinks well with other agencies – the seams of the seamless service are kept on the inside!

Discussion

You are the overall team coordinator of the Gold Standard Framework, so should ensure that everyone in your team understands what is going on and how to contribute, and will feed information back to you. You do not have to do it all yourself, but oversee it in the practice as the link person for your team (*see* Figure 13.1). You are the 'conductor of the orchestra' aiming to create a harmonious sound through effective teamworking. There are a number of options offered here but they are not all appropriate for each patient – take what works and use it to develop or adapt your own.

Check-list of the coordinator's tasks

C1 Communication

1　Maintain the Supportive Care register and collection of information (divide this into active and inactive if useful).
2　Organise regular PHCT meetings (monthly minimum, possibly weekly) to discuss all relevant patients. Keep staff updated between times. If impossible, communicate in other ways.
3　Meetings should be chaired efficiently – keep relevant and focused.
4　Be proactive and consider issues of the past, present and future – plan ahead.
5　Maintain a record of carers (this may be part of the Supportive Care register).
6　Ensure the medication cards are updated.
7　Check carers and patients receive relevant customised information of use to them (often neglected).
8　Keep a check-list of who to contact *after a death*, e.g. hospital, specialist staff (to prevent further appointments being sent), out-of-hours provider, etc.

C2 Coordinator

1　Undertake the orchestration of tasks in the practice team.
2　Check paperwork is up to date (handover form, DS1500, etc.)
3　Discuss and record advanced care planning with patient and carer and with staff.
4　Ensure good communication in the team – this may be outside meetings.
5　Organise a deputy for your absences.
6　Give your contact details as coordinator to relevant hospital and hospice staff, e.g. notify the oncology ward staff so they can contact you before a patient is discharged home.

C3 Control of symptoms

Four levels suggested – the first being used for most patients, the others optional. *The SCR sheets indicated refer to the template used in the Supportive Care Register SCR 1–7 – see www.radcliffe-oxford.com/caring and the Appendix.*

1　Ensure the summary sheet (SCR1), frontsheet (SCR2) and, preferably, problems/concerns check-list (SCR3) for each patient are updated regularly. Ensure appropriate referral is made, e.g. lead GP; specialist palliative care. Use the summary sheet at PHCT meetings to keep discussion focused. These are the main forms to use routinely – others optional as needed.

2   Additionally, use a holistic/psychosocial check-list, e.g. PEPSI COLA (SCR4), at regular intervals and track problems (e.g. using *aide-mémoire*). Take a broad view of problems, not just medical but include social, financial, housework, relationship, fears, deeper issues, sense of control – 'going to the pub, not just the pain'. Use this if found helpful only.

3   When indicated, for example when the patient is in pain, ensure accurate assessment of symptoms, using a body chart and visual analogue scales, at appropriate times. Use trigger questions for neuropathic pain and add adjuvant analgesics if indicated.

4   Spiritual and religious care discussed.

C4 Continuity out of hours

1   Send a handover form or alternative (e.g. frontsheet) to the out-of-hours provider. This should be updated at least fortnightly (longer if very stable, more frequently if many changes). Devise a system for easy update so not repeating basics, e.g. electronic format (examples can be provided).

2   Ensure the patient and carer know who to contact in an emergency (complete the section in the Home Pack) and how.

3   Ensure pre-emptive carer support is requested (see care gaps in the Home Pack). Consider early booking of respite, night sitters, Marie Curie nurses, nursing homes, etc.

4   Clarify the availability of specialists on call, medical or nursing staff, e.g. from the local hospice, and inform your team: maybe add to the handover form for the on-call doctor.

5   Ensure anticipated drugs are left in the home, where appropriate, or are readily available elsewhere. At a minimum leave enough to cover the out-of-hours period, allowing for increased dosage. PRN drugs should be written up and prescribed, plus authorisation completed for nurses. Some, for example, leave a standard four drugs in a labelled plastic box in the fridge, i.e. diamorphine, midazolam, hyoscine and haloperidol/levomorpromazine.

C5 Continued learning

1   At the organised monthly PHCT meetings to discuss patients on the Supportive Care register, ensure good proactive planning, anticipation of need and carer support – share ideas, problems and learning points.

2   Use significant event analysis, e.g. traffic lights, to discuss what aspects of care are good and what could be improved upon – either during care or after the death of the patient. Note areas of deficiency of care, e.g. lack of night sitters, drugs access, etc., for future reference.

3   Invite specialists, e.g. local Macmillan nurses, community clinical nurse specialists and hospice staff, to team meetings.

4   Organise targeted teaching related to issues brought up in case discussions – 'learn as you go' – e.g. the specialist palliative care team, videos, CD roms about, for example, hypercalcaemia, neuropathic pain, stomas, depression, etc. Use Chapters 7 and 8 to summarise brief learning points.

5   Organise six-monthly review/audit meetings to review what you have found, e.g. numbers dying at home and quality of death. Feed in specific teaching/specialist opinions here.

C6 Carer support

1   Check that the carer is asked reguarly about their own general needs and support (and that their responses are recorded as part of the PEPSI COLA or problems/concerns check-list). Note their comments on the Weekly Review sheet in the Home Pack.

2 Check each carer is given a customised information pack and that the contents are updated as appropriate with particular leaflets/information. Use websites, Cancerlink and Cancerbacup booklets plus more local information.

3 Check that each carer is listed on the carers' register/database.

4 Check that carers are given contact details for emergencies (in the Home Pack or on the yellow medication card or even as a fridge magnet).

5 Bereavement – consider the practice's policies for bereaved carers.

C7 Care in the dying phase

1 Recognise when a patient is entering the dying phase and communicate this to others, including the family. The criteria used by the Liverpool Integrated Care Pathway are when two of the following apply:
- increasing sleepiness/unconsciousness/semi-comatosed
- bedbound
- only able to take sips of fluid
- unable to take oral tablet medication.

2 Go through the check-list given in C7 (p. 253) of specific tasks relating to terminal care.

3 Introduce a protocol, e.g. the Liverpool Integrated Care Pathway for the Dying, if wanted.

Don't dismay! At the beginning it can seem like a daunting task, but slowly the pieces come together. Don't feel like your ship is sinking – do one thing at a time and when you're happy, move on. Be proud of what you've achieved rather than feeling 'down' because you haven't achieved it all. For example, what we achieved with the Gold Standards Framework after five months included better communication in the practice, a cancer register, carer support, focus on the patient agenda, improved flow of information, better forward planning and significant event analysis. What we still have to do includes improving handover forms and PHCT meetings, looking at our bereavement service, thinking about continued learning, expanding the cancer register, standardising Read codes and so on.
Jane Melvin, DN coordinator, Castlefields Surgery, Halton

Suggested evaluation and feedback

Suggested evaluation and feedback include the following.

1 The *baseline review questionnaire* (Q1) is an important baseline assessment and stimulus for thought, to undertake before commencing the Gold Standards Framework, then to send to your facilitator. The repeated questionnaire, for example six months later (Q2), allows you to measure improvements, which may be of help to your commissioning bodies, i.e. PCTs. These are being measured for the Macmillan GSF Programme at 0, 3, 6 (and ?12) months.

2 Brief monthly '*key outcomes*' *feedback sheets* are a quick assessment of progress and may be of use to you in monitoring your progress. Alternatively, a template for discussion/ SEA for patient's care after a death is suggested. This is optional in the Macmillan GSF Programme. Many of the best things cannot be measured.

3 Attend local *feedback meetings* of coordinators for support and sharing of ideas. Contribute your ideas/suggestions/feedback for others in your group and for your facilitator to report back centrally, such as adaptations or new ways you have found to improve care. Spread ideas and good practice and also share problems and lessons learned with others in the GSF, plus PCTs, Networks, etc.

4 Attend any national or regional *conferences* available, especially as part of the Macmillan GSF Programme, and share ideas.

The synergy of exploring problems together

Improvement is part of life. Watch how children learn to ride a bike: they make mistakes but keep on trying and they measure their progress by the distance covered – measuring to learn, not to feel bad. When a group of optimistic and motivated people ask the same questions they can become part of a dynamic curious team, exploring new ways of working together and bringing them home to test them out. There is a special synergy in the collective energy of people working together to explore a question. The system is important but people make the difference.

Don Berwick[2]

Ideas and suggestions – being creative!

This should be a springboard for ideas. It is likely that the more you focus on this area, the more ideas you will have on how to improve your practice for the variety of patients you come across in your own specific locality. Every area has its own flavours. The GSF should be used as a 'climbing frame' to help get you going, but the real benefit is in the way you fill in the gaps yourselves and develop your own ideas. No doubt you will already have examples of good practice and great ideas that others could benefit from trying out. *The 'networking' and collaborating aspects of this work are crucial.*

Use the collaborative model of developing new ideas – the Plan, Do, Study, Act model (*see* Figure 6.5) – learning from mistakes as well as successes, and make a point of sharing these. Ask yourself the following questions:

1 What are we trying to accomplish? (*Aims*)
2 How will we know that a change is an improvement? What measures can be made? How will we know if we get there? (*Measures*)
3 What changes can we make that will result in the improvements we seek? (*Change principles*)

This can be at your local feedback meetings, the feedback conferences, on a list-server or website, directly to the central team or through your facilitator, who will then feed them back centrally, always crediting you with your work. One person's solutions are not necessarily another's, but we may be able to find common ground by sharing the problems. A very enjoyable and creative synergy can be derived from brainstorming problems together. We're all trying to move on in the same direction. We do well but can we do even better – there's an opportunity here to 'raise our game', both individually and collectively. The GSF gives us a rare chance to think collaboratively and move services on together, with a medley of options for each signpost or gold standard: lessons learned in Scotland can be of help in Dorset or Liverpool. It presents us with a chance to share some of the good practice that is happening in the NHS today, and should be a springboard for ideas.

Other notes

PEPSI COLA check-list (used with permission)

This is a broad-brush holistic approach to trigger consideration of all areas, not a tick box. The suggested questions for each area are ways of ensuring broader issues relating to psychosocial care are covered, such as emotional, practical, spiritual and social aspects. Of course it will not be exhaustive. Planning together with patient and carers, responding to their agendas and their advanced care needs and recording this is useful, e.g. prefers home care, wants to go to hospice in last days, etc. A 'PEPSI COLA aide-mémoire' (*see* Boxes 13.1 and 13.2) was created in the feedback from one pilot practice to track problems across time

Box 13.1 PEPSI COLA check-list: summary only

Physical
symptom control, etc.

Emotional
adjustment, depression

Personal
spiritual care

Social support
services, benefits, carer support

Information and communication
between professionals, to patient, from patient

Control
choice, dignity, place of death

Out of Hours and Emergency
continuity

Late
end-of-life/terminal care

Afterwards
assessment/audit, bereavement and family support

Box 13.2 PEPSI COLA check-list for palliative care needs of patients and carers

Physical
- symptom chart, including pain diagram
- quality of life issues
- overall management plan, e.g. more radiotherapy, etc.
- medication – recorded on drug card, plus any allergies or adverse reactions, plus regular and PRN, e.g. oramorph PRN, co-prescribing of laxatives, etc.
- is a syringe driver useful
- other devices, e.g. TENS, nebuliser
- compliance – pill box?/checking
- pruning – has redundant non-urgent medication been stopped, e.g. antihypertensives in terminal phase, etc.
- complementary therapies, e.g. aromatherapy

Emotional

- emotional reaction and adjustment of patient, carers and rest of family
- understanding of diagnosis – disease process
- what might signify deterioration and what to expect
- fears discussed where possible
- relationships – unfinished business
- is the patient clinically depressed
- care for children and young people affected by a dying member of the family
- difference of opinion between patient and carer

Personal and spiritual care

- what is on the patient/carer's agenda
- religious needs identified and addressed
- spiritual issues – meaning, dignity, hope, worth, etc.
- inner turmoil or a need for forgiveness for past issues
- inner peace

Social support

- is there a care plan
- care for carers, e.g. planned respite, night sitters, home care, etc.
- benefits claimed e.g. DS1500, Macmillan grant, etc.
- social worker involved, e.g. at hospice.
- is nursing home place required/which GP will care for patient/is standard of care high/has home been informed of patient need
- physical aids, e.g. commode, handrail, mattress, etc.

Information and communication

WHAT?

- from patient to carer to PHCT, i.e. active listening, keeping a diary, what are key things that wake you up in the night, etc.
- to patient and carer – written and verbal information about what to expect, what to do, how to access help, etc.
- between professions
- within PHCT, e.g. cancer register
- labelling of notes, e.g. main GP/DN involved
- to on-call doctor – handover form faxed/sent/phoned
- to specialist palliative care, e.g. hospice, Macmillan nurse
- to hospital (secondary/tertiary)
- remembering to cancel inappropriate hospital appointments, especially after the patient has died

HOW?

- communication skills training
- use of leaflets, patient-held record, written details in DN notes, handover form, etc.

Control, choice

- have patient and carer been asked about preferred place of care/dying and has it been recorded
- are the patient and carer being consulted about treatment options
- is there some conflict between patient's and carer's wishes
- legal issues of advanced directive
- does the patient have control over who shares the end

Out of hours and emergencies

Four-point action plan (Calderdale and Kirklees out-of-hours protocol)

1 *Communication*
   - use handover form – GP/DN to on-call service and keep in DN notes
   - inform others e.g. hospice
   - does the carer know what to do in a crisis?
2 *Carer support*
   - coordinate pre-emptive care, e.g. night sitters, 24-hour DN
   - give written information to carers
   - emergency support, e.g. rapid response team
3 *Medical support*
   - anticipated management in handover form
   - crisis pack, guidelines, etc. and ongoing teaching
   - 24-hour specialist advice available from hospice
4 *Drugs/equipment*
   - leave anticipated drugs in home
   - palliative care bags in coop cars
   - on-call stocked pharmacists

Late

- end-of-life/terminal care (lasts approximately two days)
- patient is comfortable with symptoms controlled
- all inessential medication stopped and current treatment assessed
- inappropriate interventions discounted
- PRN subcut drugs prescribed, e.g. analgesic, anticholinergic, sedative
- patient and family aware of condition
- identified how family can be informed of impending death if patient worsens
- necessary verbal/written information given to relatives, e.g. what to do after a death/DSS death booklet

---

Afterwards – bereavement issue

- pre-death planning and active outreach to vulnerable
- provide information to relatives, e.g. what to do after a death
- refer to counselling agencies where appropriate
- audit/assessment/PHCT meeting/data analysis
- debriefing and team support
- inform others after a death, e.g. out-of-hours provider, hospital

---

more easily, and this is included as one of the options for use in the register, as well as a symptom chart and pain diagram (*see* SCR4 at www.radcliffe-oxford.com/caring).

Medication record card

A sample medication record card is included at www.radcliffe-oxford.com/caring – this can be kept in the Home Pack, DN notes or held by the patient to ensure current accurate information when they travel between primary, secondary, tertiary and hospice care. But it only works when kept up to date. Patient-held records might replace this, although many struggle with keeping these updated – electronic versions are eagerly awaited. The simplified medication card, piloted initially in hospices, has proved to be of great value when kept updated – a small change making a valuable difference.

Children

Dealing with children as patients is currently beyond the scope of this work, although much of it will apply. Helping *children as carers* or members of families affected by dying patients is challenging and important; for emotional support for children and young people exposed to a seriously ill or dying relative, help can be sought via local hospices, or Barnardo's Castle Project, Winston's Wish, etc. Many children act as carers for older people and have particular needs themselves. Useful books such as *The Secret C* by Julie Stokes[3] or the Cancerlink booklet *Talking to Children when an Adult has Cancer*[4] are recommended.

Benefits advice and social services

This is a complex and very important area. One survey rated concerns about money as one of the most pressing worries of patients with cancer. Specialist benefits advice should be available from social services, hospice social workers, Citizens' Advice Bureau, etc. – seek it out in your area and initiate the help for your patients. Older people especially may not feel able to ask for help in claiming the benefits they are entitled to.

Preferred place of death or place of care (see also pp. 30–1)

This is a sensitive but important subject, and one that should not be avoided if we wish to optimise care for our patients. We know that where preferred place of death has been noted it is more likely to be fulfilled.[5,6] So the point of asking is to ensure that the patient and their carer realistically plan for the future, and that we help organise as much as we can in advance around their decision. If a hospice bed is preferred it may not always be possible to realise that preference as demand for hospice beds outstrips supply, but plans can be initiated to make it more likely. Likewise, with a home death, equipment may need to be ordered in advance, night sitters booked, drugs left in the home, etc.

Asking where someone wishes to die may be a very delicate matter requiring good communication skills and sensitivity of timing and phrasing, and may not always be appropriate. Studies have shown that it may be recorded on fewer occasions than predicted.[7] The approach has to be tactful, gentle and gradual. Suggested questions might be: 'If your condition worsens, have you thought where you'd prefer to be cared for?' or 'What are your views about going into the hospice/nursing home if your illness worsens?' It's very helpful to note the answer and date it. This is the 'preferred place of death/care' (PPOD). If the person eventually dies in a place other than the stated place of choice, it may be valuable to note the reason, e.g. carer couldn't cope, difficult symptoms, etc. This might naturally lead to reflections on ways of improving service provision in your area, especially at the six-monthly review meeting, with collective data being fed back to commissioning bodies and improvements being instituted. This is the value of collecting such information: cumulatively, if there are common reasons for patients not fulfilling their preferred place of choice, then changes can be made to improve things locally.

> *It was so useful that everyone knew that John wanted to stay at home. It meant that the on-call doctor at the weekend knew the plan, that we discussed our needs for round-the-clock care every week with our nurses, and we felt more involved. John died at home and knew we'd done as much as we could for him, which helped us cope later.*
>
> MS, wife of cancer patient

It would be good to increase the home death rate eventually, moving it closer towards the estimated number who would prefer to die at home. Many patients, particularly younger patients, are very keen to stay at home. Even if home is chosen, alternatives need to be considered and planned for, e.g. nursing homes, and social services may need to be involved to help with equipment, etc. Despite much emphasis on place of death as a tangible measurement, where people actually die is not the overriding measure of our success in developing better care for our seriously ill patients; this is one factor only. The main goal is to enable patients to live and die well, to be enabled to die in their preferred setting symptom free, with fewer crisis events or admissions and a predictability and sense of security and support that reduces fear and anxiety. With most of the patient's last months of life being spent at home, how can we make a real contribution, alongside our secondary and specialist colleagues, to ensure these last months are of the highest standard of care?

There is evidence that home death is more likely if you are younger, have a carer, are male, are from a higher social class, have a shorter trajectory of illness and there is less availability of hospice admission locally. There is also evidence that carers' preferences mirror patients' but that they may be less keen on a home death (and those views change) – but is it a real choice and whose view is paramount? Despite our best efforts to fulfil patients' wishes, many will die in a hospice or hospital, often quite appropriately, as this may be the best place for them under the circumstances. But we need to get one step ahead of the reasons people are admitted, and prevent them. The main focus therefore is to *reduce the number of crisis hospital/hospice admissions* particularly, which may be deemed to be less appropriate or possibly preventable admissions. A key measurable factor in your area might be the number of cancer patients admitted to hospital who die within two days, or a week.

Much care occurs long before the moment of death – it is this we should focus on too.

References

1 More details of Macmillan primary care oncology nurse projects are available from Tonia Dawson on adawson@macmillan.org.uk or from Jane Melvin, Castlefields Health Centre, Runcorn, tel: 01928 566671.

2 Don Berwick of the Institute of Healthcare Improvement, speaking at the launch of the NHS Modernisation Agency Associate Programme, London, March 18th 2002.

3 Stokes J (2000) *The Secret C – straight talking about cancer.* Macmillan Cancer Relief. Winston's Wish, Gloucester. Order direct from the Macmillan Information Line, 9.30a.m.–4.30p.m., Monday to Friday, tel: 0845 601 6161.

4 Cancerlink booklet *Talking to Children when an Adult has Cancer.* Available directly from Cancerlink, tel: 020 7840 7840; St Christopher's Information Service, tel: 020 8776 9345 or info@his2.freeserve.co.uk and Cancerbacup, tel: 0800 181199.

5 Karlson J and Addington-Hall J (1998) How do cancer patients who die at home differ from those who die elsewhere? *Pall Med.* **12:** 279–86.

6 Carroll DS (1998) An audit of place of death of cancer patients in a semi-rural Scottish practice. *Pall Med.* **12:** 51–3.

7 Grant E and Calderdale and Kirklees Health Authority (1998) Study of preferred place of death noted for Macmillan nurses in Dewsbury. Personal communication.

CHAPTER 14

Control of symptoms: Gold Standard 3

> **C3**
>
> Each patient has their symptoms, problems and concerns (physical, psychological, social, spiritual and practical) assessed, recorded, discussed and acted upon, according to an agreed process. The focus is more on the patient's agenda.

Why

Better symptom control for patients must be one of our most important goals. Improved assessment is one of the three key processes in GSF and one that reaps much benefit in better patient-centred care. There are many choices of assessment tool, and these are suggestions to be used with your currently available tools and charts, if needed. However, remain focused on the goal of better symptom control (and communication), not more pen-pushing! Needs fall broadly into two categories of physical symptoms and psychosocial factors (emotional, spiritual, social and practical).

Physical symptoms

Good symptom control is palliative care's flagship, and the aspect of care it is rightly famous for. There have been tremendous strides in physical symptom control for people suffering from life-limiting diseases but less progress has been made in the provision of other psychosocial areas of care. There is some evidence, however, that doctors are only aware of a proportion of patients' symptoms, and some symptoms can be notoriously difficult to treat. Also, there can be some deficiencies in the management, particularly of cancer pain, in primary care. However, some patients choose a manageable level of pain in preference to perceived or real side-effects of treatment. This may be realistic, or may be an area worth unravelling to clarify fears of treatment and improve symptom control. For example, they may prefer a degree of predictable pain to the feeling of depersonalisation or 'not living in their own head'. But it is the accurate *assessment, communication and then control* of symptoms, problems and concerns that we are aiming to improve here.

Other symptoms such as nausea, agitation, dyspnoea or a rattley chest can be even more distressing than pain for patients and carers, so it is important to consider *patients' priorities*, and not just the medical aspects such as pain that tend to be addressed first. We must try to remove our medical sunglasses and view the world through the patient's glasses – what are the priorities for them? What is the impact of these symptoms on their daily lives and are there some other covert attributions they may be associating with their symptoms. Some feel that the word cancer is automatically associated with pain and there may be underlying fears about the mode of death, such as being strangled by their lung cancer or drowning in secretions. The accurate assessment of symptoms and unpacking of underlying fears and attributions may help improve the 'total pain' suffered.

Psychosocial factors

Sometimes as medically qualified professionals we think in terms of physical symptoms which require treatment and our patients' covert responses may reflect this. So a GP's question of 'how are you today' may be interpreted as 'how is your pain' and the softer but real issues that have a great impact on our perceptions of pain may be bypassed.

Psychosocial factors include the emotional, spiritual, social and practical needs of dying patients and are often provided by family and support networks as well as by GPs, DNs and others involved in community care. However there are great disparities in provision for psychosocial problems, particularly for those with non-malignant conditions or those not accessing specialist palliative care. A recent King's Fund report for primary care trusts confirmed this often neglected and inequitable area of care and offered some practical suggestions.[1] This section of the Gold Standards Framework also seeks to redress the balance towards a more holistic and accurate assessment of patient requirements, including psychosocial needs. Further resources are needed in this area and PCTs are more likely to respond if there is real evidence of need in their areas, hence accurate assessment and audits can further the case for improved local resourcing. For example, if access to equipment such as mattresses is assessed as being a significant deficiency in care in your area, following regular audit or SEA meetings primary care teams are armed with numerical ammunition to put the case to the local commissioner of services, e.g. primary care trust, leading to improvements in your own local service provision.

It may be that walking the dog, going to the pub every night, seeking financial help, healing a wounded relationship or seeking spiritual forgiveness are in fact higher on patients' agendas than we realise. The experience of 'death distress' among patients with life-threatening conditions is associated with the psychosocial–spiritual dimensions of the patient's life. Attention to these may buffer the negative effects of death distress.[2] These need to be part of the full assessment and kept in perspective, even when they may appear to be beyond our ability to help or influence.

> *The best thing she [the GP] did for me was to listen. And as she did so, I worked out my feelings about it all and it felt better.*

> Cancer patient

In many ways the outer cancer journey runs parallel with the 'inner journey', raising deeper spiritual and sometimes religious needs. Patients are gradually or dramatically changing inside along the journey, mirroring the outer tangible changes with key points of vulnerability and potential identity shifts (*see* Figure 4.2). Whilst talking at the level of aches and pains and laxatives, the undercurrent of evolving self-image and developing relationships during this traumatic time may present us with the privilege of accompanying people at a deeper level, as 'companions on the journey'. Spiritual issues should be considered as a crucial element of care, whether people express their spirituality through religious means or not. This touches on the deepest elements of our common humanity, crossing the border between 'us' as healthcare professionals and 'them' as patients. If we miss these deeper spiritual aspects we lose something very vital in our care. Much has been written on this and there is little space here to go into detail, but the reader is encouraged to seek further sources of help in spiritual care and to make contact with the local chaplain, clergy or religious leader who will be skilled in developing this theme.

The one thing that made all the difference was having the bed downstairs. It changed everything!

Cancer patient, London

Practical help in the form of commodes, mattresses, transport, help with housework, etc. can be of enormous benefit to patients but they may be unaware of available help or reluctant to ask. Delays in obtaining aids and adaptations and occupational therapy support can compound the problems. Those in primary care have long had a keen eye for the practical needs of patients and the advocacy role in applying for help on their behalf.

Informed participation in decision making (one of the stated aims of the NHS Cancer Plan) enhances patients' compliance and satisfaction with treatment and offers them the potential to reassert control over their lives. Healthcare professionals often censor information given to patients with the well intentioned but misguided desire to shield patients from reality. It is argued that this conspiracy of silence or misleading economy with the truth often leads eventually to heightened anxiety, fear and confusion and denies people the opportunity to reorganise and adapt their lives. The truth hurts but deceit hurts more – informed decision making is a key feature in the sharing of control with patients and their families.[3]

We also need to be aware of ourselves, as in Balint's model of 'the use of the drug doctor', and support each other. As we stand alongside our patients, showing simple care as one who has been this way before, we express our common humanity as 'fellow travellers'. Many are surprised how much they receive from their patients and how satisfying this dimension of care is. It is interesting to muse on what we as healthcare professionals need ourselves, to best meet the needs of our patients; how do we best care for those who care?

Much support is offered by families and non-medical carers. Within many communities there are often additional sources of support that are underused because little is known of them. Local directories that include community agencies, voluntary organisations, churches and other religious agencies may greatly increase these potential sources of psychosocial support. Examples are Befriending networks[11] and the Motor Neurone Disease Association's regional advisors (*see* Chapter 10).[12]

We need to ensure that our patients in the community are as symptom-free as possible to enable as good a quality of life as can be aspired to in the time remaining. We need to ensure that as far as possible we are aware of patients' agendas and psychosocial needs, and begin to address these by accurate assessments. Again, we need to always think and share as a team so that patients receive the benefits of complementary skills and roles.

What

Please remember the patient *is at the centre of all this, and in the interest of improving care for your patients please let no obstacle or objection be insurmountable.*

Pain is pain: it doesn't go away. Filling in forms doesn't do that alone, but filling in forms and telling others about problems may well help to alleviate suffering.

Mr RS, carer of a cancer patient, at the launch of an
out-of-hours palliative care protocol, Huddersfield

Suggested tools to improve symptom assessment and recording are included at <u>www.radcliffe-oxford.com/caring</u>. More detailed advice on assessment of pain is to be found in the excellent Scottish Intercollegiate Guidelines Network (SIGN) guideline *Control of Pain in Patients with Cancer*, available from www.sign.ac.uk, from Peter Kaye's *Decision Making in Palliative Care*[4] and from other palliative care textbooks.

The following tools should be used and adapted according to patient need and level of expediency; for example, if a patient is pain free, the pain charts are not appropriate and if a summary is up to date on the summary sheet it need not be repeated. These tools may be integrated into the pro formas in current usage in your area (and so avoid becoming additional burdensome paperwork) and should improve assessment and communication, thereby leading to better symptom control. It is worth bearing in mind the clear goal of improving care when completing any form. Too often we can become daunted and overtaken by paperwork, especially in nursing care, so these are offered only as suggestions that others have found useful. Use them intelligently and creatively as much or as little as you find helpful to improve needs assessment and symptom control for your patients. The forms are, of course, optional, but the first two (SCR1 and SCR2) have proved to be the most useful for practices, backed up by other assessment tools which improve accuracy of identification and communication of patient needs.

A suggested plan of assessment is as follows.

1 **Summary sheet (*see* SCR1)** Some find the summary sheet of the Supportive Care register, SCR1, most useful as a summary of all palliative care patients, focusing the discussions at the PHCT meetings.

2 **Frontsheet (*see* SCR2)** The summarised patient findings can be collected succinctly in the register frontsheet, SCR2, which acts as a one-page summary of most relevant information. This can be faxed or e-mailed to the out-of-hours provider, e.g. local doctors' cooperative, and used at the PHCT meetings.

Then, in addition, to be used as needed, are the following suggested assessment tools (*see* the website):

3 **Physical assessment** – body charts, scores, etc. (*see* SCR5). The use of a body chart, symptom score and pain assessment plans improves the accurate assessment of physical symptoms where present and the analysis and monitoring of symptoms. Patients may feel helped by completing the body chart themselves, improving their sense of control, and they allow easy visual modes of communicating and differentiating problems. For example, neuropathic pain becomes more distinguishable, leading to more accurate treatment.

4 **Broader holistic assessment** which includes psychosocial issues, e.g. PEPSI COLA check-list (*see* SCR4). Occasionally going through a check-list of issues with patients, such as the PEPSI COLA check-list, ensures that patients' priorities, needs and agendas are being addressed holistically and psychosocial issues are included. This is obviously only a guide not a tick-box exercise, but it attempts to be more comprehensive than the usual symptom control assessments. It can be adapted into an *aide-mémoire* (an idea which came from a district nurse in the pilot phase of the GSF) to allow easier tracking of issues, for example if a patient describes itching or relationship worries as troublesome issues there is less chance of these being lost if they are highlighted and followed

specifically, using the *aide-mémoire*. Specific key problems emerge and are summarised on the PACA sheet. Other validated assessment sheets/check-lists may already be in use in your area, e.g. The Support Team Assessment Schedule (STAS), Palliative Care Outcome Scale (POS) etc.[5]

5   **Overview of problems and concerns** – the PACA scale (*see* SCR 3). Once the key issues or priorities have been raised and assessed for the patient, these can be summarised using this problems and concerns front-sheet. This improves monitoring of symptoms and grading according to severity, 0–3, depending on how much these interfere with daily life. This score then provides a tangible measure and springboard for referral for specialist advice. The recommended action then follows, i.e. if patients score at level 2–3 for more than a week then referral to specialist palliative care services is recommended.[6] This should ensure clinical competence, and enables a tangible measure that will fit clinical governance assessments and monitoring. For example, if the patient has pain at level 2 (affecting daily life) for three days which, despite changes in treatment, then worsens to level 3 (overwhelming effect on daily life), then referral to the Macmillan nurse, hospice consultant, etc. would be normal good practice. Now it is also quantifiable, so appropriate referring or inappropriate under-referring can be measured. This also fits with current thinking on referrals to specialist services in the Supportive Care Strategy.[7] Many find specific eligibility criteria for referral to specialist palliative care helpful (*see* Chapter 10). *The carer's needs* are also noted on the sheet and included in the summary. This vital piece of the jigsaw, often overlooked, encourages constructive support for carers, one of the main factors in enabling people to remain at home.

Summary

1   Summary sheet:
    * SCR 1 for all patients
2   Front sheet:
    * SCR 2 for each patient
    * can be the handover form
    * summarises patient details
3   PACA scale:
    * quantifiable criteria for referral
    * auditable data for clinical governance
4   Holistic assessment, e.g. PEPSI COLA check-list:
    * improved agenda sharing
    * improved communication
    * tracking symptoms
5   Body chart, visual analogue scale (VAS)[5] etc.:
    * patient involvement and participation
    * more accurate assessment
    * score symptom to evaluate change.

Home Packs: patient and carer feedback sheets

In undertaking a holistic assessment of patients' needs, as well as the more physical elements of pure symptom control, we are attempting to place control back with patients and carers so that they direct proceedings wherever possible. In structuring real listening to their needs and agendas, we are more likely to be focused on, and respond to, the main issues that are important to patients. We sometimes need specific tools or skills to help with real listening and agenda sharing.[8]

The Home Pack contains feedback sheets for patients and carers to actively participate, writing about their needs, views and suggestions where appropriate. These will be more helpful for some than for others, but many use them as a vehicle to structure real listening to patients' and carers' needs and to prioritise actions. Others use 'patient diaries' or feedback pages of patient-held records – use whatever seems most appropriate for you.

How

An initial assessment and recording is recommended and is useful as a baseline, with updates at regular appropriate intervals, e.g. weekly or at appropriate consultations with the lead GP or DN for that patient. The coordinator can check each week and discuss the observations at the weekly/monthly PHCT meetings. The body charts, PEPSI COLA *aide-mémoire* and problems/concerns list (kept in the Supportive Care registers or alternatively in the DN or patient notes), contribute to the discussions by the team and form part of the significant event analysis. This also improves written communication and the transfer of information between team members between these meetings, and between patients and carers and medical staff. Electronic transfer of such forms can greatly enhance communication within teams.

Patients and carers should be given clear information and instructions about emergencies, pain and other symptom management, and be encouraged to take an active role in their own treatment; for example, with a sudden bleed, use these towels, compress the area, take this medication and call this phone number.

What if ...

What if every patient was symptom-free, where possible, and their needs and agendas prioritised and acted upon. This involves regular full assessments and needs, symptoms and concerns being noted and addressed, thereby empowering patients to play an active role in their care and decision making, and maintaining some control and good quality of life – 'to really live until they die'.

Case study – the use of assessment tools to improve patient care

Mrs Mitchell, a widowed 68-year-old lady with late-stage, left-sided fungating breast cancer, has recent onset of an intermittent sharp pain around her left chest wall and osteoarthritis of her right knee (chronic problem). She sketches in her areas of pain on the **body chart (SCR5)**, indicating a stabbing sharp pain that is suggestive of neuropathic pain and may prompt the use of adjuvant analgesics such as amitriptyline as well as her current opioid. In discussing the issues raised by the **PEPSI COLA checklist (SCR4)**, it is apparent that she is scared of the process of dying, she has some spiritual concerns and past traumas she would like to discuss and financial worries relating to her mentally handicapped daughter who lives with her.

Her main problems and concerns are assessed and graded on the **PACA scale (SCR 3)**: (1) neuropathic pain left chest (2) carer needs – daughter unable to cope alone (3) fears of process of dying (4) spiritual needs (5) financial concerns (6) osteoarthritis right knee. These are briefly noted on the **front-sheet (SCR2)** which is used as a handover form and sent to the out-of-hours provider with an updated medication list. The **summary sheet**, **SCR1**, acts as the prompt for discussions at the monthly PHCT meetings, where an appropriate action plan is agreed.

Three weeks later she requests a downstairs mattress on her **patient feedback sheet of the home pack** and a need to discuss matters that are waking her up at night: insomnia is added to her PACA list, a mattress ordered and time made to clarify her fears. A social worker visits to advise on benefits and future care of her handicapped daughter. The local Methodist minister calls at her request and she is able to deal with some of the spiritual concerns weighing heavily on her mind. After a trial of amitriptyline, her neuropathic pain continues (going from grade 2 to 3 for over a week) and specialist help is requested via her Macmillan nurse, who suggests further adjuvant therapies and possible referral for a nerve block. The downstairs mattress reduces the cause of the OA pain in her knees and she only needs anti-inflammatory medication occasionally. This is noted on her **medication form** which she keeps in the **home pack**. She wishes to remain at home if her daughter can cope (noted on the **front-sheet/handover form SCR2**) and night sitters are requested on an intermittent basis, with help from her local Crossroads scheme for household chores she can no longer manage. Her pain worsens and she receives a brachial plexus nerve block at the local hospital. A standard pack of four drugs (hyoscine, midazolam, diamorphine and cyclizine) plus 'as required' analgesics are left in the home, and this is noted on the **front-sheet SCR2**, which is sent to the out-of-hours provider. When she needs to call for help over a weekend the on-call doctor knows about her condition and manages her symptoms appropriately, without suggesting hospital admission.

With support she is able to remain at home with her daughter in the final months of her life and dies peacefully at home.

Discussion

Cancer pain

Cancer pain is a particularly unpleasant and complex pain that is frequently bound up with emotional distress and feelings of disempowerment, making it unique to each patient. It may also encompass other fears such as what the pain actually means (is the cancer taking me over) or fears of morphine.

There is much evidence that primary care can be poor at delivering good symptom relief at times[9] – we can and should do better (*see* Box 14.1). It would be no good being the amiable country GP in true Dr Findlay-style if we missed spinal cord compression and our patient became needlessly paralysed and incontinent in their final days (but we all may do it sometime!). This is the area in which we need to maintain excellent clinical competence – the 'head' knowledge to match our improved systems for delivering care – the 'hands'.

Box 14.1 Cancerbacup 'Freedom from Pain' survey, November 2000[10]

- 54% of respondents felt they had not been involved in decision making regarding pain medication.
- 67% of respondents said their doctor had not taken time to discuss with them the different types of pain medication available.
- 43% had not asked for pain control medication.
- 64% experienced side-effects from their medication.
- 10% were aware that pain control could be delivered in skin patches.
- 70% said they would consider using a patch.

Plan for assessment (adapted from Peter Kaye's *Decision Making in Palliative Care*)[4]

1 Have I set the scene?
2 Do I understand the patient's perspective?
3 Have any symptoms been missed?
4 Do I understand the patient's main concerns? The role of the professional is to be the midwife for all the patient's concerns. Ask about the patients 'ICE', which like an iceberg is usually nine-tenths hidden:
   I = ideas, beliefs, experiences – about the past
   C = concerns, worries, difficulties – about the present
   E = expectations, aims, hopes – about the future.
5 Have I written a drug card?
6 Have I interlaced the conversation with questions about feelings?
7 Have I made a plan?

Quality of life

Much work has been undertaken in attempting to assess quality of life – and quality of dying is even harder. In the end a few simple questions can reveal most, such as:

- Do you feel that your needs have been met?
- What things are concerning you most at the moment?
- If you wake up in the middle of the night is there something particularly worrying you?
- Do you feel you have retained some control?
- Do you feel you have some choices in your care?
- Have you been treated with respect and dignity?
- What is your experience of care overall?
- Do you feel depressed?

Spiritual care

This element of care is always present yet we may easily miss its importance and consequences. Some professionals experienced in palliative care reflect that as patients approach death, the 'journey home' is more of a spiritual one than a medical one. Travelling as 'companions on the journey' with patients as they approach death, it's hard not to feel challenged personally at times. We may begin to operate at a different level. This is mirrored in the patient's inner journey, the less tangible but still very real level of being, paralleling their more immediate outward journey.

> *The pain I felt inside was more real than any other bodily pain I'd known. It dominated everything and I was lost and terrified. Talking helped, and seeking out the hospice chaplain who visited me at home. Then things gradually began to fall into place. But it was very real. 'Spiritual pain' is a good description of the way it felt.*

Cancer patient, Shropshire

If we omit some form of spiritual care for our patients, we may not begin to address their real issues and they may remain in deep spiritual pain. Increasing doses of morphine will not heal a deeper pain of unresolved feelings or buried heart-searching. Spiritual care is 'grounded in the ordinary'[10] as well as touching on some of the deepest issues of life, death and meaning of existence. Again there may be issues about the past present and future (adapted from Peter Kaye[4]):

FOCUS	DISTRESS	NEED
Past issues	Regrets, guilt, fear of punishment	Acceptance of self, forgiveness
Present issues	Anger, 'Why me', disgust, isolation	Sense of unity, 'why not me', self-esteem (new role), social contact
Future issues	Fear, pointlessness, chaos	Discussion about dying, sense of meaning, order (e.g. making a will)

Many find the distinction between religious needs and beliefs and spiritual ones helpful. The religious manifestations of this spiritual journey are the tangible outer signs of the inner journey, e.g. sacraments, formalised prayers, etc. Every person, whether they have formalised religious beliefs or not, has deep spiritual needs, often relating to dignity, self-esteem, relationships, craving for real meaning 'the inner life', etc. Many healthcare professionals may find this a challenging area but awareness, listening skills and the simple act of being there are important, whilst appropriate referral to clergy or other spiritual guides is helpful. In today's multicultural society, greater awareness of the death rituals of different cultures and religions is also important.[13] Some guides to spiritual assessment are included in the Appendix.

References

1 Shipman C, Levenson R and Gillam S (2002) *Psychosocial Support for Dying People: what can primary care trusts do?* King's Fund, London. www.kingsfund.org.uk

2 Chibnall J T, Videen S, Duckro P *et al.* (2002) Psychosocial spiritual correlates of death distress in patients with life-threatening medical conditions. *Pall Med.* **16**: 331–8.

3 Fallowfield L J, Jenkins V A and Beveridge H A (2002) Truth may hurt but deceit hurts more: communication in palliative care. *Pall Med.* **16**: 297–303.

4 Kaye P (1999) *Decision Making in Palliative Care.* EPL Publications, Northampton.

5 Association for Palliative Medicine of Great Britain and Ireland (2001) *The Which Tool Guide.* APM, Southampton.

6 Ellershaw J *et al.* (1997) Developing an integrated care pathway for the dying patient. *Eur J Pall Care.* **4**(6): 203–7.

7 The draft Supportive Care Strategy can be found on the National Institute of Clinical Excellence website, www.nice.org.uk

8 Tanner G and Myers P (2002) *The Cancer Patient and their GP: a shared agenda.* Personal communication.

9 Barclay S (2000) The management of cancer pain in primary care. In: F M Hillier (ed) *The Effective Management of Cancer Pain.* Aesculapius Books, Phoenix.

10 www.cancerbacup.org.uk

11 For further details, tel: 0207 689 2448.

12 care@mndassociation.org.uk

13 Neuberger J (1994) *Caring for Dying People of Different Faiths.* Mosby Palliative Care Series. Mosby, London.

CHAPTER 15

Continuity of care out-of-hours: Gold Standard 4

C4

Practices will transfer information to the out-of-hours service for palliative care patients, e.g. using a handover form and out-of-hours protocol. This builds in anticipatory care to reduce crises and inappropriate admissions. Information should also be passed on to other relevant services, e.g. hospice/oncology department (e.g. using patient-held records/medication cards). Record and minimise the number of professionals involved, i.e. note lead GP, lead DN, etc.

Why

- Pain and fear can be a terrible combination. Physiological evidence confirms what we know, that pain is worse in the middle of the night. With additional fears of worsening symptoms, feeling unable to cope and worries about the future, many rational beings by day will panic by night. Other symptoms, notably breathlessness, agitation and vomiting, can be equally distressing causes of crisis calls. In our efforts to reduce the burden of pain suffered, we must aim to deliver round-the-clock symptom control in the home. We have made great strides in symptom relief over the last 20 years and distressing terminal symptoms could be a thing of the past; but no matter how far the boundaries of symptom control are extended in the centres of excellence, if basic levels of symptom relief are not accessed by those out in the community, then the overall burden is hardly affected.

  It was awful – I just panicked! My husband was in agony. It was three o'clock in the morning, we were at home all alone, it was dark and frightening and we didn't know what to do or who to turn to. Things all came together to make his pain seem much worse than it really was.

  Carer of cancer patient

- Many more people would like to remain at home to die than are able to do so; one of the reasons for this is crisis out-of-hours admissions in the 70% of the week outside normal working hours. Ninety per cent of the final year of life is spent at home.

- The main reasons for urgent admission are *symptom control* and *carer breakdown*, with *poor communication and lack of anticipation of problems* major contributory factors.

- Many healthcare professionals consider continuity out of hours to be a substantial problem in the organisation of palliative care services. Indeed, the Department of Health now confirms that any consideration of the organisation and standards of palliative care services is incomplete without the mention of providing adequate out-of-hours care. The NHS Cancer Plan recommends examination of this issue,[1] and points to the Macmillan Report on *Out-of-Hours Palliative Care in the Community*.[2]

- GP out-of-hours arrangements have changed over the last decade and may be changing further in the near future if the new GMS contract comes into being. There are many new factors, e.g. the growth of co-ops and NHS Direct, and many feel that the service given to palliative care patients has been significantly affected by these changes.
- Almost 50% of our cancer patients die in hospital, and only 26% at home. Crisis 'inappropriate' hospital admissions are a contributory factor to the high hospital death rate.
- Winter pressures, Friday discharges and rapid turnover of hospital beds may all exacerbate the problem. Patients in private hospitals can receive the worst of care at times, and miss their rightful NHS benefits.
- By introducing a few initiatives and agreed changes in your area, this problem can be significantly reduced; patients are less likely to be admitted to hospital, carers feel better supported and healthcare staff can feel more comfortable with out-of-hours care of the seriously ill. Current evidence is emerging of the impact of out-of-hours protocols on crisis hospital admissions, staff satisfaction and improvements in patient care.[3]
- Developing an **out-of-hours protocol** in your area can make a real difference, by assembling an agreed plan for helping seriously ill patients out-of-hours.
- Sending handover forms to the out-of-hours service with information about palliative care patients can improve care and reduce crisis admissions. (Use SRC2, the front-sheet of the Supportive Care register if no local handover form has been developed.)

What

At minimum, the practice coordinator is being asked to complete a **handover form** for every palliative care patient on the register and to keep it updated – perhaps a regular Friday afternoon job. You may devise your own, use an adapted version, e.g. from the Macmillan *Out-of-Hours* Report,[2] or you can use the front-sheet from the Supportive Care register to act as a summary and handover form, faxed or e-mailed to your out-of-hours provider. (This may be a task for the practice administration if the coordinator is a district nurse.)

For those interested in taking it further, an **out-of-hours protocol** for palliative care or vulnerable patients can be developed.[4] The first step is to gather round a table all those interested in out-of-hours palliative care, e.g. out-of-hours providers (cooperatives, deputising services, etc.), primary care representatives, PCT Cancer Leads or intermediate care representative, palliative care specialists, district nurse managers, social services managers, hospital representatives such as bed managers, etc., to discuss the issues in your area. As an example, in my previous area of Calderdale and Kirklees Health Authority, West Yorkshire, whilst visiting many GP practices as Macmillan GP Facilitator, there was an over-riding impression of deficiencies in out-of-hours palliative care. With the advent of a new GP cooperative linked with NHS Direct, and the lack of transfer of information to on-call services previously demonstrated, there was an obvious need and a great opportunity to do something to improve the out-of-hours care for palliative care patients. (More details of the protocol are included on the Macmillan website and in the Macmillan *Out-of-Hours* Palliative Care Report.[2]) The impact of the protocol has been evaluated[3] and early findings confirm that definite improvements have been made. Pendoc, the local co-op, was given an exemplar award by the National Association of GP Cooperatives, in part for their palliative care work.

Simplistically, this was an attempt to better use what we already had with the addition of a few initiatives, specifically the handover form, crisis pack and guidelines in the newly assembled palliative care bags ('Bearder' bags – named after a local patient who died in pain and whose charity wished to prevent such a sad situation recurring). By attempting to improve access to carer support, medical support and drugs out of hours, plus the vitally important proactive role of the handover form, we hoped to reduce the number of crisis 'inappropriate' admissions, thereby enabling more people to die in their place of choice.

Box 15.1 Summary of four-point plan for out-of-hours palliative care, Calderdale and Kirklees Health Authority Protocol

1   Communication
   • use handover form – GP/DN to write and fax to on-call service; keep in DN notes
   • inform others, e.g. hospice
   • does the carer know what to do in a crisis?

2   Carer support
   • coordinate pre-emptive care, e.g. night sitters, 24-hour district nursing service
   • give written information to carers
   • emergency support, e.g. rapid response team

3   Medical support
   • anticipated management in handover form
   • crisis pack, guidelines, etc. and ongoing teaching
   • 24-hour specialist advice available from hospice

4   Drugs/equipment
   • leave anticipated drugs in home
   • Bearder palliative care bags in coop cars
   • on-call stocked pharmacists

Communication

Handover form

The handover form has two important functions: (1) to improve information transfer and (2) to build in anticipatory care. The process of completing it is part of the benefit; if, for example, you think that a patient might become agitated or develop a rattley chest over a weekend, then leave some midazolam or hyoscine in the home for administration either by the on-call doctor or district nurse. If the on-call doctor presented with the handover form notes that the patient has stated a preference to remain at home, then there is more chance that they will be enabled to do so.

The Home Pack

The Home Pack contains an emergency section to be completed by the primary care team, to help patients and carers know what to do and who to call in a crisis. This information can be standardised, e.g. surgery and co-op number, with customised information for the patient. For example, a patient's wife who was concerned about epileptic fits was shown how to place her husband in the recovery position, how to give rectal diazepam, which number to call and where in the home the midazolam was stored should one occur. With this information written down, they felt reassured and less anxious.

Another suggestion to improve communication is a fridge magnet with important phone numbers immediately to hand. If it has been agreed, some have added 'not for CPR (cardiopulmonary resuscitation)' so that ambulance staff are aware of this request, preventing the distress of inappropriate attempts at resuscitation.

Carer support

Twenty-four hour access to district nursing or alternative nursing care is a basic prerequisite for good palliative care out of hours. The Audit Commission reported in 1999 that 32% of community trusts had no service after midnight,[5] and many areas have an inadequate evening provision. This is being seen as a major area of deficit nationally and one that the Community and District Nursing Association are campaigning to remedy; the hope is that this may be addressed through the implementation of the Supportive Care Strategy in time. It has an impact on GP out-of-hours care also, where the only on-call service in the middle of the night is that of the GP service. Some have likened it to a hospital ward where the nurses switch off the lights at six o'clock and go home, leaving the patients to fend for themselves!

Some areas have rapid response teams, an excellent needs-based, crisis-only service for use by patients who would otherwise be admitted to hospital. When used appropriately this can be invaluable in preventing admissions. There are examples of good coordination of care across the UK with one single contact 'phone number accessing all other services. Some hospice-at-home services also provide an emergency service to patients at home.

Medical support

The handover form informs the visiting on-call doctor of the GP's care plan for the patient and the current medication and proposed changes. When faced with a difficult medical symptom, the crisis packs in the palliative care bags (kept in the on-call cars) have crisis symptom sheets, guidelines and booklets on symptom control to refer to. Most specialist palliative care services are available for on-call advice, either from a nurse or on-call doctor, often via local hospices, although this may be an unrecognised and underused service.

Drugs and equipment

Drug access, may be improved by:

1 leaving anticipated drugs in the home, prompted by the handover form
2 the stock of palliative care drugs in the 'Bearder' palliative care bags kept in co-op cars and out-of-hours provider base (Healthcall base)
3 and there is also the on-call pharmacist, stocked with an approved list of drugs.

Further details and other examples of good practice are in the Macmillan Report on *Out-of-Hours Palliative Care*.[2]

Other aspects of continuity, e.g. across the boundary to specialists and hospital staff, use of the medication card, etc. have been discussed in Chapters 12 and 13. The handover form or its equivalent could be completed by hospital or hospice staff before discharge, especially before a weekend. Improved links between the practice coordinator and hospital staff can ease patient discharge home. There is much that still needs to be done here to improve cross-boundary and discharge management and the sense of continuity of care for patients.

How/who/when

The coordinator should ensure that the updated handover form is complete for each patient. It can be completed by the district nurse, Macmillan nurse or other admin member of the team, but it is important that the GP sees it, prescribes as prompted and signs the form. It then becomes a legal document and, importantly, may avoid the possibility of the patient becoming a coroner's case in future, with all the ensuing distress that causes (contact your local coroner to discuss this).

Updating the forms can become a regular Friday afternoon and pre-holiday job (*see* Box 15.2). Do remember to inform the out-of-hours provider when the patient has died.

Box 15.2 The coordinator's tasks

The tasks of the coordinator are to ensure:

- the handover form is completed for every patient on the register
- that written information is given to the patient and carers about what to do, who to contact out of hours and how, using the Home Pack, patient-held record, leaflet or other method
- pre-emptive carer support is requested, e.g. Marie Curie nurses, Macmillan Carers scheme, night sitters, respite
- that anticipated drugs are left in the home where appropriate, and enough drugs are always left to cover the out-of-hours periods at current dosage.

What if ...

What if patients and carers receive a continuity of service across the boundaries of care, both day and night (*see also* Box 15.3).

- Crisis admissions are averted and more are enabled to remain at home, if that is their wish.
- GPs and district nurses feel confident that their seriously ill patients will receive excellent care when left in the hands of the co-op or other on-call service. They may choose to give their home phone number if available (but they shouldn't feel compelled to do this) – if not they feel comfortable that they have handed care on as well as possible, left necessary drugs at home and that patients and carers know what to do if worried.
- Out-of-hours providers feel more comfortable that they can deal professionally with a dying patient at home, and are less likely to admit them to hospital in their final days.
- Patients and carers feel supported and confident in their home team, and better enabled to remain at home. Carers feel satisfied that they were able to fulfil the wishes of their dying relative at the end.

Discussion/ideas

Breathing space box

The Motor Neurone Disease Association developed what they termed a 'breathing space box', a small cardboard box with a drawer on either side (thanks to Dr David Oliver, Medical

---

Box 15.3 Model of a good palliative care service in and out of hours[2]

- Good anticipatory care and proactive planning by the PHCT.
- Efficient transfer of information between those working in hours and out of hours.
- Appropriate advice, information and support to patients and their carers from health professionals, who are well informed about their condition, medication and future management needs.
- Quick responses to requests for help, with information being passed on to relevant colleagues and revisits when necessary.
- Carer support in the form of 24-hour availability of district nurses and access to night sitters.
- High-quality symptom control with access to specialist palliative care advice when needed.
- Easy availability of appropriate drugs and equipment in and out of hours, without the need for the carer to leave the patient.
- Easy access to, and good coordination of, the provision available, so that all palliative care patients have equity of access to services.

Director, Wisdom Hospice, Rochester). One drawer holds the patient's medications to use in a crisis, e.g. sevredol or diazepam tablets, and the other holds the medication for use by the on-call service, e.g. ampoules of diamorphine, midazolam, hyoscine or cyclizine, etc. On the central section is a place to write emergency contact details and in the lid are relevant leaflets related to the patient's condition. The box is kept in the fridge and used as a central place to keep emergency medication, ensuring all drugs are kept safely in one place, rather than in a disorganised state under the bed!

Further reading

- the Macmillan report *Out-of-Hours Palliative Care*[2]
- the out-of-hours chapter in *Primary Palliative Care*[6]
- the website for the National Association of GP Cooperatives, www.nagpc.org.uk

References

1 The NHS Cancer Plan (2000) *A Plan for Innovation, A Plan for Reform*. Department of Health, London.

2 Thomas K (2001) *Out-of-hours Palliative Care in the Community*. Macmillan Cancer Relief. Available from Macmillan suppliers, tel: 01344 350310, ref no. OOHFR/01.

3 King N, Thomas K *et al. Evaluation of the impact of an out-of-hours palliative care protocol in Calderdale and Kirklees Health Authority*. Research ongoing, personal communication.

4 Thomas K (2000) Out-of-hours palliative care: bridging the gap. *Eur J Pall Care*. **7**: 22–5.

5 Audit Commission (1999) *First Assessment: a review of district nursing services in England and Wales*. Audit Commission, London.

6 Munday D (2002) Out-of-hours and emergency and palliative care. In R Charlton (ed) *Primary Palliative Care*. Radcliffe Medical Press, Oxford.

CHAPTER 16

Continued learning: Gold Standard 5

> **C5**
>
> The primary healthcare team is committed to continued learning of skills and information relevant to patients – 'learn as you go'. Using practice-based or external teaching, lectures/videos, significant event analysis or other tools, the practice and personal development plans are implemented. A practice reference library resource is assembled. Learning is clinical, organisational/strategic and also attitudinal/personal, e.g. communication skills. At least six-monthly, practice review/audit meetings are held to reflect on past patients, current practice and future needs, including the implications for service provision by commissioning groups.

Why

Learn as you go

Reflective learning, or learning rooted in specific patient care, has a deeper impact on the development of skills and knowledge, and is more likely to change practice. We learn best from our experience of looking after patients; we learn most from our mistakes.

The commitment to continued lifelong learning has recently changed within general practice. The previous system of rather passive attendance at lectures to accumulate points for post-graduate education allowance (PGEA) payments has moved on to more integrated, rooted, ongoing learning from experience, attempting to meet the perceived learning needs of the individual. Both personal and practice development plans are means of clarifying and meeting these educational needs, and palliative care lends itself excellently to the model of multidisciplinary learning and self-improvement. The NHS Modernisation Agency is keen to stress the value of 'measuring for improvement, not measuring for judgement', building audit into routine care to clarify areas for further development. The trick is to find the 'key levers of change', according to the Pareto theory, the 20% of factors that have 80% of the effect.

Staff support and morale

Support for staff involved is a neglected but important area. Hospices are often better developed in this area than we are in primary care. This is particularly relevant when we deal with patients of our own age, with circumstances that may chime with ours, or when something appears to go badly wrong. If staff have a sense of there being a 'bad death', or after a traumatic event, the team can greatly benefit from some 'unravelling' of feelings, both to prevent a recurrence where possible and to defuse suppressed tensions and feelings of guilt.

Stress and burn-out are potentially real issues for any members of staff and have been well researched amongst healthcare professionals. Burn-out can be described as having three components:[1]

1 *emotional exhaustion* – wearing out, depletion of emotional resources, loss of energy, debilitation, fatigue
2 *depersonalisation* – negative, callous, excessively detatched attitude towards other people, loss of idealism, irritability.
3 *reduced personal accomplishment* – reduction in self-confidence, low productivity, poor morale, inability to cope.

There are a number of factors that enable us to classify work stressors in healthcare environments.[2] These are:

1 *relationships* – communication problems with managers, lack of teamwork, conflict with colleagues
2 *tasks* – difficult patient groups, role ambiguity, role conflict, low sense of autonomy
3 *system management* – inadequate resources, poor physical environment, old equipment, work overload.

Interestingly, some qualitative work on the main stressful events experienced by doctors and nurses revealed that incidents related to death and dying top the list, with interpersonal intimacy and problems with colleagues following closely.[3] Complaints of work overload and lack of management support may be used to mask other underlying tensions of intimacy, death and suffering. A predictable situation of a team coping with a difficult death, some personality issues between colleagues and some deep involvement with relatives could potentially cause enormous stress to healthcare staff; this may lead to stress-related sickness – a familiar picture in today's NHS.

We need to look after ourselves too! A key finding from both the pilot practices and those in Phase 2 of the Gold Standards Framework has been the coincidental building up of morale and teamworking that ensued from joint working and structured sharing. In gathering a group of primary care staff together for a meeting, other things were happening imperceptibly that enabled higher levels of support, job satisfaction and team-building. This has consequences for ourselves as healthcare professionals in our enjoyment of our work and obviously for our patients – happy teams function better.

And do tell them what fun it is – we've really enjoyed it!

JS, district nurse, GSF Phase 1

There is a better sense of teamwork and we are planning better for patients since starting the project.

District nurse, GSF Phase 1

It improves morale and team functioning and is very rewarding for all the team.

CM, GP, GSF Phase 1

It was a morale booster for the whole team – we felt we were providing a better service for our patients and felt better about ourselves as healthcare professionals. We functioned better as a team and this had an effect beyond this work.

OD, GP, partner in GSF Phase 1

What

Significant event analysis *(see Chapter 6)* and 'traffic lights'

During the course of managing every patient's illness there will be notable learning points which are, good, bad and indifferent. These can be reflected upon using standard significant event analysis techniques for the palliative care patients in a practice, i.e. those on the register, creating an opportunity to establish more reflective practice and team-building as a means of improving care. The 'traffic lights' system has been used widely and can be applied here to reflect the good, the bad and the indifferent in a no-blame culture, focused on improving care not attributing blame. You can use a page with red, orange and green sections, or separate cards of these colours.

We can learn from experience of things that have gone well or not so well; but we may be too quick to point out deficiencies and too slow to celebrate successes as a team. The coordinator or key personnel involved in these patients' care could track all such learning points and note them in colour-coded sections: the things that were not so good (red), the things that went well (green) and the near misses (amber). These should then be discussed openly, during the monthly multidisciplinary meetings. Pendleton's rules apply, i.e. this is a non-judgemental, non-critical and supportive approach in which positive successes are celebrated and 'development needs' or stretches are suggested rather than imposed. We work from a baseline of mutual trust and respect, and belief that we are all trying to do a good job. The key is to find which aspects of the system of care can be improved upon and which have proved their worth. So by collecting rather ordinary situations, e.g. a difficult conversation with a relative or a mismatch of services, we develop more insight into areas of need.

Review meetings

Regular six-monthly practice reviews of patient care using cumulative real evidence from individual patient cases allows reflection on the practice team's overall care and targeted action plans. Recurring 'red' issues should lead to action planning, both for the practice and perhaps also the commissioning of services beyond the immediate practice remit; for example, problems accessing night sitters is a regular complaint, and with detailed patient examples and collated figures, stronger cases can be made for further funding. This might reveal some of the strengths of the new primary care-led NHS, where fully assessed local needs will determine the prioritising of spending by primary care organisations. A suggested plan for a review meeting is included at www.radcliffe-oxford.com/caring.

> *Doctors were the most difficult group to influence. The thing that eventually persuaded my medical colleagues of the benefits of improving palliative care was the use of stories with statistics – real patient examples backed up by accumulated figures.*
>
> Dame Cicely Saunders on the growth of the modern hospice movement,
> Radio 4 Interview, June 2000

After a death, it might be appropriate to review the patient's journey as a whole, as a significant event analysis. Realistically speaking, some practices find it hard to have regular monthly meetings, so a compromise that some find useful is for the coordinator to undertake a mini-SEA using the 'traffic lights' page after a patient's death, with the GP and DN involved. Collected reflections can then feed into the six-monthly review meetings.

Personal development plan: targeted learning

It is important to structure learning to meet individual needs and to build in review at regular intervals. In prioritising our learning needs we need to consider safety (first do no harm), national directives such as the National Service Frameworks or guidelines from the National Institute of Clinical Excellence, ideas for practice development and our own personal learning needs, such as computer skills, etc.[4] If the team feels it has only a limited knowledge of, for example, use of adjuvant therapy in cancer pain, it may pursue this as a learning need, related to specific patients. A palliative care specialist, Macmillan nurse or team member may present a brief résumé of current thinking at the next PHCT meeting. Videos, tapes, case analysis, even quizzes or games of 'consequence' can be used.

Specific learning needs in palliative care

There are a limited number of specific 'tripwires' in palliative care for the competent GP – certain treatments or modes of care that are more specific to care delivered at this stage of life and commonly seen in hospices but infrequently encountered in day-to-day general practice (*see* Chapter 8). For example, hypercalcaemia is relatively rare in ordinary general practice, but is a more commonly seen tripwire in palliative care patients, especially in certain cancers. So learning about Mrs Bloggs with breast cancer who developed hyper-calcaemia, received rapid treatment with a pamidronate drip and thus relief from her symptoms links the condition with the person and ensures that the team are more likely to recognise the symptoms again: 'You remember Mrs Bloggs' nausea and confusion that improved with those infusions? Is it worth checking Mr Green's calcium, just in case?'

How/who/when

Tasks of coordinators in the Gold Standards Framework

These include:

- having monthly PHCT meetings with discussion of patients on the Supportive Care Register, using significant event analysis, in a non-blame supportive culture of continued learning and improving
- inviting specialist, e.g. Macmillan nurses/hospice consultants, to team meetings to discuss patients on the register
- directing specific teaching to the needs clarified by this kind of regular discussion – this may include factual or skills-based teaching. If an issue comes up, e.g. neuropathic pain, this could be the subject of a 10-minute teaching session from the specialist related to the patient care discussed
- imaginative use of other resources such as videos/CD-ROMs, tapes, presentations from textbooks, etc. Use hospice/hospital libraries
- significant event analysis during care or after a death
- feeding back learning needs to your Macmillan GP Facilitator/palliative care team/PCT education facilitator/continuing medical education (CME) tutor.

What if ...

What if:

- learning in primary palliative care is rooted and 'real', focused on patients seen, so that primary care staff become aware of recent developments, of what they know and what they don't know and new knowledge is effortlessly absorbed
- significant event analysis is used as an instrument of change and constructive action plans devised
- 'stories and statistics' are used to persuade commissioners to direct their expenditure on areas that truly reflect the community's needs
- staff roles, both generalist and specialist, doctors and nurses are mutually respected and a greater sense of teamwork and practice morale evolves
- staff support is inbuilt so that 'thinking team', the patient and carers feel the benefit of a united team approach and staff protect themselves from the stresses of their demanding roles
- you really enjoy your work!

References

1 Maslach C, Jackson S E and Leter M P (1996) *The Maslach Burn-out Inventory*. Consulting Psychologist Press, Palo Alto, CA.

2 Davidson R (2000) Stress issues in palliative care: caring for the community professional. In J Cooper (ed) *Stepping into Palliative Care*. Radcliffe Medical Press, Oxford.

3 Firth-Cozins J (1996) Stress in health professionals. In A Baum *et al.* (eds) *Cambridge Handbook of Psychology, Health and Medicine*. Cambridge University Press.

4 Rughani A (2001) *The GP's Guide to Personal Development Plans* (2e). Radcliffe Medical Press, Oxford.

CHAPTER 17

Carer support: Gold Standard 6

C6

- *Emotional support*. Carers are supported, listened to, kept fully informed and encouraged and educated to play as full a role in the patient's care as they wish. Where appropriate, they are regarded as an integral part of the team.

- *Practical support*. Practical hands-on support is supplied where possible, e.g. night sitter, respite, benefits advice, etc.

- *Bereavement*. Practices plan support, e.g. practice protocol, visits, notes tagged, others informed, etc.

- *Staff support* is inbuilt and nurtured, leading to better teamwork.

Why

Carer support

This is one of the most important aspects of the care provided by primary healthcare teams. Carer breakdown is THE key factor in prompting institutionalised care for dying patients. This is the experience of most healthcare professionals and is reflected loudly and clearly in the literature.

Some suggest that the impact of cancer (or other serious illness) on the carer can be even greater than that of the patient. Certainly, there is resounding evidence that without support from family and friends it would be impossible for many patients to remain at home. Those without carers are less likely to be able to remain at home to die – they present particular difficulties for us in primary care.

***Carers' anxiety is rated alongside patients' symptoms as the most severe problems by both patients and families.*[1]**

> *I get no freedom. He is very loving and caring but very demanding. I have one day off a week.*
> Carer of cancer patient[2]

> *I was terrified when they said they would discharge him home – I didn't think I could cope.*
> Widow of cancer patient

Despite their natural feelings of trepidation beforehand, there can be a great sense of satisfaction for the carer in having fulfilled the wishes of their loved one who expressed a preference to stay at home during their final days. However, it places a great strain on carers, both emotionally and physically.

My husband didn't want to go to hospital at all. But the weekend doctor sent him in to the hospice after he had coughed up blood, and he died 8 hours later. I felt guilty that I hadn't done more for him at home.

Wife of lung cancer patient

There are things I would like to ask, but I always have my husband there. I would like to ask questions about the bleeding and just what is going on, but I feel I can't. I can never see any of his carers alone.

Wife of cancer patient[2]

The family will usually be registered as patients of the practice as well, so may continue under the care of the GP. Often a special relationship remains between the family and the primary care team, who together have looked after the dying patient, and that relationship may be therapeutic in their grieving process. This remains a very rewarding part of general practice. Derek Doyle writes:

It is worth reminding ourselves that the principal providers of care are actually the relatives. We are still not doing nearly enough to empower, strengthen, educate and support carers and to use imaginative means to help and support them through this ghastly time.[3]

National support for carers

The number of carers in the community is rising. There are currently thought to be up to six million carers in the UK providing degrees of care – almost one in eight of us – and nearly one million are providing at least 50 hours of care per week.[4] Informal carers, as they are termed, span all age groups and social classes but are most commonly female and aged between 50 and 70,[5] although 33% of care for people over 65 is provided by people over 70. Among cancer patients, a third receive care solely from one close relative and half from two or three relatives, typically a spouse and an adult child.[1] Half of all carers are in paid work. A smaller proportion of non-cancer patients than cancer patients have access to such informal care, reflecting their older age at death.

It makes humanitarian and financial sense for the Government to support carers as they look after people at home, and reduce the expensive burden on hospitals and other state-funded institutions. There are hidden costs to carers such as loss of work, travelling, expensive drugs, etc., and in other countries such as the USA the financial burden of paying for care can be crippling. Since the 1980s it has been estimated that nearly half of Medicare expenditures are for the care of eventually fatal illnesses.[6] Some interesting initiatives, for example in Motala, Sweden, have reimbursed family members choosing to remain at home for loss of income and in that group the home death rate has reversed from 15% to 89%.[7]

Since the NHS Plan of July 2000 and the gradual phasing out of Community Health Councils, we now have the Patient Advisory and Liaison Service (PALS) in England, offering support to patients and carers and an advocacy position in strategic planning.

Help from social services

Having cancer and caring for someone with cancer or other end-of-life conditions can lead to real impoverishment. Advice on finances and ensuring maximum claiming of entitled benefits is a crucial part of care. The convolutions of the benefits system mean that few are competent in this area but help can be found from social workers and other benefits advisors.

This is an area of overlap between health and social services boundaries and we need to work closely with local authorities to provide social benefits to carers. There are statutory obligations that local authorities are asked to fulfil related to, for example, the continuing care funds, and new measures are being devised to link with the National Service Framework for the Elderly Assessment procedures. Consult your local social services for details. Some local authorities run centres for carers (such as the Kirklees Gateway Centre in Huddersfield), which provide in emotional and practical ways. Macmillan Cancer Relief have long been giving patient grants and are improving the availability of benefits advice. Hospice social workers specialise in this area and can be very helpful, well-informed resources.

DS1500

Special rules apply to those with terminal illness for fast-tracking Attendance Allowance claims to support home care. For patients whose prognosis is considered to be six months or less, the GP has to complete a standard form (the DS1500) and send it to the local Benefits Agency office. This can be Read coded in most practice systems and a small fee is due. It has been used as a helpful trigger for entry onto the Gold Standards Framework pathway and adoption onto the Supportive Care register; it is only a trigger not a barrier, but as yet there is no other significant indicator of a limited prognosis available. Therefore once the GP considers, or has been informed, that the patient is in the last six months or so of life, the DS1500 form is completed and the patient adopted onto the Framework.

Also, many patients at this stage would be unable to collect prescriptions unaided, so would qualify for exemption of prescription fees – a considerable expense for already impoverished families. So check for each patient on the register whether they might qualify for exemption also.

Carers as partners in the team

The ideal model appears to be that the carer should be treated as an integral member of the team, taught or enabled to do as much or as little as they wish for the patient, informed and consulted at every stage. Advice on practical matters such as lifting and handling, bathing, etc. comes high on the list of needs from user groups, such as Carers UK.[8] (Some advice is included in the home packs but personal demonstrations are of most value.)

The NHS Executive White Paper *Caring about Carers: a national strategy for carers*[9] describes the difficulties that carers face, and emphasises that carers should be treated as partners in the team but with specific, and sometimes unmet, needs of their own:

> We intend to make progress so that more carers – and eventually all carers – feel adequately prepared and equipped to care if that is what they choose to do, feel cared for themselves, and feel their needs are understood.[9]

PHCTs are asked to keep a carers' register to enable full support to be provided. For those using the Supportive Care register, this then becomes a carers' database, computer coded to form the basis of the carers' register.

Carer's needs

More than half of informal carers find the caring 'rewarding', 10% find it a burden and the rest find it both in equal measure. In the year before death of a cancer patient, the estimated prevalence of anxiety and depression among informal carers is high, reported to be about 46% for anxiety and 39% for depression. About half of carers report problems sleeping, and about a third report weight loss during the year.[1] Many informal carers also feel isolated, particularly after the patient's death, when suddenly must sources of support are withdrawn.

> *There must be an acknowledgement of the fundamental and very special role family members can play in care – it's more than supporting the carer, it's recognising their key role in providing a loving and supporting relationship for the patient.... Spiritual peace may come if they have a close and trusting relationship with someone within which they can make sense of their life and approaching death.*

> J Bradburn, daughter of cancer patient and Cancerlink Lead Manager

---

Box 17.1 Main needs of the carers[10]

Main needs of the carers include:

- recognition of their value and importance
- being involved in devising care plans (one in three carers felt their comments and concerns were not taken into account)
- information – sources of support, decision making about medical care, relevance of symptoms, what to do in an emergency, etc.
- support – practical, emotional, social, financial, spiritual
- training, e.g. in lifting, giving medication, etc.
- confiding in and being listened to – needs expressed and supported, often outside the home
- coping strategies, both internal (faith, positive attitude, etc.) and external (social networks)
- personal health – time out to sleep, socialise, eat well, etc.

Intermediate care

Intermediate care is a whole system approach high on the political agenda since the NHS Plan. It aims to be a bridge between hospital and home 'as a transient stage in patient care, not a new location for long-term care'.[11] The aims are promoting independence by reducing avoidable admissions, facilitating discharge, promoting effective rehabilitation, minimising dependence on long-term care institutions and employing clear admission and discharge criteria for the use of specialised intermediate beds.[12] Partners of patients sometimes have to be admitted to hospital, reminding us how finely balanced our services are. Community hospitals play a vital role, particularly in rural areas, involving to some extent a quarter of all GPs. There is much good work on the development of palliative care within community hospitals, especially in Scotland and Cumbria, where Macmillan GP Facilitators have helped develop guidelines and improve standards of care.

Primary care can make a difference

This is an area where evidence confirms that primary care can make a real and very valued difference. The Griffiths Report[13] highlighted the importance of general practice in providing support for carers, and the National Strategy for Carers formally recognised that for many carers the most important initial point of contact is with their GP or other member of the PHCT. On average, 88% of informal carers have seen their GP and 51% their DN within the past year, and when asked who has the most important power to improve their life, 72% of carers rank their GP top of the list. However, many carers feel that GPs do not understand their needs and in turn many GPs and DNs feel they lack the relevant time, resources and training to take a more proactive role. But primary care is in the best position to help and there are many things that we can improve upon that are much appreciated by carers.

Staff support

Caring for dying patients or those undergoing traumatic life events has a significant impact on the healthcare professionals involved. Doctors and nurses have high rates of psychological and physical morbidity (*see* Chapter 16, p. 234), and primary care and palliative care professionals have particular risk factors – we must not add to the already overwhelming burden. There are strategies to improve the teamworking of professionals. By encouraging primary care to fulfil its potential, and by reducing the burden of extraneous pressures, we can better serve ourselves and our patients.

All the team are responsible for staff support – this may require a little 'blurring of the role boundaries' and better mutual respect for each others' roles and commitment. Support is generated through the PHCT meetings, individual support and through the significant event analysis reflecting on a team's performance. A no-blame culture encourages honesty and constructive suggestions (*see* Chapter 6).

What

Four levels of support for carers are suggested:

- *emotional support* – informed, listened to (very important), encouraged – the 'getting alongside' and attempting to meet some of their needs
- *practical support* – hands-on support, e.g. dressings, night sitter, bathing, respite, commode, etc., usually provided by the DNs and greatly appreciated
- *bereavement support* – planned support, open listening and initiated care
- *staff support*.

What can primary care teams do?

The important contribution of general practice in providing support for carers has been well highlighted, underlining the key role played by the primary healthcare team in supporting carers, many of whom otherwise might receive little support from elsewhere.[14] Box 17.2 contains measures that GPs can take to improve the quality of life of carers. Many of these will be part of standard good practice but using the systems of reporting and noting care suggested in the Gold Standards Framework, it is hoped that others could easily become integrated into the routine care for carers.

Box 17.2 Measures GPs can take to improve the quality of life of informal carers

- Acknowledge carers, what they do and the problems they have.
- Flag the notes of informal carers so that in any consultation you are aware of their circumstances.
- Treat carers as you would other team members and listen to their opinions.
- Include them in discussions about the person they care for.
- Give carers a choice about which tasks they are prepared to take upon themselves.
- Ask after the health and welfare of the carer as well as the patient.
- Provide information to the carer about the condition the patient suffers from.
- Provide information about being a carer and the support available.
- Provide information about benefits available.
- Provide information about local services available for both the person being cared for and the carer.
- Be an advocate for the carer to ensure services and equipment appropriate to the circumstances are provided.
- Liaise with other services.
- Ensure staff are informed about the needs and problems of informal carers.
- Respond quickly and sympathetically to crisis situations.

Sources of support to enable informal carers to look after dying patients at home include:

- *symptom control* – general practitioners, district nurses, clinical nurses, specialists such as Macmillan nurses
- *nursing* – community nurses
- *night-sitting service* – Marie Curie nurses, district nursing services
- *respite care* – hospices, community hospitals
- *domestic support* – social services
- *information* – general practitioners, district nurses, clinical nurse specialists, voluntary organisations such as BACUP
- *psychosocial support* – general practitioners, district nurses, Macmillan nurses, bereavement counsellors
- *aids and appliances* – occupational therapists
- *financial assistance* – social workers.

How/who/when

Open questions

Supportive, listening and counselling skills are a necessary part of emotional support. One way of monitoring this is to regularly ask and note carers' views, what are their own needs and what other things or improvements would they suggest. The PACA scale allows recording of this to be brought to the PHCT meetings and the Weekly Review sheets from the Home Pack may be helpful as prompts. It may enable you to focus on their key problems and help address them, if possible.

Carers' register and link with the Local Authority Carers' Strategy Group

The Supportive Care register sheets can provide the basis of the carers' register, recommended by the National Strategy for Carers, to prompt referral to appropriate local and national agencies. Lists of local and national self-help groups should also be available.

Information, knowledge and wisdom

Some practices have produced their own information package to include advice on symptoms. A suggested package is included in the GSF Home Pack. Other information such as Cancerlink's booklets, Cancerbacup's leaflets and *The Secret C*[15] are also available for carers. Information about benefits should be available from social services or hospice social workers.

Often it is particular information about the patient's condition that is required. The GP or a coordinator/key worker acting as advocate for a patient can sometimes discover and interpret the necessary information from hospital sources. Without specific details of the patient's condition, explained in a meaningful way, there is likely to remain a feeling of constant low-grade anxiety – described as 'fear spread very thin'. It is hard to feel safe or secure without personalised information. Interpretating that information as appropriate advice or wisdom for the patient is a vital and often unacknowledged skill, and one that GPs are often particularly adept at.

> I don't know because nobody will tell us what the situation is. She is on chemotherapy now because the radiotherapy failed. How do you discuss dying when you don't know when and how? Nobody has talked to us about dying.[2]
>
> Husband of cancer patient

Practical support for carers

This is a valuable part of the DN's role, and a regular monthly check on carers' practical needs (part of the PEPSI COLA check-list) should be performed, recorded and addressed. The 'planning for care' list in the Home Pack could be used to clarify gaps in care in the week. Check the Home Pack regularly for responses on the Weekly Review sheets. Note deficiencies in accessing equipment or other services in the traffic lights, SEA sheets or elsewhere for later action.

The support and teaching of carers on self-care

This also applies to patients living alone and includes, for example, how to massage feet, put on support stockings, give a bed bath and lift the patient from the sitting position. It is important that carers are seen as part of the team and helped to care for their loved one, rather than feeling de-skilled by uniformed professional strangers who take over the care and then suddenly disappear again. Some areas run courses in simple skills for carers.

Preferential treatment for carers

Respond quickly and sympathetically to crisis situations. All reception staff should be aware of those patients and families on the register and respond to them appropriately. Staff should be informed about the needs and problems of informal carers. Tag the notes so that in any consultation you are aware of their circumstances. Many practices keep these patients' names on a 'white board' in a private part of the reception area, allowing them preferential treatment for prescriptions, visit, etc.

Bereavement *(see Chapter 9)*

This is optional but you might feel you wish to introduce a system into your practice for bereavement care. Various protocols have been suggested:[16]

- referral to other agencies or use the local church (discuss with local clergy as to whether a bereavement support group is run by the local church)
- put the date the patient died on the bereaved person's notes and send a card or letter of sympathy a year later (or at Christmas)
- ensure the bereaved person's notes are completed with an entry concerning the relative's death
- planned appointments/visits for the bereaved at various intervals (i.e. not waiting for them to have to come with a 'medical ticket')
- setting up of a self-help group – an informal practice-based supportive group for carers of patients with any diagnosis such as cancer, dementia or any debilitating disease.

The role of coordinators

Coordinators should be responsible for ensuring that these processes are underway, to assemble responses from carers gleaned from conversations, the problems/concerns list and the Weekly Review sheets, etc. to report back at the PHCT meetings (*see* Box 17.3). By regularly raising the issue of carers' needs, these may become higher on the agenda for possible actions. GPs and DNs should continue to be aware of their key role in supporting carers.

Box 17.3 The coordinator's tasks

1 Check that, at least monthly, the carer has been asked (and recorded) about general needs and support. Look at Weekly Review sheets.

2 Check that, at least monthly, the carer has been asked what one thing is bothering them most or would they like to change, and where possible address this.

3 Check that each carer is given an information pack from the Local Authority Carers Group.

4 Check that each carer is listed on the carers' register/database.

5 Check that each carer is given a copy of relevant booklets in the Home Pack. Add others where appropriate.

6 Check that the carer is informed of contact details in an emergency (on the yellow medication card or in the Home Pack).

7 Bereavement – *see* Chapter 9.

Q. *Do you think there has been any benefit to the carers with having the register?*

A. *The carers need to be taken into account more ... I do think yes, we have to look at their needs because the paperwork forces us to, so we can't forget the carers. They are important.*
                                                                    DN, Coordinator, GSF Phase 2

What if ...

What if:

- carers feel supported and cared for themselves as they look after the dying patient
- their confidence and ability to cope at home is improved so more are enabled to remain at home
- family and carers are looked after into bereavement as they adjust to life without their loved one
- staff feel good about the care they are able to provide and respect the mutually complementary roles of different members of the team. Should a difficult or traumatic event occur, staff will support each other – including the doctors!

Discussion

Specific areas of need

Children (*see also* Chapters 9 and 13)

Witnessing the deterioration of family members may be distressing and children may need particular support and counselling. Although parents may believe that children should be dealt with openly, frequently many do not disclose information about a life-threatening illness to their children even when they are obviously deteriorating.[17] The natural protective instinct of parents may prevent them from overtly discussing the situation, and yet children's innate sense of something being wrong creates more anxiety and distress. Where there is open communication within families the level of anxiety in children is lower.[18] Many parents struggle to know how to help their children and would welcome help from health professionals. It is therefore recommended that parents are offered help in disclosing information about their illness to children, appropriate to their age and level of understanding.[19] Similar advice applies to children with life-threatening illnesses themselves and the Association for Children with Life-threatening or Terminal Conditions (ACT)[20] suggests that discussions with children should be 'sensitive and appropriate to age and understanding'. The report of the Joint Working Party on Palliative Care for Young People[21] makes many constructive recommendations for improving services.

The main message is not to overlook children, but to include them wherever possible in your communication with the family. Children need clear, repeated explanations of the simple, but not bald, truth. Using euphemisms can be very misleading and lead to entrenched fears and problems later. Never bypass the parents or replace explanations with books, but giving a book such as *The Secret C*[15] can be helpful once shown to their parents. Adults often find the clear language of children's books helpful too (the average reading age in this country is estimated at seven), so children's books can help anyone.

Children need to be reassured that someone will continue to look after them when the parent has died. They need to know about the illness, how they can help or what they should do, permission to say how they really feel, acknowledgement that it is very sad and explanation if things change. Older children may appreciate straight talking about dying itself (e.g. the skin colour may change, breathing may be noisy, the heart eventually stops and the brain stops working and they do not move any more). Family meetings may occur naturally but skilful orchestration is often required (*see* Peter Kaye's *Decision Making in Palliative Care*).[22]

Young carers

There is a growing body of young carers looking after older relatives, with specific needs of their own that may go unrecognised. Self-help groups for this age can be useful in providing extra support.

Lifting and handling techniques for carers

This is an often ignored area but carers do struggle with the practical aspects of caring for patients in sometimes awkward home circumstances, and may undergo severe back strain following regular handling or after a fall. In a self-sacrificial way, some may feel this is part of the care offered but as so many will be elderly themselves with osteoporotic spines and tendencies to imbalance, the potential for disaster is enormous. The situation can suddenly develop into a crisis call for help and a possible urgent admission. Not every problem is preventable but many may benefit from simple instructions or leaflets on lifting patients, basic rules for coping, plus occupational therapy assessment or other practical advice on adaptations, stair lifts, aids, etc. For example, moving a bed downstairs can be the simplest and most revolutionary of measures and one that might not have crossed the mind of the family. One website with further advice on this is www.pallcareqld.com/lifting&handling.htm. Their advice sheet is printed in the Home Pack.

> *The reason my husband had to go into a nursing home in the end was quite simply that I couldn't lift him to the commode. It all came to a head after a fall and I felt I couldn't cope on my own any more. We were both heartbroken.*
>
> Elderly carer of cancer patient

Information

Carers want to know:

1   what is happening
2   what is going to happen
3   what they need to help (*see* Box 17.4).

Planning ahead increases their sense of security (like reading the road ahead and knowing what to expect) which reassures as well as prepares them, for example so knowing how to deal with emergencies, i.e. what they could do and who to phone, also promotes a sense of safety and security. There is also a need to translate clinical language and to humanise complex terms, without patronising or over-simplifying.

Box 17.4 Needs of informal carers[1]

Carers need information and education about:

- the patient's diagnosis
- causes, importance and management of symptoms
- how to care for the patient
- likely prognosis and how the patient may die
- sudden changes in the patient's condition, particularly those which may signal that death is approaching
- what services are available and how to access them (including emergencies).

Assessment of carers' own needs

It is sometimes difficult to assess carers' needs as they may 'wear the same face' whether depressed or happy. They may be so focused on the patient that they may not feel they have permission to express their own needs, fears and concerns. Like the iceberg, much goes on beneath the surface (*see* Figure 17.1).

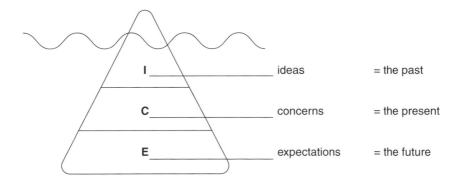

I _____	ideas	= the past
C _____	concerns	= the present
E _____	expectations	= the future

Figure 17.1: The iceberg of needs.[22]

Carers may be frightened that there will not be the care available when it is needed or that they will not be able to cope. This anxiety about the future magnifies fears and the resultant inability to cope and carer breakdown may mean the patient is unable to stay at home. Financial help is important – income may be cut considerably and this may not be expressed openly, so routinely offering help in every case and making carers aware of benefits advice is important.

Carers' perspectives on place of death

Sometimes carers' views on the preferred place of care may differ from that of the patient's, although they often mirror them. Many carers struggle and may feel unable to look after the dying patient at home for reasons of severity of symptoms, lack of nursing support or night sitters, absence of equipment or just the horror of having someone die in the bed next to you. However, carers have been reported retrospectively to invariably be satisfied with the place of death when it is at home. Many patients feel concern about not being a burden to others and this often triggers admission. There may always be the potential for a conflict of views between patient and carer, which we in primary care may find difficult to handle and have to respectfully observe. However, we can attempt to 'unpick' the reasons and underlying fears, the 'attributions',[23] and offer a plan of management, written information of what might happen and what to do and the availability of open access and support. Once fears have been clarified, many will be dispelled, but not in every case. Sometimes there is no more that we can do to help, but we should not allow ourselves to feel guilty at the breakdown of a home situation and certainly not allow carers to feel the burden of guilt as well as grief after a death.

Example of a local authority carers' scheme: Kirklees Carers' Gateway[24]

This initiative supports carers to enable them to continue in their caring role. The aims of the strategy are to:

- support carers in their own right
- support carers in their ability to care
- involve carers in the planning and monitoring of services.

In December 1999, a carers' centre opened, the Kirklees Carers' Gateway, funded by social services and the health authority. It provides information, support, office equipment and training. The Kirklees Carers' Information Pack which accompanies this also provides information and help with assessment and care arrangements for the person being looked after. There is a Carers' Project Officer, based at Kirklees Social Services, an awareness of the needs of carers from black and ethnic minorities, advice on benefits, a young carers' service, and short-break respite care can be provided. A Carers' Gateway newsletter is provided quarterly. It is linked with the rapid response team and intermediate care group of Huddersfield Central PCT. Those in primary care are asked to identify carers to link them up to this service. Carers should be made aware of what is available should they wish to pursue it, and information packs given.

References

1 Ramirez A, Addington-Hall J and Richards M (1998) ABC of palliative care: the carers. *BMJ*. **316**: 208–11.

2 Meads J, Coe N and Davies D (2002) *A qualitative evaluation of community palliative care nurse specialists', patients' and carers' views.* Avon, Somerset and Wiltshire Cancer Network User Group. [Personal communication.]

3 Doyle D (1998) *The Way Forward in Promoting Partnership: planning and managing community palliative care.* National Council for Hospice and Specialist Palliative Care, London.

4 General Household Surveys, 1985 and 1990.

5 Travers A F (1996) Caring for older people: carers. *BMJ*. **313**: 482–6.

6 Lynn J, Scuster J L and Kabcenell A (2000) Medicare reimbursement. In J Lynn (ed) *Improving Care for the End of Life.* Oxford University Press, Oxford.

7   Beck Frus B and Strang P (1993) The organisation of hospital-based home care for terminally ill cancer patients: the Motala model. *Pall Med.* **7**: 93–100.

8   Carers' National Association, www.carersuk.demon.co.uk

9   NHS Executive (1999) *Caring about Carers: a national strategy for carers.* NHS Executive, Leeds.

10 Piercy J (2000) The plight of the informal carer. In R Charlton (ed) *Primary Palliative Care.* Radcliffe Medical Press, Oxford.

11 Department of Health (2000) *The NHS Plan.* DoH, London.

12 Garry A (2002) Palliative care. In M Baker (ed) *Modernising Cancer Services.* Radcliffe Medical Press, Oxford.

13 The Griffiths Report (1988) *Community Care: agenda for action.* HMSO, London.

14 Simon C (2001) Informal carers and the primary care team. *Br J Gen Pract.* **51**: 920–3.

15 Stockes J (2000) *The Secret C – straight talking about cancer.* Macmillan Cancer Relief. Winston's Wish, Gloucester.

16 Charlton R and Dolman E (1995) Bereavement protocol for primary care. *Br J Gen Pract.* **45**: 427–30.

17 Benson J and Britten N (1999) Respecting the autonomy of cancer patients when talking with their families. *BMJ.* **319**: 479–82.

18 Nelson E, Sloper P, Charlton A *et al.* (1994) Children who have a parent with cancer: a pilot study. *J Cancer Educ.* **9**: 30–6.

19 Fisher J and Barnett M (2002) Communication with the dying and their loved ones. In R Charlton (ed) *Primary Palliative Care.* Radcliffe Medical Press, Oxford.

20 The Association for Children with Life-threatening or Terminal Conditions (ACT) offers information on support services for families on www.act.org.uk or e-mail: info@act.org.uk

21 Elston S and Thornes R (2001) *Palliative Care for Young People aged 13–24. Report of the Joint Working Party of the Association for Children with Life-threasatening or Terminal Conditions (ACT).* National Council for Hospice and Specialist Palliative Care Services and the Scottish Partnership Agency for Palliative and Cancer Care.

22 Kaye P (1999) *Decision Making in Palliative Care.* EPL Publications, Northampton.

23 Dunlop R [Personal communication.]

24 Kirklees Carers' Gateway, contact via Huddersfield Central PCT, St Luke's House, Blackmoorfoot Road, Huddersfield HD5 5AP. Tel: 01484 466000.

CHAPTER 18

Care of the dying (terminal phase): Gold Standard 7

C7

Patients in the last days of life are cared for appropriately, for example by following a protocol such as the Liverpool Integrated Care Pathway.[1] This includes stopping non-essential interventions and drugs, symptom control, psychological and religious/spiritual support, bereavement planning, communication and care after death being assessed, recorded and acted upon.

Why

For patients entering the terminal phase (last hours/days of life) there are a few specific needs and challenges. If not well addressed, there may be a lasting sense of dissatisfaction with care from both the carers and staff involved, and a yearning for what might have been. By undertaking a few measures in the last days of life using an agreed protocol or pathway, patients may be enabled to die well and peacefully, there may be improved confidence in the professionalism and thoroughness of the community team and the carers' lasting memories, imprinted forever on their minds and hearts, will be as positive as it is possible to be.

What

The Liverpool Integrated Care Pathway for the Dying Patient[1] presents a very thorough guided pathway which can be followed by community teams and is recommended as a further development for those who are interested (*see* Figure 18.1). An abbreviated version is given below:

Box 18.1 Minimal protocol for care of the dying

1 Diagnosis of dying – awareness of signs of the terminal phase.
2 Current medication assessed, non-essentials discontinued, essential treatment converted to subcutaneous route via a syringe driver.
3 PRN drugs written up as per protocol including pain, agitation, respiratory secretions and nausea and vomiting.
4 Ensure the carers know the patient is dying.
5 Spiritual and religious needs assessed and met regarding patient and carers.
6 There is an agreed plan of ongoing assessment and care, including symptom control (pain, agitation, respiratory tract secretions, mouth care, pressure areas, psychosocial support).
7 Relatives are aware of what to do when the patient dies at home.
8 Communication with others – handover form for out-of-hours providers updated, secondary/specialist services informed and hospital appointments cancelled after a death, etc.

How

This can be undertaken by:

- development of a practice check-list/protocol, informed by nationally agreed criteria[2] – at minimum use the eight criteria listed in Box 18.1
- use of the full Liverpool Integrated Care Pathway (*see* Figure 18.1).[1,3,4] Core outcomes of care and prompts accompanying goals can be modified to make them specific to the care setting, e.g. the Welsh Collaborative Care Pathway.[5]

What if ...

What if:

- patients were enabled to die peacefully, retaining dignity and control to the end, in the place of their choice
- relatives/carers were enabled to provide as much care as they wished themselves, were kept informed as active members of the team and felt that everything possible had been done in the care of the dying patient
- PRN medication was available in the home when the patient needed it and unnecessary admission to hospital was therefore prevented
- staff involved had a sense of satisfaction that a 'good death' had been achieved.

Discussion

Suggested minimal protocol for care of the dying *(see* Box 18.1)

1 *Diagnosis of dying* – awareness of signs of the terminal phase. The multiprofessional team agree that the patient is dying if two of the following four criteria apply. The patient is:
   - increasing sleepiness/unconsciousness/semi-comatosed
   - bed-bound
   - only able to take sips of fluids
   - no longer able to take tablets.

2 *Current medication* is assessed, non-essential medication discontinued, essential treatment converted to subcutaneous route via a syringe driver. Discontinue any inappropriate interventions, e.g. blood tests, intravenous infusions, antibiotics, turning of patients, etc.

   The debate about cardiopulmonary resuscitation: consider whether 'not for CPR' is appropriate for this patient, discuss this with relatives/carers and record it clearly in the notes. Ensure that ambulance/emergency staff know of this decision, and that carers know what to do when the patient deteriorates and that calling 999 is inadvisable.

   One patient my DN colleague dealt with died suddenly as she was giving him some hyoscine for his bronchial secretions. The family had no idea he was dying, so called 999. The ambulance staff attempted to resuscitate him, the police were called and the poor nurses were kept under suspicion whilst the family were thrown into total confusion. This was not a good way to die and much of it could have been prevented.

   District nurse, Yorkshire

3 *As required (PRN) drugs are written up,* including drugs for pain, agitation, respiratory secretions and nausea and vomiting. A standard pack of four drugs may be agreed,

such as diamorphine, midazolam, hyoscine butylbromide and haloperidol/cyclizine/levomorpromazine (additionally, rectal diazepam in specific cases where an epileptic fit is likely). These may be assembled in a pack to be left in the home of any patient entering the dying phase. If there is local agreement with palliative care specialists, local medical committees or PCT leads, district nursing managers, pharmacists, etc., authorisation for administration by nursing staff may be included. The drugs remain the patient's property, and thought should be given to their appropriate storage and later disposal in the home. The local pharmacy committee may advise you on locally agreed criteria.

Though some may argue that providing drugs in anticipation of need is wasteful, they are relatively inexpensive and may prove invaluable in a crisis. There is always the potential for abuse by others, such as a member of the family seeking opioids, but the team must weigh up the potential risks and advantages in symptom relief for the patient in each case. Living now in the 'post-Shipman' era of medical accountability, due care and attention must be paid to the accurate usage and recording of any drugs, especially opioids. However, proactively leaving a few drugs in the home seems a small price to pay to counter the potential crisis of unremitting pain and distress experienced by patients unable to access appropriate symptom relief, especially during the long out-of-hours periods. There is physiological evidence that most humans have a lower pain threshold in the night-time hours, and the distress caused by severe symptoms or the fear of their recurrence to both patients and carers must be balanced against the appropriate precautions taken to prevent abuse. As advocates for our patients, there may be times when, whilst agreeing to the appropriate methods of accountability, we have to argue this case against the rising tide of litigious precautionary form-filling that we are faced with.

One thing that has particularly improved since starting this GSF project in our practice is that now we leave a supply of the anticipated drugs in the home of those palliative care patients we have identified on the register; having assessed their particular problems and likely needs, the drugs are already in the home in case they are needed out of hours by the visiting doctor (who also has information on them in a handover form). There have been no crisis calls for drugs and no 50-mile round trips, chasing chemists at weekends, since we started doing this.

DN, coordinator, Shrewsbury, GSF Phase 2

4   *Ensure the carers know the patient is dying*:
   - It is a very important duty of the GP and district nurse to assess when the patient is in the terminal phase and allow proper preparation, both clinically as described and by informing the relatives/carers.
   - It is essential that family and carers, including any children involved, are informed that the patient is likely to die soon. This is something that relatives often say in retrospect they would have appreciated being specifically told but it may not have been clearly communicated. Medical and nursing staff may feel reticent about discussing this, are not always aware of the importance of informing extended family (including children) and do not always feel confident or courageous enough to voice this in gentle terms. Relatives can be left with a sense that if only someone who knew the territory, and had seen this before, had had the courage to tell them there were only a few days/weeks remaining, they would have been better prepared. Family members may need to be recalled from far-off parts, practical arrangements may need to be discussed and final goodbyes made. Frequently, bereaved carers, especially after a sudden deterioration, feel they were cheated of time at the last, and those unspoken words hang heavily in the air, sometimes forever. Helping patients and relatives voice their heartfelt final messages is a particular skill and a special privilege.

It was very brave and helpful of our GP to tell us that she only had days to live. It helped us prepare, to say goodbye and to cope with the long nights of vigil. It would have been dreadful if we'd missed that moment.

MC, carer of cancer patient, Shropshire

5 *Spiritual/religious needs* are assessed with patient and carer:
- chaplain/minister/religious leader informed
- religious observances addressed
- spiritual needs discussed
- space made to discuss deeper issues with patient and carer.

6 *There is an agreed plan of ongoing assessment and care*, e.g. four-hourly assessments:
- symptom control – particularly bronchial secretions, agitation as well as pain relief
- mouth care – regular oral hygiene to relieve dryness and discomfort
- pressure areas – reduce turning of the patient if not appropriate or distressful
- regular assessment – but avoiding excessively disruptive interventions.

7 *Relatives are aware of what to do when the patient dies at home*:
- 'not for CPR' discussed
- Plan of care discussed (999 not called in panic)
- information/leaflet on what to do after a death is given
- removal of body and funeral director discussed
- leaflet on bereavement given.

8 *Communication with others*:
- handover form for out-of-hours providers updated and provider informed after patient's death
- secondary/specialist services informed of likely death, and afterwards
- hospital appointments cancelled after a death
- remainder of team informed.

Funeral directors

Funeral directors or undertakers are specially trained to deal with bereaved relatives, giving some counselling and support in the immediate period after death. As well as making the practical arrangements necessary they will often help with details such as obituary notices, contacting relatives, death registration, etc. There are a few independent trained funeral advisors in institutions where deaths occur, such as hospitals and nursing homes, supported by the National Funerals College's Independent Funeral Advisors.[6]

References

1 The Liverpool Integrated Care Pathway for the Dying Patient Project Beacon resource pack. The Marie Curie Centre, Liverpool and Broadgreen University Hospitals NHS Trust, September 2000.

2 National Council for Hospice and Specialist Palliative Care Services (1997) *Changing Gear: guidelines for managing the last days of life in adults*. NCHSPCS, London.

3 Ellershaw J (2003) *Care of the Dying: a model for excellence*. Oxford University Press, Oxford.

4 Ellershaw J (2000) Integrated care pathways. In J Cooper (ed) *Stepping into Specialist Palliative Care: a handbook for community professionals*. Radcliffe Medical Press, Oxford.

5 wccpp.manager@nww-tr.wales.uk

6 For more details contact rheatley@blueyonder.co.uk

COMFORT MEASURES	**Goal 1: Current medication assessed and non-essentials discontinued**	Yes ☐ No ☐
	Appropriate oral drugs converted to subcutaneous route and syringe driver commenced if appropriate	
	Inappropriate medication discontinued	

Goal 2: PRN subcutaneous medication written up for list below as per protocol   Yes ☐ No ☐

Pain	Analgesia
Nausea and vomiting	Anti-emetic
Agitation	Sedative
Respiratory tract secretions	Anticholinergic

Goal 3: Discontinue inappropriate interventions   Yes ☐ No ☐
Blood test
Antibiotics

Goal 3a: Decisions to discontinue inappropriate nursing interventions taken   Yes ☐ No ☐
Routine turning regime (turn for comfort only)
Taking vital signs

Goal 3b: Syringe driver set up within four hours of identified need   N/A ☐ Yes ☐ No ☐

| PSYCHO-LOGICAL/ INSIGHT | **Goal 4: Ability to communicate in English assessed as adequate** | Yes ☐ No ☐ |

Goal 5: Insight into condition assessed		Comatosed	Yes ☐ No ☐
Aware of diagnosis	(a) Patient	☐	Yes ☐ No ☐
	(b) Family/Other		Yes ☐ No ☐
Recognition of dying	(c) Patient	☐	Yes ☐ No ☐
	(d) Family/Other		Yes ☐ No ☐

RELIGIOUS/ SPIRITUAL SUPPORT	**Goal 6: Religious/spiritual needs assessed with patient/carer**	Yes ☐ No ☐
	Formal religion identified:	
	Special needs now, at time of and after death identified: (please state)	

COMMUNI-CATION WITH FAMILY/ OTHER	**Goal 7: Family/other given information on:**	Yes ☐ No ☐
	Not to call emergency ambulance	
	Not to attempt to resuscitate	
	Contact numbers for 24-hour cover	

COMMUNI- CATION WITH PRIMARY HEALTH- CARE TEAM	**Goal 8: GP and practice are aware of patient's condition** GP and practice to be contacted if unaware patient is dying	Yes ☐ No ☐

SUMMARY

Goal 9: Plan of care explained and discussed with:
(a) Patient ☐   (b) Family ☐   (c) Other ☐   (d) No ☐

Goal 10: Family/other express understanding   N/A ☐ Yes ☐ No ☐
of care plan
Family/carer involvement in physical care

CARE AFTER DEATH

Goal 1: GP and practice contacted re patient's death   Yes ☐ No ☐
Date: —/—/—

Goal 2: Procedures for laying out followed   Yes ☐ No ☐

Goal 3: Procedure following death discussed or   N/A ☐ Yes ☐ No ☐
carried out
(If yes, please indicate)
Patient had infectious disease   ☐
Patient has religious needs   ☐
Post-mortem discussed   ☐

Goal 4: Necessary documentation and advice given to   Yes ☐ No ☐
the appropriate person
- Information leaflet on bereavement/support groups given
- Advised to contact registrar to make an appointment
- Contact number for care practitioner involved

Figure 18.1: Initial assessment and care for patients in the dying phase (adapted from the Liverpool Care Pathway for the Dying Patient).

CHAPTER 19

Getting going: tool kits and the next steps for the Macmillan Gold Standards Framework Programme

We used to pride ourselves on giving most of our patients a very high standard of palliative care. Gold Standards have ensured that we give everyone that high standard.

GP, Northern Ireland, GSF Phase 2

This chapter includes:

- tool kit for **coordinators** and next steps, including an introduction to the Framework
- tool kit for **facilitators** and next steps
- getting going and suggested roles
- evaluation of the first two phases of the GSF.

Tool kit for coordinators and next steps

With many thanks to Dr Hong Tseung, the Halton PCT GP Facilitator, for this helpful introduction to the GSF Handbook for the coordinators of his project. He wrote this as a précis for the coordinators (mainly DNs but some practice managers) as they were about to undertake the GSF. It is a useful, succinct introduction and could be given as a stand-alone document to practices considering taking part. (Therefore there may be a few points repeated from previous pages.)

Tell me and I will forget,
Show me and I might remember,
INVOLVE ME and I will understand.

Old Chinese proverb

Community palliative care – what a mess!
The Gold Standards Framework – an opportunity to organise it!

What is the Gold Standards Framework?

It is an ongoing and developing framework, piloted in 12 practices in Yorkshire and now rolled out to others across the UK, attempting to help primary care to improve their current palliative care provision for their terminally ill/palliative patients. It is jointly funded by Macmillan and the Cancer Services Collaborative (NHS Modernisation Agency). We are part of a group of a number of practices simultaneously undertaking this work across the UK, and we will benefit from shared learning together. It is targeted specifically at primary healthcare teams (GPs, district nurses, practice staff, social workers, associated Macmillan nurses, etc.).

What will it hope to achieve?

The aim is to develop a practice-based system to improve the organisation of care of cancer patients in their last 6–12 months of life. This may later be extended to those with non-malignant conditions and those from diagnosis or with more chronic cancer.

What will it improve?

1   Teamwork and continuity of care.
2   Advanced planning, including out of hours.
3   Symptom control.
4   Patient, carer and staff support.

Who is going to benefit?

1   The PHCT:
   • better teamwork and practice morale
   • better communication, which will also benefit other areas in their work

- fewer crisis calls and admissions with more proactive care
- better organisation of care for most seriously ill patients – more efficient practice to reduce workload, visits, waste less of our limited time
- satisfaction that we are providing our patients with the best service available
- resources in the form of educational materials (books, CD-ROMs, educational meetings) for the PHCT
- fits Personal Medical Services (PMS) and clinical governance agendas and may be of use in new BMA GPC contract quality awards.

2 The patient:

- reassurance that there is good support at hand
- better symptom control
- better rapport with PHCT
- choice of where to die
- support for carers.

Evaluation

This is not just for the sake of another audit. Evaluation is for our own purpose so we can see what we are doing and what we can do to improve. Following the baseline questionnaire or other evaluations will enable us to assess the success of the project, and also how we can improve/identify problems for the future. We hope to use these figures to rally our PCTs and Networks to improve services locally for our patients and for our future patients.

The key players

GP lead
A nominated GP, whom the practice can refer to with regard to the project.

Coordinator
A district nurse or practice manager who can organise Gold Standards activities within the practice. This person can be compared to the 'conductor' (coordinator) of an 'orchestra' (the PHCT).

Key GP/DN
Seeing a multitude of professionals is a problem for many patients (whom it's estimated may see an average of 75 different healthcare professionals during the course of their illness) – we don't need to add to this in primary care. For every patient clinically, there will be a key GP and deputy and a key nurse and deputy, thereby trying to reduce the numbers of professionals involved to four, if possible.

What needs to be done?

1 A team decision
Practice and PHCT to agree to undertake the project.

2 Nominate
Nominate a GP lead and a coordinator.

3 Fill in the baseline questionnaire
It will form the basis for us to compare whether what we do will make a difference.

4 Create a Supportive Care register (palliative care register)
This is to identify these palliative care patients better and keep relevant documents in one place. Include patients who are entering the last 6–12 months of life. As a minimum, all patients who have had a DS1500 completed can be identified and put on the register. However, we all have patients who have had a DS1500 for more than 12 months and some who are ill but not needing much help at present, so discuss amongst the PHCT who is appropriate to include or exclude. Keep some in the 'active' section and others in the 'inactive' or quiet – 'the poorlies and the pendings'! For computerised practices, make sure the data inputter enters DS1500 (Read code is 9EB5) whenever it is completed. IT versions of the register are welcomed. The criteria for entry in the register is based on need not stage – add the patients who you feel would benefit from more input or who have problems which require our help. It is envisaged that the register will not be massive but is a tool to improve care and to keep us focused on why we are doing this, not how!

5 Hold monthly PHCT meetings
These are not expected to be additional to the existing PHCT meeting, but for the routine meeting to set a small portion of time aside to discuss the patients on the Supportive Care register. Updates can then be given more frequently as needed.
   At these meetings, for each patient on the register:

- Invite all relevant members – DNs, Macmillan nurses, practice manager (all definitely), but optionally also social workers, occupational therapists, physio-therapists, etc. (as required). They might be interested in coming to the six-month review meeting at minimum.

- Discuss those patients that you have already identified on the register. Note also the key GP and key nurse who is looking after each patient mainly, with one back-up for absences.

- *Assess* your patients using the suggested tools provided, but only those that are relevant for your patients. Prepare your updated register – needs, problems, etc. – ready to present for discussion with the PHCT. Go through the summary sheet as a focus, backed up by the PACA scale regularly and the PEPSI COLA check-list if useful for each patient (once as an initial assessment and then only as needed). Relevant members of the PHCT to implement any recommendations.

- *Plan* for the future care of these patients. Think what you might predict possibly happening and ensure that you have reduced the chance of an unanticipated emergency taking place. Consider support for carers, leaving drugs in the home, how their condition might worsen, etc.

- Discuss if it is appropriate for each patient to be given a Home Pack, and who should introduce it with the patient and family before giving it to them. This is not always easy and requires good communication skills. Add the relevant information, e.g. phone numbers, predicted problems and what to do. Add the booklets that you think are most relevant to the stage and needs of the family – don't be put off by titles. More booklets are available on different subjects to make the Home Pack very personal for that family (*see* Macmillan's *Directory of Patient Resources* or the Cancerbacup website www.cancercup.org.uk).

- Every six months hold a review meeting or significant event analysis on patients looked after – you can use the 'traffic lights' in the Gold Standards handbook to help. Relay your findings to the facilitators and to your PCTs – use your findings as collective evidence to make improvements in your area.

- Agree the time of the next monthly meeting. Keep momentum going! The time set aside for all this should only be around 15–20 minutes, except that the six-monthly review meeting may take longer. This could be part of your practice and personal development plans.

In summary

It is not expected that the regular members of the PHCT (GP, DN, etc.) need to do much extra work, other than attempt to assess patients more fully and discuss their findings as they would ordinarily do at the PHCT meetings. However, the coordinators and GP leads will have extra administrative duties (see later), but even then, once the system is in place, the whole set-up should run by itself. Also, coordinators and GP leads can delegate some of the admin to supporting receptionists/secretarial staff.

Specific roles of the PHCT

The lead GP

- Highlight Gold Standards Framework within the practice.
- Support and assist the GSF coordinator as necessary.
- Develop any initiatives/ideas with the coordinator and PHCT.
- Attend local GSF support meetings arranged by the facilitator.
- If possible, attend coordinators' national conference.
- Feedback to PCT, maybe via cancer or clinical governance lead.

The coordinator ('the conductor of the orchestra')

- Create and keep up to date a Supportive Care register.
- Arrange and coordinate monthly PHCT meetings.
- Invite relevant members of PHCT to meetings.
- Record the key GP and key nurse for each patient.
- At each meeting, ensure issues that have arisen from the Problems and Concerns/PEPSI COLA check-list are raised for each patient on the register.
- Ensure each patient summary sheet is completed and kept up to date, and the out-of-hours handover form is sent to the out-of-hours provider (co-op).

- Ensure the monthly key outcome sheet is completed and returned to the facilitator regularly. Attend local Gold Standards Framework support meetings arranged by the facilitator.
- *If necessary, delegate some of the administrative duties* (e.g. booking meetings, form filling, sending back evaluation sheets, etc.) to practice admin staff – discuss with your practice manager. This is particularly important for district nurses who are nominated as coordinators, and who are also responsible for their daily clinical case load – don't get yourself overwhelmed!

The patient's key GP
- May be first port of call for the patient.
- Holds clinical responsibility for the patient.
- Responsible for management decisions and prescribing.
- Makes accurate assessment of symptoms, e.g. using body charts/PACA/other templates suggested.
- Discuss Home Pack with patient/family if nurse has not done so.
- Pass on clinical information to the rest of the PHCT.
- Assess carer's needs and support independently.

The patient's key nurse
- This is usually the district nurse.
- Provide practical nursing care.
- Communication and counselling for the patient.
- Provision of equipment.
- Terminal care.
- Liaison with other agencies/multidisciplinary team.
- Documentation (care plan).
- Attend PHCT meetings; offer appropriate advice on management.
- Discuss home care pack with patient/family if GP has not done so.
- Assess carer's needs and support independently.

Macmillan nurse/clinical nurse specialist in the community
- Attend PHCT meetings where possible.
- Advice to PHCT on management of patients' symptoms.
- Involved in education of the PHCT.

Practice manager
- Attend PHCT meetings.
- Liaise with coordinator to provide admin support, e.g. data collection/evaluation forms, faxing out-of-hours handover forms, customising practice information or leaflets.

Receptionist
- Access point for patient to practice.
- Be aware of patients on Supportive Care register so problems can be fast-tracked to GP/nurse – use of a 'care board' such as names on a discreet white board in the practice?

Other PHCT members
Other professionals who may be involved at some point in the patient's care:
- occupational therapist, physiotherapist, health visitor (for elderly visits or, rarely, child cancer) tissue viability nurse, lymphoedema nurse, social worker, etc.

Final tips

DO	let your facilitator know if you have any problems.
DO	communicate and work with your PHCT, and clarify each others' roles.
DO	introduce changes at the pace and in the way you see fit in your area. Rooted and realistic changes make more difference – we are not seeking flashes in the pan here but a system of change that will improve long-term patient care.
DO	expect resistance and pull back from some – if they see an improvement for their patients and an easier system for them, they are likely to come round.
DO	copy, modify, change, add, customise for your area anything on the templates.
DO	attend the local Gold Standards feedback meetings, where problems and possible solutions can be shared. You'll find great encouragement and have fun!
DO	undertake the baseline questionnaire and other evaluation sheets and send these back on time to the facilitator.
DO	try to attend the conferences if available – you will enjoy being energised by the sense of others moving in the same direction.
DON'T	suffer in silence and allow obstacles to stop you implementing the Framework.
DON'T	get overloaded – share your workload and keep in mind the goals.
DON'T	feel disheartened, especially if the team is struggling or there are staff changes – this is real life!
DON'T	lose your sense of humour or your perspective.
DO	take care of yourselves –the most precious resource of the health service.
DO	remember that all this will help us as well as our patients!
DO	have fun! Enjoying your work is allowed!

Next steps for those interested in becoming GSF coordinators

1 Agree as a primary healthcare team to take part in the GSF for at least six months' trial.
2 Nominate a coordinator, often a district nurse or could be a practice manager/practice nurse.
3 Nominate a lead GP for the project.
4 Send confirmation and contact details to your facilitator.
5 Enter all cancer patients for whom you write a DS1500 form, i.e. those you would expect to be in the last six to nine months of life, into the pilot.
6 Assemble a Supportive Care register and complete for all relevant patients (standardised sheet and resources provided).
7 Hold monthly meetings to discuss these patients – these can be part of your regular PHCT meeting. Invite specialists if possible, e.g. Macmillan nurses, to hold special relevant teaching sessions or provide 'learn as you go' input, related to the patients discussed.
8 Follow the seven Cs.
9 Attend training and feedback sessions run by your facilitator.
10 Receive resources at these sessions, e.g. Supportive Care register, home packs, etc.
11 Complete baseline and post-project questionnaires.
12 Hold a review/audit meeting after six months, then regularly at six-month intervals. Communicate this with others, e.g. PCT cancer lead/clinical governance lead and Cancer Network.
13 Develop, agree and record your own practice protocol.

Tool kit for facilitators and next steps

Training sessions, templates and resources, etc. (*see* the website for details) will be available and there will be contact via e-mail, list-serve, conference calls, conferences, etc. The aim is to help you as you develop changes in your area, so sharing areas of difficulty as well as successes is essential. Please contact the central team at any time and we hope you will feel well supported in this valuable work.

Your contribution as facilitator

The extra items you may need to provide yourself are:

- a list of the practices and coordinators involved on a spreadsheet
- your own *local information*, e.g. local contact details, guidelines, formulary, etc. to add to the information going to practices
- *resources* – you may need extra funding for lunch-time meetings, suggested books, resources, etc.
- to organise *teaching sessions* and later feedback sessions (dates, venue and lunch), plus invite palliative care specialists to contribute if possible. Past experience suggests having a lunch-time session (12.30–2pm) for GPs, coordinators, DNs, practice managers, specialists, etc. to introduce the whole project is useful, then for the coordinators to stay on after the others have gone to go through each point in more detail. Then four- to six-weekly feedback meetings ensure that people are kept buoyed up and can hear how others are doing, go through good things, not so good things and share ideas, etc. The important skill of listening is greatly valued here, involving everyone and listening to concerns and issues in a constructive, problem-solving way. This builds support and a sense of moving on together, one of the greatest benefits of this work.
- *feedback/evaluation* – in order to assess progress in your practices and project area, some kind of measurement is valuable. We ask the facilitator to be responsible for chasing any errant practice feedback sheets. Therefore some administrative back-up for distribution of questionnaires, chasing any non-responders and organising meetings is especially helpful.
- *continuation* – many will only just be getting going after 6 months. Sustainability and empowerment are key factors in this and worth pondering over, but if good ideas are well rooted they shouldn't be dependent on your enthusiasm to continue. However, building in six-monthly reviews for individual practices and regular meetings for the GSF teams together, holding open conferences to present their findings to others, etc. are all im-portant ways in which ideas are maintained and spread. This is long-term work.
- *extension to non-cancer patients and from diagnosis* – as previously discussed, the GSF programme began mainly with cancer patients for whom a DS1500 was thought applicable, but palliative care obviously extends beyond the boundaries of cancer care to all patients with any end-stage illness, including end-stage heart failure, HIV, COPD and so on. So many practices have extended to patients with non-malignant conditions and also to those more chronic cancer patients from diagnosis onwards. Some have different coloured folders for patients with differing needs and many have divided the register into 'active' and 'inactive' patients, but maintaining an overview of all. Patients need support from diagnosis onwards and many offer this (*see* the Supportive Care Strategy of the NHS Cancer Plan). Improving the care of patients with non-malignant conditions to the same standard as those with cancer is one of the challenges of the coming years.

- *working with specialist palliative care colleagues* – it is important to affirm your local contacts with palliative care specialists, i.e. consultants based at the hospice or hospital and Macmillan/community CNS nurses, and involve them as much as possible in the development of this work. Effective patient care depends on the close working together of generalists and specialists, and the knowledge of when to refer is an important skill. The specific guidelines of the PACA model used in C3 can become a suggested guide for specialist referral, to audit if required as part of clinical governance. Eligibility criteria for referral to specialists are of use to some. Most are keen to work together in partnership with GPs and DNs, so referral can be for advice, admission or practical support such as day care, without losing the continuity of patient care. The fears of a takeover of care which may have lingered with some GPs are usually unfounded now. Some areas still have no palliative care specialist available or use them mainly for back-up telephone advice, whereas others, such as parts of London, appear to use specialists in a particular way and seem more likely to take over full care if requested. Where there is no hospice or specialist palliative care service, improving generalist services is even more important. It is vital to dovetail generalist and specialist care as appropriate, integrating whatever specialist service is available in your area. Many specialists say they are used more appropriately after the introduction of the GSF.

Gains to you as facilitator

You will have the opportunity to learn more about various skills and techniques, such as the improvement methods employed by the NHS Modernisation Agency, the PACA assessment tool, etc. You will gain experience in group working for a specific purpose, across boundaries and roles. You will help to develop and inform local strategic changes in your area. You will be well supported, with many other benefits, and enjoy being part of a wider team across the UK with a common intent. Your main contribution to make this work is your *enthusiasm and inspiration* plus your original ideas on how to improve what is on offer for others.

Our hope is that you enjoy being part of this project and that together we can make a difference in improving primary palliative care and thereby the quality of patient care in the community.

Next steps for those facilitating a project

1   Agree to facilitate a project in the GSF programme for your area and complete the form (*see* www.radcliffe-oxford.com/caring) to register your interest with the central GSF team.
2   Develop interest in improving community palliative care in your area. Enlist a group of practices and provide contact details for the central team. It is important that all the PHCT should agree to undertake this work and that it should not rely on the enthusiasm of just a few.
3   Undertake a baseline questionnaire for each participating practice *before* commencing any changes – it is easy to miss this baseline point but important to capture the baseline initially. Asking the questions also stimulates change.
4   Plan teaching sessions/meetings. Help practices set up Supportive Care registers. Discuss the coordinators' roles. Plan feedback meetings.
5   Keep connected with the central team – attend any available conference and facilitators' meetings.

Getting going: the Macmillan GSF Programme

Moving from something being a good idea to becoming a real improvement in everyday life takes a team effort. We need skills, support and resources: both the paperwork and the people.

- The *skills* are those of good primary care, change management, as described, focusing on aims, measures and change principles, plus the necessary optimism.
- The *support* is from the Macmillan central team via local facilitators, as described.
- The *resources* are:
  - **Paperwork/tools** – the tools are supplied in the form of the Macmillan Gold Standards Framework tool box, backed up by resources available on websites, by e-mail, post and from the central GSF team, e.g. Supportive Care register templates, Home Packs, etc. Resource packs of textbooks, articles and CD-ROMs to kick-start your practice library may be available.
  - **People factors** – this is the key factor. A developing momentum of people moving forward together in practice teams (led by coordinators) and local project areas (led by facilitators) and nationally as a collective movement. Most importantly the will and enthusiasm to make it happen. Both the facilitators of projects and the coordinators within practices are vitally important for the running of this programme. The GSF central team will support you and are available by phone, e-mail, list-serve, website, etc.
  - **Plan** – a planned support programme of workshops, visits, etc. and collective evaluation of the changes made (anonymously) is organised.
  - **Funding** – this may be available in a variety of ways (more details are available on the website) such as local development schemes, new opportunity funding, network primary care bids, the new BMA contract (still under review as we go to press) and others. Funding is used mainly to kick-start the first two–three months of this work, with the introduction of the register or the payment of the local facilitator.

The mode of delivering change is important, developing change in a relationship-based 'physiological' way,[1] i.e.:

- 'top-down support is needed for bottom-up change': the GSF programme, with central support but localised adaptation via facilitators and coordinators
- you need a plan to set direction but must be flexible: the GSF feeding into practice protocols
- objectives must be set and the team congratulated when each objective is achieved, but improvement never ends: the seven Cs standards and their ongoing evaluation, plus six-monthly review meetings
- correct use of improvement tools and techniques should be planned and monitored but gaining the commitment of people is vital: teaching sessions for facilitators but ongoing contact and support by the central team.

Plans for roll-out of Macmillan GSF Programme

Plans for future phases of the Macmillan GSF are still to be confirmed at the time of going to press, but those registered with the GSF programme will be informed of details directly. For any other enquiries, please contact us via e-mail at gsf@macmillan.org.uk or the website and more details will be available soon.

The same structure will continue in future phases, i.e. a central team to support facilitators who run the work in their areas with their practice coordinators. The project areas for each facilitator have been approximately the size of a PCT or about 100 000 population.

There will be three conferences for each phased roll-out with a launch, an intermediate and a finale six months later. The tool kit will be given at the launch and evaluation commenced over the 6–12 month period.

Box 19.1 Suggested roles

The central GSF team

- direct and oversee the programme, including future phases, following evaluation and modifications
- write, produce and distribute materials, including templates, register, etc.
- train, encourage and support facilitators of projects
- support with visits, phone calls, conference calls, list-serve, etc.
- feedback ideas and share examples of good practice to a wider group
- commission, coordinate and fund evaluation
- interlink phases 1, 2 and 3
- interlink with other agencies.

The suggested role of the **facilitator** (and admin support) is to:

- nurture an interest in developing community palliative care in their own area
- raise awareness – from 'pre-contemplation and contemplation to preparation' stages
- enlist practices wishing to make changes and undertake the GSF
- visit, encourage and discuss the introduction of the GSF
- run teaching sessions for teams – set up four- to six-weekly feedback meetings in advance (venue and drug company-sponsored lunches planned for every six months) – for coordinators and others interested
- organise the collection of evaluation from practices which is then sent to an information analyst – baseline questionnaire, and follow-up and other measures if used
- be the link to the central team
- link locally to the PCT, Cancer Network, hospice/specialist palliative care teams, social services, pharmacist, etc.
- share good practice examples and encourage and support any struggling practices.

The suggested role of the **coordinator** is to:

- encourage all of the PHCT to agree to undertake the GSF programme for six months at least
- undertake baseline evaluation and follow-up measures
- orchestrate tasks (as in C2) and appoint a deputy and admin help
- set up the Supportive Care register (C1)
- set up monthly PHCT meetings and briefly go through the list of patients in the summary
- discuss problems individually with other staff, e.g. GPs, after a death if needed
- attend local project feedback meetings for support and sharing of information and, if possible, national conferences
- link with others, e.g. Macmillan nurses/hospice staff – invite to PHCT meetings regularly or for occasional teaching sessions on agreed topics
- add in C3, C4, C5, C6 and C7 at an appropriate pace
- feed queries back to the facilitator/central team.

Evaluation of the first two phases of the Gold Standards Framework: does it make a difference?

Phase 1 evaluation

The pilot was undertaken by Calderdale and Kirklees Health Authority, with the Macmillan GP Facilitator based in Huddersfield.

Phase 1 was evaluated in traditional quantitative and qualitative terms by the author. There were three questions:

1 Is it acceptable to the practice? (*structure*) – time taken, staff workload, efficiency, input/output, resources supplied, useful, etc.
2 Does it change practice? (*process*) – are they doing things now not done before, e.g. PHCT meetings, Supportive Care registers, handover forms, assessment tools, etc.
3 Does it make a difference to patients and carers? (*outcome*) – numbers dying in their preferred place of death, reduced number of crises/admissions, 'bed days' in hospital per cancer patient per year, number of cancer patients admitted to hospital who die within 48 hours, proportion of patients whose care follows evidence-based guidelines of care, patient/carer satisfaction improved, staff satisfaction with care improved, etc.

These were measured by:

1 *quantitative methods*, using a questionnaire before and six months after undertaking the GSF for:
   - the 12 intervention practices
   - 12 matched non-intervention practices (purposive matching)
   - an end-point sample of 18 other practices to assess 'background noise'.
   This revealed that all intervention practices were able to improve the standard of care to differing degrees. They achieved the 'Gold Standard' in most categories after six months (following then six standards, not seven), and there was a difference between the GSF practices and the non-intervention practices. This confirmed the impression that this was achievable and that practices undertaking the GSF had improved their levels of appropriate interventions and care. Also, incidentally, asking certain questions in the baseline questionnaire triggered some practices to initiate changes.
2 *qualitative methods* – 'action research' – which included:
   - a focus group, involving GPs, district nurses and practice managers discussing the barriers and key issues in community palliative care, before the start of the GSF and afterwards. In the latter, the group was asked to vote on a scale of 1–10 on the issues they had brought up before and after the introduction of the project. Four areas were highlighted: teamwork/continuity, advanced planning, symptom control and carer and staff support. The resulting discussion was recorded, transcribed and analysed using an agreed template and standard qualitative methods.
   - semi-structured telephone interviews one year on with the GPs from the 12 practices, using a standard template of questions.
   - other 'softer' data, e.g. quotes from staff, patients and carers and some anonymised letters and feedback. These include the impressions the staff have about teamwork, morale and acceptability within the already heavy primary care workload.

Full evaluation will be available later (www.modern.nhs.uk/www.macmillan.org.uk) (*see* Box 19.2).

Box 19.2 Brief summary of Phase 1 pilot evaluation

1 *Was it acceptable?* Yes.

  Time not excessive, saves some GP time; took more DN time initially, then easier to maintain; affirms roles; teamwork better; communication better – all continuing in some form one year later

2 *Does it change practice?* Yes.

  All had Supportive Care registers (seen as crucial); nine out of 12 had PHCT meetings, three for the first time when they began GSF; raises awareness; patient focused with handover out-of-hours forms and use of SEAs

3 *Does it make a difference and is the change an improvement?* Yes.

  Teamwork/communication improved (greatly in some); advanced and improved planning; symptom control – assessments better; carer support better; staff morale better; FUN! Still improving and developing.

More details available in the future from www.modern.nhs.uk and www.macmillan.org.uk or by e-mail gsf@macmillan.org.uk.

Acceptability of time and workload

One key element was that although there was an increase in 'administrative' time for the coordinators, there was little or negligible extra GP time involved; in fact, four out of 12 GPs felt that there was a saving of time because of centralised information. Most felt that the early weeks setting up the register took most time, but that once established and integrated there was less extra time involved, as long as they avoided becoming overwhelmed with form filling. Workload was easier as there was less crisis management.

Phase 2 evaluation

At the time of going to press this information is still being collected and analysed. More details will be available later on the website. An interim report is available at www.modern.nhs.uk.

The emphasis is on measuring for improvement not for judgement, to allow practices feedback on their developments and indicate areas where the central team can help with support or improvement. Again, the measuring is by:

1 *quantitative methods*, involving from each practice team:
   • baseline and after intervention questionnaires (Q1 and Q2), noting change in behaviour after six months
   • monthly key outcome sheets relating to the seven C's, and noting specifically numbers of patients who die whilst on the programme and numbers who die in their preferred place of death.

   These are analysed by the Cancer Services Collaborative information Analyst.

Early results confirm an increase in identification of palliative care patients, in noting and attaining the preferred place of death, in carer information given and in using a protocol for terminal care, plus a possible decrease in crisis admissions in some areas.

Phase II plan of GSF

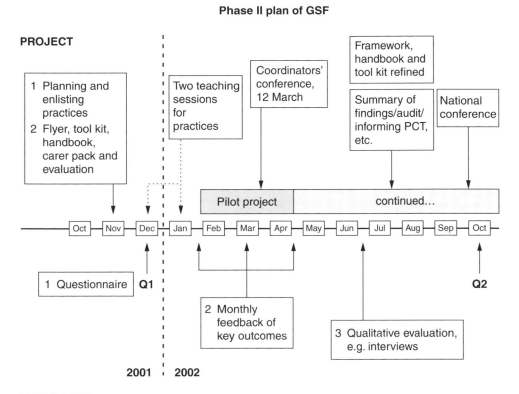

Figure 19.1: Time-line plan.

2   *qualitative methods*, involving a full qualitative analysis, using an independent university research team plan to interview GPs, DNs, carers and others interested, in eight GSF practices compared with eight non-GSF practices, in four areas undertaking the GSF Phase 2 work. It is hoped this will capture some of the more intangible but very valuable elements such as staff satisfaction, empowerment and communication levels, as well as some of the other factors of workload and acceptability.

Early results confirm improved levels of satisfaction, communication and organisation of care compared with non-GSF practices.

For planned Phase 3 evaluation contact the Macmillan GSF Programme. The plan for Phase 3 and further evaluations is to conduct a baseline questionnaire, repeated at 3, 6 and 12-month intervals, tailoring the questions more specifically to the global outcomes required, via the seven Cs. Other research projects will look at some smaller issues in more detail.

Box 19.3 The five Global Outcomes (GO) of the Gold Standards Framework

GO 1   **Patients:** symptom control, holistic (psychosocial), dying phase, etc.

GO 2   **Patients:** customised care, needs-based, preferred place of care/death, services and responses shaped to needs.

GO 3   **Patients:** security and support, advanced care planning, fewer crises, information well communicated, good access with prompt response, smooth transitions across care boundaries.

GO 4   **Carers' needs met:** information provision, communication, carer assessment and support, education, social/financial help.

GO 5   **Staff:** teamwork, coordination, morale, confidence, co-working with specialists/hospital staff.

Box 19.4 Specific measurables relating to the seven Cs (* denotes the most important)

1	Identification of palliative care patients and use of the register	C1*, GO2
2	PHCT meeting to discuss advanced care planning	C1
3	Co-working with specialists	C1
4	Coordinator named, cross-boundary communication	C2
5	Care plans, including advanced care planning noted	C2
6	Preference for place of care/death noted	C2*, GO2
7	Preferred place of death attained	C2*, GO2
8	Staff teamwork/satisfaction/confidence	C2*, GO5
9	Assessment tools used, e.g. PACA	C3
10	Confidence in assessment of symptoms	C3*, GO1
11	Out-of-hours handover form sent	C4*, GO3
12	Drugs left in home	C4*, GO3
13	Crises reduced, e.g. fewer admissions in last days	C4*, GO3
14	Six-month review meeting and audit	C5
15	In-house learning/library use/SEA	C5
16	Information given specifically to carer	C6*, GO4
17	Carer assessed and supported	C6*, GO4
18	Staff support and teamwork	C6*, GO5
19	Use of protocol for end-of-life	C7*, GO1
20	Overall quality of care and confidence of team	Other*, GO5

Reflection so far

Different practices and project areas of the GSF programme have responded in different ways, with various levels of 'successes' and also some problems, although all have had some very significant achievements in their own ways. The waves of enthusiastic positive feedback, and the potential numbers wishing to take part, affirm that this is an area that primary care really wishes to excel in and many feel extremely committed towards. The fact that so many practices in such a variety of situations have undertaken this work with such gusto, and have continued to make great strides in their level of care, is great testimony to the quality of our NHS healthcare professionals. It also demonstrates that with protected time to pick out and consider this subject, and with certain levels of support, encouragement and resourcing, practice teams can hardly fail to make some improvements in their organisation of care of the dying.

On reflection, it seems that those practices and projects which fare better:

- are well supported by their primary care organisation/Network
- have some extra resources in some cases, e.g. DN time, GP facilitator time, etc.
- have good administrative back-up, especially in the initial stages
- are well facilitated – those with protected time, e.g. Macmillan GP Facilitators
- have few staff changes in the practice team
- have all the practice informed and all are in agreement with the work
- make steady progress, with a long-term view, rather than a quick fix
- have keen innovators within primary care – GPs, nurses and managers.

The initial, unconfirmed impression is that projects having more problems tend to have a higher level of changing staff, there is less 'buy-in' from all the team, there is greater resistance to holding meetings and some were overwhelmed initially by the perceived amount of paperwork (something which has to be watched constantly – it is only there to further the goal of better communication and assessment and must be integrated into the assessment system already in place, without adding to the burden). Alternatively, a few jump at the work initially and then may not be able to sustain interest, perhaps partly because changes are not embedded as standard practice procedures and a lack of teamwork means they are too dependent on the keenness of a few individuals, who may become overwhelmed.

Specific clinical outcome measures are still being clarified, but increased noting and attaining preferred place of death, increased carer information and decreased crises are some tangible improvements worth pursuing.

> The GSF is really more about 'hearts and minds', so collecting data is only a small part of it. It represents much deeper changes that cannot be easily defined or measured and may not be represented by data. But in fact these changes are the more important ones.
>
> Specialist Palliative Care, Northern Ireland

However, the important question must always be whether it has benefited patients. If DNs and GPs feel that their care of the dying has improved since the introduction of this Framework together with the provision of protected time for these patients, this is likely to be reflected by those on the receiving end of care. It is also an achievement if the practice team feels a greater sense of satisfaction in their work and in the service provided.

It is our responsibility to take the initiative and ensure we provide the highest quality service for our patients, not the patients' role to have to request it. In a theatrical analogy, it is up to us to ensure the 'backstage' organisation is functioning well and efficiently so that what the audience see gives satisfying confidence and security, whilst they cope with the progression of their illness. These things are hard to capture in evaluations, but the enthusiasm of the staff involved (with examples quoted in this book) is the greatest tribute we can achieve and the strongest testimony to this work.

> *As a district nurse, I have been providing palliative care to my patients for over 20 years and it is an area I am particularly keen on. But this work has helped us so much to organise ourselves and communicate better, and to provide much more personalised care for our patients. We now all feel better able to continue giving our best to those in our community who are dying.*
>
> DN, Northern Ireland, GSF Phase 2

Reference

1 NHS Modernisation Redesign Team *Managing the Human Dimension of Change*, www.modern.nhs.uk/improvementguides/human

Further reading

- Addington-Hall J and Higginson I (2001) *Palliative Care for Non-Cancer Patients*. Oxford University Press.
- Back I (2001) *Palliative Medicine Handbook* (3e). BPM Books. A useful and detailed pocketbook with handy facts, drug information and check-lists. It is well referenced with clinical, organisational and factual information.
- Baker M (ed) (2002) *Modernising Cancer Services*. Radcliffe Medical Press.
- Bosanquet N and Salisbury C (1999) *Providing a Palliative Care Service*. Oxford University Press.
- Cancerlink (2000) *Directory of Cancer Self-Help and Support, 2001*. Cancerlink.
- Charlton R (ed) (2002) *Primary Palliative Care: dying, death and bereavement in the community*. Radcliffe Medical Press. A valuable discussion on all topics of relevance to this area.
- Clark R with Jefferies N, Hasler J and Pendleton D (2002) *A Long Walk Home*. Radcliffe Medical Press. A moving book written by a dying cancer patient, which details her experiences of the healthcare systems in the UK and Australia.
- Cooper J (ed) *Stepping into Palliative Care: a handbook for community professionals*. Radcliffe Medical Press. Geared mainly for nurses but all will find it a useful workbook.
- Diamond J (1999) *C: Because Cowards Get Cancer Too*. Vermilion. The moving account of his personal experiences as he approaches death.
- Doyle D, Hanks G W C and Macdonald N (eds) (1998) *Oxford Textbook of Palliative Medicine* (2e). Oxford Medical Publications. The major reference book on palliative care with sections covering all topics.
- Doyle D and Jeffrey D (2000) *Palliative Care in the Home*. Oxford University Press.
- Fallon M and O'Neill B (1998) *ABC of Palliative Care*. BMJ Books. Includes helpful sections on all subjects.
- Faull C, Carter Y and Woof R (1998) *Handbook of Palliative Care*. Blackwell Science.
- Higginson I (1997) Palliative and terminal care. In: A Stevens and J Raftery (eds) *Health Care Needs Assessment: the epidemiologically based needs assessment reviews. Second Series*. Radcliffe Medical Press.
- Jeffrey D (2000) *Cancer: from cure to care*. Haigh and Hochland. Description of GPs' views of palliative care.
- Jeffrey D (ed) (2002) *Teaching Palliative Care: a practical guide*. Radcliffe Medical Press.
- Kaye P (1998) *A–Z of Palliative Care Pocketbook*. EPL Publications. An invaluable guide that has always been popular with GPs and DNs.
- Kaye P (1999) *Decision Making in Palliative Care*. EPL Publications. Easy to read with helpful flow diagrams. Easy to refer to and very practical.
- King N and Anderson N (2001) *Managing Innovation and Change: a critical guide for organisations*. Thomson.
- Lee E (2002) *In Your Own Time: a guide for patients and their carers facing a last illness at home*. Oxford University Press.
- Lynn J and Harrold J (1999) *Handbook for Mortals: guidance for people facing serious illness*. Oxford University Press.

- Lynn J (1999) *Improving Care for End of Life: a sourcebook for health managers and clinicians.* Oxford University Press. Includes details of the American Institute of Healthcare end-of-life developments (<u>www.ihi.org</u>).
- Macmillan Cancer Relief (2001) *A Directory of Information Materials for People with Cancer, 2000/2001* (2e). Macmillan Cancer Relief.
- Macmillan Cancer Relief (2002) *Directory of Complementary Services in UK Cancer Care, 2002.* Macmillan Cancer Relief.
- Mayne M (2001) *Learning to Dance.* Darton, Longman & Todd. A spiritual journey rich with quotations.
- NHS Modernisation Agency *Improvements Leaders Guides* on *Process Mapping, Analysis and Redesign; Measurement for Improvement; Matching Capacity and Demand; Involving Patients and Carers; Managing the Human Dimensions of Change; Sustainability and Spread* – available from the NHS Modernisation Agency or via <u>www.modern.nhs.uk/ improvement</u>
- Regnard C and Kindlen M (2002) *Supportive and Palliative Care in Cancer: an introduction.* Radcliffe Medical Press.
- Regnard C and Tempest S (1998) *A Guide to Symptom Relief in Advanced Disease.* Haigh and Hochland.
- Robbins M (1998) *Evaluating Palliative Care: establishing the evidence base.* Oxford University Press.
- Speck P (1988) *Being There: pastoral care in time of illness.* SPCK.
- Stokes J (2001) *The Secret C.* Winston's Wish/Macmillan Cancer Relief. A straight-talking children's guide about cancer.
- Sweeney K and Griffiths F (eds) (2002) *Complexity and Healthcare: an introduction.* Radcliffe Medical Press.
- Thomas K (2001) *Out-of-Hours Palliative Care in the Community: continuing care for the dying at home.* Macmillan Cancer Relief.
- Twycross R and Wilcock A (2001) *Symptom Management in Advanced Cancer* (3e). Radcliffe Medical Press.
- Twycross R, Wilcock A and Thorp S (2002) *Palliative Care Formulary 2.* Radcliffe Medical Press. Invaluable for checking drug details and addressing problems.

Appendix

Contents

Vision of a better service for dying patients

These seven promises to patients from the *Vision of a Better System of Care for Dying Patients*, promoted by Dr Joanne Lynn, Director at the RAND Center to Improve Care of the Dying, Arlington, VA and President of Americans for Better Care of the Dying, Washington, DC are worth pondering and, if possible, emulating.

Source: Lynn J (2000) *Collaborative on Improving End-of-Life Care: 'Accelerating Change Today'*. National Coalition on Healthcare (www.nchc.org) and Institute of Healthcare Improvement (www.ihi.org).

Making Promises
Vision of a better system

For patients with advanced stages of serious illnesses, it is not possible to promise cure or restoration of health. However here are seven promises that really seem to make a difference to such patients. In each case, we define the promise, its core statement, and list a few examples of what it might mean to put practices in place to deliver on that promise.

1 *Good medical treatment.* You will have the best of medical treatment, aiming to prevent exacerbation, improve function and survival, and ensure comfort.
   - Patients will be offered proven diagnosis and treatment strategies to prevent exacerbations and enhance quality of life, as well as to delay disease progression and death.
   - Medical intervention will be in accord with best available standards of medical practice and evidence-based when possible.

2 *Never overwhelmed by symptoms.* You will never have to endure overwhelming pain, shortness of breath or other symptoms.
   - Symptoms will be anticipated and prevented when possible, evaluated and addressed promptly and controlled effectively.
   - Severe symptoms, such as shortness of breath, will be treated as emergencies.
   - Sedation will be used when necessary to relieve intractable symptoms near the end of life.

3 *Continuity, coordination and comprehensiveness.* Your care will be continuous, comprehensive and coordinated.
   - Patients and families can count on having certain professionals to rely upon at all times.
   - Patients and families can count on an appropriate and timely response to their needs.
   - Transitions between services, settings and personnel will be minimised in number and made to work smoothly.

4 *Well-prepared – no surprises.* You and your family will be prepared for everything that is likely to happen in the course of your illness.
   - Patients and families come to know what to expect as the illness worsens, and what is expected of them.
   - Patients and families receive supplies and training needed to handle predictable events.

5   *Customised care, reflecting your preference.* Your wishes will be sought and respected, and followed wherever possible.
- Patients and families come to know the alternatives for services and expect to make choices that matter.
- Patients never receive treatments they refuse.
- Patients who want to live out the end of their life at home, usually can.

6   *Use of patient and family resources (financial, emotional and practical).* We will help you and your family to consider your personal and financial resources, and we will respect your choices about the use of your resources.
- Patients and families will be aware of services available in their community and the costs of those services.
- Family care-givers' concerns will be discussed and addressed. Respite, volunteer and home aid care will be part of the care plan when appropriate.

7   *Make the best of every day.* We will do all we can to see that you and your family will have the opportunity to make the best of every day.
- The patient is treated as a person, not a disease, and what is important to the patient is important to the care team.
- The care team responds to the physical, psychological, social and spiritual needs of the patient and family.
- Families are supported before, during and after the patient's death.

Medico-legal considerations

Death certification and referral to the coroner

The doctor who attended the patient during their last illness will normally issue a medical certificate of the cause of death or report the death to the coroner. If the body is to be buried there is no legal requirement for it to be seen by a doctor after death, although it is advisable for the doctor who issues the certificate to do so. Some funeral directors refuse to move a body until it has been seen by a doctor and the death confirmed. In many institutions, including nursing homes, hospices and hospitals, appropriately trained nurses can verify a death and agree to the removal of the body (the Royal College of Nursing has issued guidance on this).

If the body is to be cremated it must first be seen by the certifying doctor and by a second independent medical practitioner, whose registration is of at least five years' standing and who is not a partner or a relative of the first doctor or of the deceased.

Circumstances in which a death must be reported to the coroner

- When the certifying doctor has not seen the patient professionally in the 14 days leading up to the death.
- Cause of death is unknown.
- If there is any doubt about natural cause – suggestions of violence, neglect or other suspicious circumstances.
- Death was due to industrial disease or poisoning, including alcoholism.
- Death occurred during surgery or before recovery from anaesthesia (often interpreted as within 24 hours).
- Death was due to an abortion.
- Death occurred in prison or in police custody.

Some coroners advise which deaths which occur within 24 hours of admission to hospital and those where there is any allegation of negligence should also be reported.

(Adapted from Knight B (1992) *Legal Aspects of Medical Practice*. Churchill Livingstone, Edinburgh.)

NB. Some coroners have accepted the presence of an out-of-hours palliative care handover form, signed and dated by the GP, as evidence that death might be expected. This avoids patients becoming coroners' cases if the form is completed within two weeks of death.

Advanced directives or living wills

Living wills or advanced directives have a legal force in Britain and should be respected by all. It is vital to check that the statement presented is that of the patient being treated and has not been superceded or withdrawn. It is advisable to contact persons nominated by the patient and the usual GP if there is any doubt whether circumstances may have changed since the writing of the directive; and if there is doubt, the law requires the exercise of a best interests judgement.

With good communication by all and the dispelling of fears about treatments and terminal events, there may be less need for advanced directives which can be limited by inflexibility and difficulties recording a change of mind. However, helping a patient and their family go through the details of an advanced directive is an excellent opportunity for real discussion on patient choices and underlying needs and may help assuage many of the concerns that led to its request in the first place.

The BMA Code of Practice on Advanced Statements about Medical Treatment – Code of Practice, 1995 – is available from the British Medical Association or via www.bma.org.uk.

Spiritual care

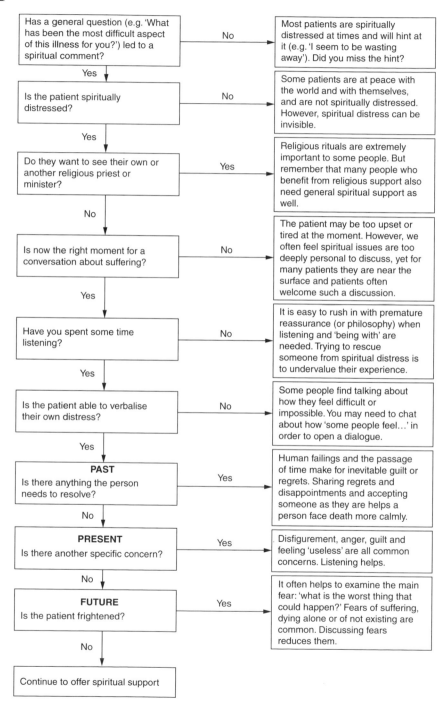

Has a general question (e.g. 'What has been the most difficult aspect of this illness for you?') led to a spiritual comment?	No	Most patients are spiritually distressed at times and will hint at it (e.g. 'I seem to be wasting away'). Did you miss the hint?
↓ Yes		
Is the patient spiritually distressed?	No	Some patients are at peace with the world and with themselves, and are not spiritually distressed. However, spiritual distress can be invisible.
↓ Yes		
Do they want to see their own or another religious priest or minister?	Yes	Religious rituals are extremely important to some people. But remember that many people who benefit from religious support also need general spiritual support as well.
↓ No		
Is now the right moment for a conversation about suffering?	No	The patient may be too upset or tired at the moment. However, we often feel spiritual issues are too deeply personal to discuss, yet for many patients they are near the surface and patients often welcome such a discussion.
↓ Yes		
Have you spent some time listening?	No	It is easy to rush in with premature reassurance (or philosophy) when listening and 'being with' are needed. Trying to rescue someone from spiritual distress is to undervalue their experience.
↓ Yes		
Is the patient able to verbalise their own distress?	No	Some people find talking about how they feel difficult or impossible. You may need to chat about how 'some people feel...' in order to open a dialogue.
↓ Yes		
PAST Is there anything the person needs to resolve?	Yes	Human failings and the passage of time make for inevitable guilt or regrets. Sharing regrets and disappointments and accepting someone as they are helps a person face death more calmly.
↓ No		
PRESENT Is there another specific concern?	Yes	Disfigurement, anger, guilt and feeling 'useless' are all common concerns. Listening helps.
↓ No		
FUTURE Is the patient frightened?	Yes	It often helps to examine the main fear: 'what is the worst thing that could happen?' Fears of suffering, dying alone or of not existing are common. Discussing fears reduces them.
↓ No		
Continue to offer spiritual support		

Extract from Peter Kaye's *Decision Making in Palliative Care* (1999, EPL Publications).

An aid to spiritual care

Here are some questions which may touch on the holistic and spiritual needs of patients. When exploring them with a patient, a greater sense of aliveness may come which may enhance the healing process and add to their sense of well-being.

1   **Being valued:**
   - What is the extent of family, home care and the quality of relationships?
   - Ask about significant family, friends and neighbours; who is the closest?
   - Comment if appropriate on the number of cards, flowers, gifts, etc. Name of partner or closest friend?
   - The degree of self-esteem of the person?

2   **Finding meaning:**
   - The patient's most frequent topic of conversation?
   - What do they most want at that moment to ease their situation?
   - What brings them aliveness, happiness and contentment?
   - What is it that makes them feel healed, even for a moment?
   - What hobbies and interests do they have?

3   **Having hope:**
   - What does the patient 'live' for or look forward to?
   - Major anniversaries and future events?
   - What gives hope and what is there to look forward to?
   - Are they hopeful about their prognosis?

4   **Dealing with emotions:**
   - What is their greatest dread or fear?
   - Can you tell what the patient's inner feelings are?
   - Can they express fear, anger, guilt, anxiety, despair, loneliness and isolation?
   - Does the patient need time, help or privacy to express them?

5   **Dignity:**
   - Is the patient receiving the amount of privacy and confidentiality needed?
   - Are you addressing them in the way they prefer, e.g. Mr, Mrs, 'Jack', 'Daisy', etc.?
   - Is the patient's toileting private and to their liking? Do you detect hidden fears of smell, bodily noises, etc.? Is the patient receiving undivided attention?
   - Does the patient feel in control or are choices made for them by other people?

6   **Truth and honesty:**
   - How much does the patient want to know?
   - Are their wishes being granted?
   - Is there a sense of conspiracy of silence?
   - Is anything being kept from the patient or family?
   - How much have they understood of their prognosis?
   - Is denial apparent here?

7   **Language and communication:**
   - What is the degree of understanding between significant people; family, nurse, etc.?
   - Are there deafness or speech difficulties here? Is the patient always understood?
   - Does the patient feel rejected or ignored?
   - Are there things the patient finds difficulty in talking about?

8 Death, dying and bereavement:
- Is there unresolved grief or anticipatory grief at present?
- Has there been much loss in the patient's life?
- Is there evidence of great disappointment, unfulfilled hopes, etc.?
- Is there an absence of significant relatives?
- What 'loss' might they be wrestling with, e.g. mobility, bodily functions, independence?

9 Religion:
- Has the patient been asked if they have a religious need?
- What is the patient's faith/denomination? Is religion important to them?
- Would they like to see a chaplain or faith representative?
- Can you personally help in trying to answer a religious need?
- Is there evidence on the locker of a bible or a prayer card?

10 Culture:
- Have cultural (background) needs been considered?
- Do you have contact names of faith representatives?
- Is the patient offered the right diet?
- What is the protocol about visiting and when a person has died?
- Have any cultural needs (artistic appreciation), interests or pursuits been recognised, e.g. reading, music, art, drama, etc.?

From Cressey R (1999) *An Aid to Spiritual Care*. Pinderfields Hospital Trust, Wakefield.

Summary of Palliative Care Patients

Name of patient Name of carer	Diagnoses (+code)	G P	D N	Problems/concerns	Anticipated needs	Information given/carer issues	DS 1500 date	Macmillan nurse/CNS	Hospice	OOH handover form: date sent	Preferred place of death stated + date	Actual place of death + date	Bereavement care	Notes

Summary Sheet © Gold Standards Framework. Keri Thomas 2002. Macmillan

Supportive Care Register Front Sheet

SCR2

Name	Diagnosis
....	
Comp. No.	**Secondaries**
DOB	
Hosp. No.	

Date of diagnosis	DS 1500 date/Ca registered...........

Address

Tel No.

Family/carer contacts

Personnel involved

Oncologist ....

Other specialists ....

Macmillan/Nurse/SPC ☐   Hospice ☐

Others e.g. SS ....

Key GP	Key DN
, ...	. . . . . .
. . . .	. . . .

Other conditions

Treatment

Surgery   Radiotherapy   Chemotherapy

Current medication

Priorities (Problems and concerns – physical, psychological, social, spiritual)

Other issues (incl. care plan, out-of-hours care, drugs left at home, before considering admission try, etc.)

Preferred place of death (dated)	Date of death	Place of death	Comments

Supportive Care Register Front Sheet/Out-of-hours Handover Form
© Gold Standards Framework, Keri Thomas 2002, Macmillan

Supportive Care Register Front Sheet

Date	Initials	Notes/important events

'Reactive' and 'proactive' patient journeys

A 'reactive' patient journey – BEFORE GSF
- Patient in last months of life.
- GP and DN *ad hoc* arrangements.
- Problems with symptom control – high family anxiety.
- Crisis call, e.g. out-of-hours, no plan or drugs available.
- Dies in hospital.
- Carer given minimal support or help in grief.

A 'proactive' patient journey – WITH GSF
- Patients in last months of life on SC Register and discussed at PHCT meeting.
- DS1500 and information given to patient and carer.
- Patient and carer given regular support, visits/phone calls.
- Assessment of symptoms – referral to specialists if needed.
- Carer assessed including psychosocial needs.
- Preferred place of care and arrangements made.
- Handover form written and drugs issued for home.
- End of life pathway/protocol used.
- Patient dies in preferred place – bereavement support offered.
- Staff reflect/SEA – review gaps, audit and constantly improve.

With thanks to Rosie Norbury, DN, Huddersfield

There was a real shift towards anticipating problems, rather than trying to cope and patching up when they did happen. In hospitals and hospices, there can be more planning of care but we don't do it much in general practice because we have patients with us long term. These few minutes a month got us into the habit of 'horizon scanning' for likely problems and doing what we could to prevent them. Proactive care feels better, is less panicky and saves time in the end.

GP, Huddersfield, Phase 1

Index